PHARMACOTHERAPY

ENCYCLOPAEDIA OF PHARMACEUTICAL TECHNOLOGY - 5

PHARMACOTHERAPY

By

Dr. G.P. Garg

&

Dr. M. Prakash

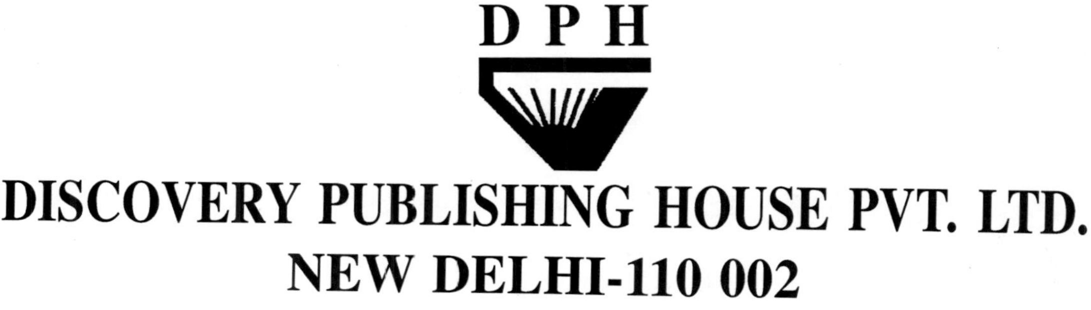

DISCOVERY PUBLISHING HOUSE PVT. LTD.

NEW DELHI-110 002

Published by:
Tilak Wasan

DISCOVERY PUBLISHING HOUSE PVT. LTD.
4383/4B, Ansari Road, Darya Ganj
New Delhi-110 002 (India)
Phone : +91-11-23279245; 23253475; 43596065
E-mail : discoverybooksindia@gmail.com
discoverypublishinghouse@gmail.com
namitwasan9@gmail.com
web : www.discoverypublishinggroup.com

***First Published:* 2011**

ISBN: 978-81-8356-595-0 (Set)

ISBN: 978-81-8356-742-8

Pharmacotherapy

Printed at:
Infinity Imaging Systems
Delhi

Preface

The present title "Pharmacotherapy" has been written for those in the pharmaceutical research and those responsible for the education and training in pharmaceutical science and technology of graduate and undergraduate students. Medicine is an ever changing science. As new research and clinical experience broaden our knowledge, changes in treatment and drug therapy are required. This branch of life science has progressed enormously in recent years and the significant advances in therapeutics and an understanding of the need to optimize during delivery in the body have brought about an increased awareness of the valuable role played by the dosage forms. This statement is as true as it was back in ninteenth century and perhaps more so, given the increasing emphasis being placed on discovery, development, and use of large molecular entities as therapeutic and diagnostic agents. Development of these abilities requires an integration of knowledge, skills, attitudes, and values that can be acquired only through structured learning process including independent study, hands on practice and the availability of advanced literature. This tittle has designed to meet such needs of learners in the health professions.

In the last two decades, the pharmaceutical industry has experimented and successfully adopted several integrated and multidisciplinary approaches in the research areas of dring compound screening, toxicological evaluation, and pharmaceutical product development. The book is written in a concise style that facilitates an in-depth level of understanding of the essential concepts. The objectives of the present title are three folds: (i) to serve as a useful tool to help guide scientists in research and development by out-lining the theory and successful practice of in vitro - in vivo correlation, (ii) to help formulators apply the tool in designing and developing prototypes that enable selection of clinical formulations, and (iii) to help formulate strategy(ies) for product life-cycle management.

To make the work more comprehensive and informative, the author has consulted many authoritative books, research journals, abstracts, monographs etc., so there can be no claim to originality except in the manner of treatment.

The author expresses his thanks to his friends and colleagues whose continue inspirations have initiated him to bring out this book.

The author expresses his gratitude to Mr. Wasan and staff of M/s Discovery Publishing House Pvt. Ltd. for their whole hearted co-operation in the publication of this book.

Author

CONTENTS

1

INTRODUCTION

The U.S. Food and Drug Administration defines "*bioavailability*" as "the rate and extent to which the active ingredient or active moiety is absorbed from a drug product and becomes available at the site of action." Because, in practice, it is rare that drug concentrations can be determined at the site of action (e.g., at a receptor site), bioavailability is more commonly defined as "the rate and extent that the active drug is absorbed from a dosage form and becomes available in the systemic circulation." Usually bioavailability refers to the absorption of a drug from the gastrointestinal tract following oral administration of a dosage form. The dosage form may be any type of product, including a solution, suspension, tablet, capsule, powder, or elixir. Bioavailability can also refer to the absorption of a drug from other routes of administration, such as intramuscular (IM) injection, transdermal patches, ointments and other topical preparations, and implants, which also require absorption prior to reaching the systemic circulation. As these routes of administration (e.g., oral, IM, and topical) deliver the drug to a site outside the vascular system, they are often referred to as routes of extravascular administration. The only route of drug administration that will always result in a bioavailability of 100% is an intravenous injection, in which the amount of drug reaching the systemic circulation is equal to the total administered dose. The term "*relative bioavailability*" refers to a comparison of two or more dosage forms in terms of their relative rate and extent of absorption. If an intravenous injection is employed as the reference dose, one can determine the absolute bioavailability of the test dosage form. Two dosage forms that do not differ significantly in their rate and extent of absorption are termed "*bioequivalent*."

In general, bioequivalence evaluations involve comparisons of dosage forms that are "*pharmaceutical equivalents*." Such dosage forms are defined as "drug products that contain identical amounts of the identical active drug ingredient, i.e., the same salt or ester of the same therapeutic moiety, in identical dosage forms, but not necessarily containing the same inactive ingredients, and that meet the identical compendial or other applicable standard of identity, strength, quality, and purity, including potency and, where applicable, content uniformity, disintegration times, and/or dissolution rates." Bioequivalence determinations may also be made for "*pharmaceutical alternatives*," defined as "drug products that contain the identical therapeutic moiety, or its precursor, but not necessarily in the same amount or dosage form or as the same salt or ester. Each such drug product individually meets either the identical or its own respective compendial or other applicable standard of identity, strength, quality, and purity, including potency and, where applicable, content uniformity, disintegration times, and/or dissolution rates." In some instance, two pharmaceutical alternatives exhibit markedly different bioavailability, for example, a rapidly absorbed elixir vs. a more slowly absorbed capsule. In other cases, two different dosage forms (e.g., a tablet and a capsule) may or may not exhibit very similar bioavailability.

Factors Affecting Drug Bioavailability

Extravascularly administered drugs must traverse several barriers to reach the systemic circulation and/or their site of action. Many studies illustrate that differences in manufacturing procedures as well as the composition of the dosage form can affect the bioavailability of a drug product. In addition, the bioavailability of a drug product can also be influenced by the physiology of the patient and other factors, such as the content of the gastrointestinal tract.

A major factor determining the bioavailability of an orally administered drug product is the dissolution rate of the drug. A drug must be in solution to be absorbed from the gastrointestinal tract. Even if the drug product is administered as a solution, some dissolution process may be required in the event the drug precipitates as a result of low solubility in the fluids of the gastrointestinal tract.

Drug Product Formulation

Most drugs are not taken as pure chemicals, but are formulated into a pharmaceutical dosage form. Such drug products may be a relatively simple solution, a compressed tablet-containing binders, fillers, lubricants, a coloring agent, and the like, or a controlled-release product. The following are a few of the formulation and manufacturing variables that could influence the bioavailability of a drug product:

1. The properties of the drug (salt form, crystalline structure, formation of solvates, and solubility).
2. The composition of the finished dosage form (presence or absence of excipients and special coatings).
3. Manufacturing variables (tablet compression force, processing variables, particle size of drug or excipients, and environmental conditions).
4. Rate and/or site of dissolution in the gastrointestinal tract.

Physiologic and Other Factors Affecting Bioavailability

The rate and extent of drug absorption can also be affected by a wide variety of factors related to the characteristics of the subject/patient receiving the drug product. These factors are important to consider, because they can contribute to intrasubject and inter- subject variability in the treatment of patients. Further, if not well controlled during the course of a bioavailability study, these factors can bias the study results and confound interpretation of the data. Examples include the following:

1. Contents of the gastrointestinal tract (fluid volume and pH, diet, presence or absence of food, bacterial activity, and presence of other drugs).
2. Rate of gastrointestinal tract transit (influenced by disease, physical activity, drugs, emotional status of subject, and composition of the gastrointestinal tract contents).
3. Presystemic drug metabolism and/or degradation (influenced by local blood flow; condition of the gastrointestinal tract membranes; and drug transport, metabolism, or degradation in the gastrointestinal tract or during the first pass of the drug through the liver). Age, sex, race, disease, body size, time of day, and physical activity.

Other factors related to the subject or patient, if not recognized or controlled, can also influence the assessment of drug bioavailability and product bioequivalence. For example, bioavailability studies typically involve the collection of blood and/or urine specimens to determine drug appearance in the systemic circulation. Thus, physiologic and pharmacokinetic perturbations that affect the concentration of drug measured in these fluids can potentially influence the results and interpretation of the study. Examples include changes that alter: (i) the rate, extent, and/or route of metabolism (e.g., coadministered drugs that compete for or induce drug-metabolizing enzymes); (ii) the rate and/or extent of drug elimination by the kidney (e.g., kidney disease and/or competition and changes in urine pH that affect renal transport mechanisms); (iii) the degree of binding of the drug to plasma or tissue proteins (e.g., age-related changes in plasma-binding proteins or protein-binding displacements); and (iv) distribution of drug into the erythrocytes. Genetic polymorphisms in the drug-metabolizing enzymes of the liver may also contribute to large differences in the pharmacokinetics of a drug and the interpretation of bioavailability studies. A well-designed bioavailability study must either control or account for the influence of such variables.

Characteristics of Drugs with the Greatest Potential for a Bioavailability Problem

The total number of marketed drug products known to exhibit a significant bioavailability problem is relatively small. Thus, one point of view is that the bioavailability has been overemphasized and that for most drug products, it is not a matter of concern. Another point of view is that those products that exhibit a bioavailability deficiency in a carefully controlled study provide ample evidence of the potential for many drug products that have not yet been studied to present a bioavailability problem.

With minor exceptions, the US Food and Drug Administration has required that bioavailability and bioequivalence of a drug product be demonstrated through in vivo studies. However, a "*Biopharmaceutics Classification System* (BCS)" was recently proposed, which divides drugs into classes based on their solubility, permeability, and in vitro dissolution rate. This classification system could be used to justify the waiver of the requirement for in vivo studies for "rapidly dissolving drug products containing active moieties/active ingredients that are highly soluble and highly permeable." If adopted by the Food and Drug Administration, the bioavailability and bioequivalence of drug products meeting these requirements could be demonstrated using in vitro solubility, permeability, and dissolution studies. On the other hand, drugs that are poorly permeable, poorly soluble, and/or formulated in slowly dissolving dosage forms would be considered as more likely to demonstrate a bioavailability problem, and would not be candidates for the waiver of in vivo bioavailability studies.

To provide some guidance as to which drugs have the greatest potential for a bioavailability problem, the US Food and Drug Administration published a summary of the type of evidence that may be employed to assess the importance of establishing the bioavailability of a given drug:

1. Data from clinical trials or bioequivalence studies that indicate a bioequivalence problem.
2. The drug has a narrow therapeutic range, and the concentrations of the drug in the patient must be carefully adjusted.
3. A lack of bioequivalence could have serious medical consequences.
4. Physicochemical evidence that:
   (a) The drug has low solubility in water and/or the dissolution rate of the dosage form is slow.
   (b) The particle size, crystalline structure, and other factors of the drug can affect the dissolution and bioavailability.
   (c) The drug product contains a high ratio of excipients to active ingredients, or the product may require excipients to enhance absorption or contain excipients that inhibit absorption.
5. Pharmacokinetic evidence that:
   (a) The absorption of the active drug is limited to a specific region of the gastrointestinal tract.
   (b) The extent of absorption is low.
   (c) There is rapid metabolism such that rapid dissolution and absorption are required for effectiveness.
   (d) The product required special formulations to stabilize the drug in the gastrointestinal fluids.
   (e) The drug exhibits dose-dependent pharmacokinetics.

Drugs that meet one or more of the criteria given above and have been shown to exhibit significant differences in the bioavailability of marketed dosage forms include digoxin, quinidine, furosemide, nitrofurantoin, prednisone, chloramphenicol, theophylline, chlorpromazine, phenytoin, amitriptyline, and phenylbutazone.

BCS

The goal of correlating in vitro drug dissolution and in vivo bioavailability data engendered the BCS. The BCS permits classification of drug substances based upon the key determinants of rate and extent of drug absorption from immediate release solid oral dosage forms—aqueous solubility, gastrointestinal permeability, and dissolution. The BCS provides four distinct classes of drug substances:

Class 1: High Solubility High Permeability

Class 2: Low Solubility High Permeability

Class 3: High Solubility Low Permeability

Class 4: Low Solubility Low Permeability

Solubility class is assigned on the basis of the volume of an aqueous medium required to dissolve the highest dose strength in the pH range of 1–7.5. A drug is classified as highly soluble, if the drug can be dissolved in a volume of ≤ 250 ml of aqueous media. A volume of 250 ml estimates the amount of water (approximately 8 ounces), administered to fasting human volunteers during a typical bioequivalence study.

Systemic bioavailability is the product of fraction of dose absorbed (f_a), fraction of dose escaping gut metabolism (f_g), and fraction of dose escaping first- pass metabolism (F^*). Permeability class is based upon f_a, which may be estimated either in vivo or in vitro by direct measurement of mass transfer across human intestinal epithelium. In vivo methods include: (i) mass balance studies using unlabeled, stable-isotope labeled, or a radiolabeled drug substance; (ii) oral bioavailability using a reference intravenous dose; or (iii) intestinal perfusion studies either in humans or an acceptable animal model. Suitable in vitro methods involve the use of either excised human/animal intestinal tissues or cultured epithelial monolayers. All of these methods are deemed appropriate for drugs whose absorption is controlled by passive mechanisms.

However, drug substances for which f_a may be affected by active transport processes [e.g., the efflux transporter P-glycoprotein (P-gp)] may require further model characterization to prevent misclassification of their permeability class. For example, functional expression of efflux transporters must be determined in cultured human or animal epithelial monolayers. At this time, the FDA recommends limiting the use of non-human permeability test methods to drug substances whose absorption is controlled by passive mechanisms. When applying the BCS, an apparent passive mechanism may be inferred when one of the following conditions is satisfied: (i) a linear pharmacokinetic relationship between dose and a measure of bioavailability (e.g., area under the plasma concentration–time curve, AUC) is demonstrated in humans; (ii) in vivo or in situ permeability in an animal model is independent of drug concentration in the initial perfusion fluid; or (iii) in vitro permeability is independent of initial donor fluid concentration and transport direction using an in vitro cell culture model known to express functional efflux transporters. Finally, if evidence of gastrointestinal instability is lacking, a drug substance is classified as highly permeable if its extent of absorption in humans is ≥ 90% of an administered dose based on either mass balance determination or comparison to a reference intravenous dose.

Immediate release solid oral dosage forms are classified as either having rapid or slow dissolution rates. Immediate release dosage forms are those for which ≥ 85% of the labeled amount dissolves within 30 min. Dissolution testing must be performed with US Pharmacopeia (USP) Apparatus I at 100 rpm (or Apparatus II at 50 rpm) in a volume of ≤ 900 ml of each of the following: (i) 0.1 N hydrochloric acid or simulated gastric fluid USP without enzymes; (ii) a pH 4.5 buffer; and (iii) a pH

6.8 buffer or simulated intestinal fluid USP without enzymes. Test (T) and reference (R) product dissolution profiles may be compared using a similarity factor (f_2)

$$f_2 = 50 \times \log\{[1 + (1/n) \times \sum_{t=1}^{n} (R_t - T_t)^2]^{-0.5} \times 100\} \qquad ...(1)$$

Values of f_2 > 50 (or closer to 100) ensure sameness or equivalency of the two dissolution profiles and thus performance of the test and reference products being compared. The profile comparison using f_2 is unnecessary if ≥ 85% of the labeled amount of both the test and the reference products dissolve in 15 min using each of the aforementioned dissolution media.

Biowaiver

In vivo differences in drug dissolution may explain observed bioavailability differences between two pharmaceutically equivalent solid oral dosage forms. However, for high permeability drugs with rapid dissolution relative to gastric emptying, bioavailability is likely independent of the dissolution rate and/or gastric emptying time. Thus, for immediate release solid oral dosage forms with rapid in vitro dissolution, the BCS may be used to justify a waiver (i.e., biowaiver) of in vivo bioavailability/ bioequivalence studies for Class 1 drug substances, with the caveat that inactive ingredients found in the dosage form must not significantly affect absorption of the active moiety. Moreover, the test and reference products should have similar dissolution profiles. For prodrug biowaiver requests, permeability must be determined either for the prodrug, assuming that the conversion to the active moiety occurs after intestinal permeation, or for the drug if conversion occurs prior to intestinal permeation. Drugs with narrow therapeutic indices or those designed for absorption from the oral cavity do not qualify for BCS-based biowaivers. Biowaivers for immediate release solid oral dosage forms may also be granted for Level 3 scale-up and postapproval changes (SUPAC). For example, a full bioequivalence study may be waived when an acceptable in vivo/in vitro correlation (IVIVC) has been demonstrated. In general, the likelihood of an IVIVC is low for Class I, III, and IV drug products, as defined by the BCS. For high solubility drugs (BCS Classes I and III), dissolution is assumed to be rapid. Thus, the rate of drug absorption will be controlled by either gastric emptying (Class I) or permeability (Class III).

Experimental Determination of Bioavailability

Types of Studies

Several methods can be used to determine the bioavailability or bioequivalence of a drug product. The vast majority of bioavailability studies involve the administration of the test dosage form to a group of healthy human subjects, followed by collection and assay of drug concentration in blood (plasma or serum) samples. The second most frequent type of study utilizes urinary excretion measurements. Occasionally other types of biologic material such as saliva, cerebrospinal fluid, bile, or feces are also collected. For a few drugs, for which assay methods are not available for the determination of drug concentrations in biologic fluids, a pharmacologic response may be measured. Finally, some bioavailability assessments have been made on the basis of a determination of the therapeutic response of patients to a given dosage form. However, this type of study is usually restricted to drugs that are active at the site of administration (e.g., topical) but are not intended to be available in the systemic circulation. For approval by the US Food and Drug Administration, pharmacokinetic, pharmacodynamic, clinical, and in vitro studies are recognized (in descending order of preference) as acceptable approaches to document the bioavailability or bioequivalence of a drug product.

Blood level studies

The primary basis for blood concentration studies is the assumption that two dosage forms that exhibit superimposable blood concentration–time profiles in a group of subjects should result in identical therapeutic activity in patients. The key parameters to note from this figure are the maximum blood concentration (C_{max}), the time (T_{max}) of occurrence of the maximum blood concentration, and the total area under the blood concentration–time curve (AUC). The value of Tmax provides a means to assess the rate of absorption of the drug. The T_{max} is independent of the amount of drug absorbed, but is inversely related to the absorption rate. Thus, the faster the absorption of a drug, the shorter will be the T_{max}. The value of T_{max} is also influenced by the rate of elimination of the drug from the body. However, if one assumes elimination rate does not change during the period when two or more dosage forms are being tested in a given subject, then observed differences in T_{max} will reflect absorption rate differences among the test products. The interpretation of C_{max} is somewhat more complicated because it is a function of both the rate of absorption and the extent of absorption, as well as the elimination rate. Thus, as the amount of drug absorbed increases and/or the rate of absorption increases, the C_{max} also increases, assuming no change in elimination rate. A determination of the extent of drug absorption is usually based on a measure of AUC, which is directly proportional to the fraction of the administered dose that reaches the systemic circulation and is independent of the rate of absorption. The blood concentration–time curve is divided into a series of geometric sections, and the area encompassed by each section is determined from the trapezoidal rule:

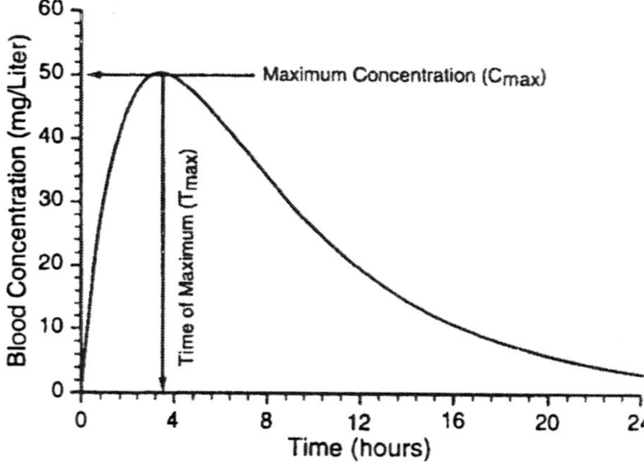

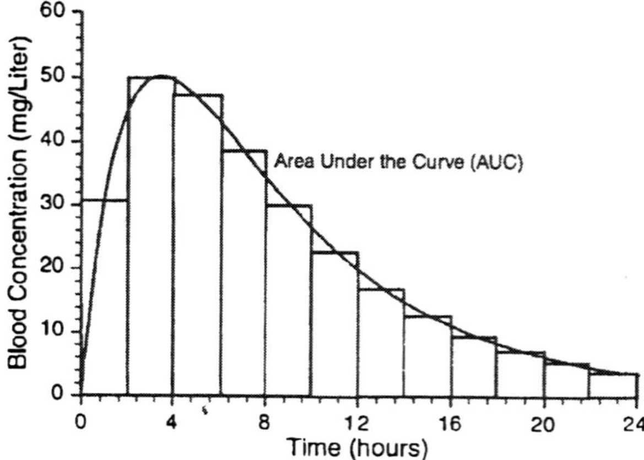

Fig. 1.1. Drug concentration in blood vs. time plots illustrating calculation of C_{max}, T_{max}, and AUC.

$$AUC = 1/2 \times (\Delta t) \times (C_1 + C_2) \qquad \ldots(2)$$

where Δt is the time interval between the collection of two blood samples of concentrations C_1 and C_2. The units of AUC are given as the product of concentration and time (e.g., mg/L × hr). If blood samples are not obtained for a sufficient period of time to result in a zero drug concentration in the final sample, it is necessary to estimate the portion of the AUC remaining after the final sample. Eq. (3) gives the relationship between the AUC (0–t) for the portion of the curve to the last sample taken at time t, and the total AUC (0-∞)

$$AUC(0 - \infty) = AUC(0 - t_{last}) + C_{last}/K \qquad \ldots(3)$$

where C_{last} is the last measurable drug concentration, tlast is the time at which it was collected, and K is the apparent first-order elimination rate constant estimated from the terminal slope of the log-linear plot of concentration vs. time. In studies involving blood sampling intervals after the peak that are relatively long compared with the half-life of the drug, the use of the logarithmic trapezoidal method has been recommended to estimate the postpeak AUC. The value of AUC (0–∞) may also be expressed as given in Eq. (4) for a drug whose disposition in the body can be described by a one-compartment pharmacokinetic model.

$$AUC(0 - \infty) = F \times D/CL \quad ...(4)$$

where F = the fraction of dose absorbed

D = the administered dose

CL = the total body clearance of the drug

Thus, a comparison may be made between two different dosage forms on the basis of the ratio of their respective AUC (0–∞) values. Assuming equivalent doses are given and the clearance of the drug remains constant during the time the two doses are administered, the ratio of the AUCs will be directly proportional to the ratio of the fraction of each dose absorbed, that is, the extent of absorption. Fig. 1.2 illustrates the types of plasma concentration time data that might be obtained during the testing of three different bioinequivalent formulations of a drug. Products A and C are absorbed at the same rate, based on identical T_{max} values, but B is more slowly absorbed, as shown by the longer time required to achieve C_{max}. Products A and B appear to be absorbed to the same extent on the basis of very similar values for AUC. However, product C is obviously less completely absorbed, as shown by the lower AUC.

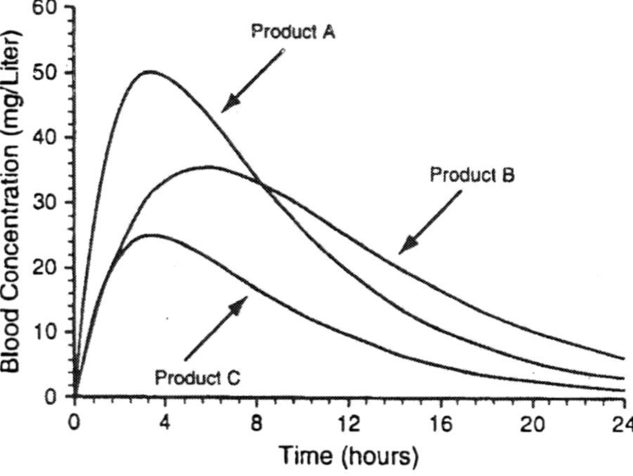

Fig. 1.2. Drug concentration in blood vs. time after single doses of product A, product B, and product C.

All of the foregoing discussion assumes the absorption and elimination of the drug do not exhibit dose-dependent pharmacokinetics. For example, if the metabolism of a drug is a saturable process, the total AUC may be significantly increased for a rapidly absorbed dosage form, because the initial blood drug concentrations exceed the metabolic capacity of the body to eliminate the drug. Non-linear pharmacokinetics may also be caused by changes in the clearance of a drug owing to factors such as non-linear drug binding to plasma and/or tissue proteins. Thus, for a drug such as disopyramide, the AUC does not increase in proportion to the administered dose. This is the result of a decrease in drug binding as drug concentration increases. Thus, it is necessary to measure free drug concentration in the plasma, rather than total drug concentration (free + bound), for disopyramide bioequivalence studies. Other mechanisms that can contribute to non-linear pharmacokinetics and complicate the interpretation of bioequivalence data have been reviewed by Tozer and Tang-Liu. The interpretation of non-superimposable blood concentration–time profiles for drugs that exhibit non-linearity must be done with caution. Further, bioavailability and bioequivalence studies of such drugs may need to include multiple-dose protocols to further define the effect of differences in the rate and extent of absorption on the steady-state drug concentrations.

Urinary excretion studies

The estimation of bioavailability on the basis of appearance of drug in the urine is an attractive alternative to blood sampling, because it represents a noninvasive method. This approach is particularly useful for drugs that have the urine as the site of activity (e.g., urinary tract antiseptics such as nitrofurantoin and methenamine). The method is also useful for drugs that are extensively excreted unmetabolized in the urine, such as certain thiazide diuretics and sulfonamides. Often a less-sensitive analytical method is required for urine concentrations compared with blood concentrations. If the urine concentrations are low, assaying larger sample volumes is relatively easy. The primary disadvantage to urinary excretion studies is that they require the collection of samples for a longer period of time to ensure complete recovery of absorbed drug. In addition, the subjects must be careful to completely void at each collection time and to avoid accidentally discarding any samples. As with the assessment of bioavailability from blood levels, urinary excretion studies also generally assume the pharmacokinetics are not dose dependent. If renal excretion is a saturable process, the percentage of drug excreted unmetabolized in the urine may not reflect the rate and extent of the drug absorption.

The three major parameters examined in urinary excretion bioavailability studies are the cumulative amount of drug excreted unmetabolized in the urine (ΣXu); the maximum urinary excretion rate (ER_{max}); and the time of maximum excretion rate (T_{max}). In simple pharmacokinetic models, the rate of appearance of drug in the urine is proportional to the concentration of drug in the systemic circulation. Thus, the values for T_{max} and ER_{max} for urine studies are analogous to the T_{max} and C_{max} values derived from blood level studies. The value of T_{max} decreases as the absorption rate of the drug increases, and ER_{max} increases as the rate and/or the extent of absorption increases. The value for ΣXu is related to the AUC and increases as the extent of absorption increases.

The calculation of ER is based on Eq. (5)

$$ER = \left(\sum Xu_2 - \sum Xu_1\right) / (t_2 - t_1) \qquad \ldots(5)$$

where ΣXu_1 and ΣXu_2 represent the cumulative amount of drug recovered in the urine samples obtained at sampling times up to t_1 and t_2, respectively. When constructing a plot of ER vs. time, or for the determination of ER_{max}, the values for time are taken to be the midpoint of the urine collection period, that is, the midpoint between t_1 and t_2. Thus, estimates of Tmax and ER_{max} from urinary excretion data provide less information on the rate of drug absorption than can be obtained from analysis of the blood concentration–time profile, largely because of the fact that there is a limit to frequency at which urine can be readily collected.

When sufficient urine samples have been collected to ensure that no significant amount of drug remains to be excreted, the cumulative urinary recovery is symbolized as ΣXu^{∞}. The relative extent of absorption of drug from two dosage forms may then be expressed as the ratio of the ΣXu^{∞} values. However the value of ΣXu^{∞} is a function of the fraction (F) of administered dose (FD) absorbed, the renal elimination rate constant (k_e), and the rate constant for overall elimination (K) from the systemic circulation, as expressed in Eq. (6).

$$\sum Xu\infty = F \times D \times k_e / K \qquad \ldots(6)$$

Assay of other biologic material

For a few drugs such as theophylline, saliva drug concentrations have been employed to supplement the collection of blood samples. However, the intersubject and intrasubject variability in saliva/plasma ratios have generally precluded the sole use of saliva drug concentrations to assess bioavailability. For some drugs such as cephalosporin antibiotics, clinical studies may also include a determination of appearance of drug in other body fluids such as the cerebrospinal fluid and bile.

One might initially think that assessing the extent of drug absorption after oral administration would be possible by simply quantitating the amount of drug excreted in the feces. Such determinations occasionally provide useful data. For example, if subjects receive the drug as an enteric-coated tablet or some other solid dosage form and the product is recovered intact in the feces, there is little question regarding the lack of bioavailability. However, the data obtained from fecal recovery studies must be carefully interpreted. If drug is analytically measured in a fecal sample, this does not establish that the drug was not absorbed. For example, certain drugs undergo extensive enterohepatic recycling and/or excretion in the saliva. Thus, a drug could be fully bioavailable, and yet a portion of the administered dose could be found in the feces. Further, the absence of intact drug in the feces is not proof of absorption because the drug may be degraded during its transit through the gastrointestinal tract.

Assessment of bioavailability from pharmacologic response

Topical application of a corticosteroid does not generally result in measurable blood concentrations of the drug. Thus, bioavailability and bioequivalence determinations for these drug products may involve measurement of dermatologic vasoconstriction (i.e., skin blanching), a pharmacodynamic response. A few studies have attempted to relate quantitatively a pharmacologic response to the oral bioavailability of a drug. For example, a relationship between the extent and duration of serum glucose concentration reduction and the bioavailability of two dosage forms of tolbutamide were demonstrated. Others have employed pharmacologic end points that were not necessarily related to the therapeutic activity of the test drug. For example, attempts have been made to relate pharmacologic responses such as changes in pupil diameter, electrocardiogram readings, or electroencephalogram readings to the time course of a given drug in humans and animals. However, pharmacologic data tend to be more variable, and demonstrating a good correlation between the measured response and the amount of drug available from the dosage form may be difficult. Further, the potential exists that the measured response may be owing to a metabolite whose concentration is not proportional to the concentration of the parent drug responsible for therapeutic activity.

Assessment of bioavailability from therapeutic response

Because the ultimate goal of drug therapy is to achieve some therapeutic response in a patient, ideally the assessment of drug product efficacy should be studied in patients requiring the drug. Unfortunately, the quantitation of patient clinical response is too imprecise to permit anything approaching a reasonable estimation of the relative bioavailability of two dosage forms of the same drug. Thus, there are good reasons to utilize healthy volunteers rather than patients. Bioequivalence studies are usually conducted using a cross-over design in which each subject receives each of the test dosage forms. It is assumed that the physiologic status of the subject does not change significantly over the duration of the study. If patients were utilized, this assumption could be less valid because of changes in their disease state. Further, unless multiple-dose protocols were employed, a patient who might actually require the drug for the disease would be able to receive only a single dose of the drug every few days or perhaps each week. To avoid such problems, one could test each product in different groups of patients, but this would require the use of a large number of subjects and careful matching of the various patient groups. Another problem is that many patients receive more than one drug, and the results obtained from a bioavailability study could be compromised because of a drug–drug interaction. Finally, an ethical question would arise in the case in which a particular product was believed to be defective. Thus, a patient requiring treatment with a given drug would need to consent to receive a product that might not provide sufficient drug to result in adequate treatment. Because of these considerations, the general conclusion is that most bioequivalence studies should be carried out with healthy subjects. However, for drugs that are not designed to be absorbed into the systemic circulation, and are active at the site of administration, clinical studies in patients are the only means to determine bioequivalence. Such studies are usually conducted using a parallel rather than a crossover design. Examples include studies of topical antifungal agents, drugs used in the treatment of acne, and agents such as sucralfate used in ulcer therapy.

Other experimental approaches

The current bioequivalence regulations of the US Food and Drug Administration describe several types of experimental approaches in addition to those involving human testing.

Use of experimental animals

Animal studies are not acceptable for bioequivalence determinations unless data obtained with animals have been correlated with data obtained in human studies, ensuring that the bioavailability of a dosage form in animals is closely related to that in humans. Animals are known to differ from humans in terms of gastrointestinal tract characteristics, metabolism, distribution, and excretion. For the study of solid dosage forms, relatively large animals such as dogs or monkeys must be employed. Although such studies can provide useful data during the development stages of a drug formulation and may provide useful alternates to human studies for drugs that are quite toxic to humans (e.g., cancer drugs), in general, animal studies are not acceptable as the final assessment of the bioavailability of a dosage form.

In vitro methods

In recent years, there has been great interest in the development of laboratory test systems that can simulate the disintegration and dissolution of a drug product in the human gastrointestinal tract. The development of such devices is desirable as a means to reduce the need for human testing. One of the early approaches to relate in vivo bioavailability data to in vitro measurements employed testing based on the time required for a solid dosage form to disintegrate in a particular solvent. The official apparatus employed for such testing is described in the USP XXIV. However, the problem with this method is that the measurement of the time required for a dosage form to break into small particles may not necessarily relate to the dissolution rate of the drug. The current USP XXIV describes one official in vitro disintegration apparatus (i.e., basket-rack assembly) and two official dissolution apparatus (i.e., one with a paddle and one with a basket-stirring element) for the evaluation of solid dosage forms. Although these methods are well established and used extensively, few in vitro/in vivo correlations between dissolution data and human bioavailability data have been established. In vitro dissolution testing is useful as a standard for monitoring product quality and can be used to distinguish between dosage forms for which a bioavailability problem is known to exist. However, the USP acknowledges that many of the formulation factors that affect the performance of a drug product during in vitro dissolution testing may only sometimes affect the in vivo bioavailability of the drug (i.e., dissolution testing may identify subtle differences in the characteristics of the dosage form that are not relevant to its in vivo performance). Thus, in vitro dissolution testing cannot necessarily be assumed to relate to the in vivo bioavailability of a given dosage form. In conducting dissolution studies, the choice of an appropriate solvent is very important. Dissolution experiments should be conducted using conditions that mimic the environment in the gastrointestinal tract. Typical dissolution studies employ 0.1 N hydrochloric acid, water, or a buffer as the dissolution media. Simulated gastric fluid (pH 1.2) with or without pepsin and simulated intestinal fluid (pH 6.8) with or without pancreatin are also commonly employed for in vitro dissolution testing. It is widely recognized that the dissolution of controlled-release dosage forms may be pH dependent. Thus, the US Food and Drug Administration recommends that dissolution testing for controlled-release dosage forms be conducted over a wide range of pH values, including 1-1.5, 4-4.5, 6-6.5, and 7-7.5, with multiple time determinations to better characterize the dissolution properties of the dosage form. Bioequivalence determinations for products containing cholestyramine resin (used to control cholesterol) represent a novel in vitro approach to bioequivalence testing. Generic versions of such drug products are evaluated in vitro by determining the rate and extent of the interaction of different bile salts with the resin.

Experimental Design

The proper design of a bioavailability or bioequivalence study is essential to the collection of meaningful data. Studies must include a sufficient number of subjects and collect blood or urine samples at appropriately spaced intervals to accurately characterize the pharmacokinetics of the drug product(s) and make statistically relevant conclusions regarding their bioavailability and bioequivalence. Amongst other factors, study design must consider the characteristics of the study population (e.g., age, weight, gender, race, and health), the timing of dose administration, meals, and blood sample collection, and the time interval (i.e., washout period) between consecutive administrations of the drug products. In a bioequivalence study involving two or more dosage forms, the sequence of product administration must also be carefully considered to minimize experimental bias. The purpose of these rigorous controls on experimental design and conduct is to minimize the variability associated with pharmacokinetic (e.g., clearance, volume of distribution, and absorption) and physiologic (e.g., gastric emptying and pH) factors, such that the variability observed during the study is more closely related to the performance of the drug product(s) under consideration.

Crossover designs vs. other designs

The most common type of study uses a crossover design in which each subject receives each of the test products. In such a design, differences among dosage forms, subjects, and sequences of administration can be readily estimated. In essence, each subject serves as his own control. Crossover designs have also been developed to minimize the effects of residual or carry-over effects, which could occur if the administration of a given dosage form had an influence on the bioavailability of a subsequently administered product.

Table 1.1. Three-way crossover design for bioequivalencestudy

	Dosing Period		
Subject	*Period 1*	*Period 2*	*Period 3*
1 and 2	A	B	C
3 and 4	A	C	B
5 and 6	B	A	C
7 and 8	B	C	A
9 and 10	C	A	B
11 and 12	C	B	A

Note that there are six possible sequences for the administration of each of the three products. Further, each subject receives each of the three products, and each dosing period contains all three products. The value of such a design is that it minimizes any bias relating to subject and dosing sequence effects. Replicate study designs, in which each subject receives the test and reference drug product on more than one occasion, are currently being evaluated as an alternative method to examine the bioequivalence of drug products.

Single-dose vs. multiple-dose studies

Bioavailability studies intended to determine the disposition of a drug, particularly those involving new chemical entities, must include both single-and multiple-dose administration. However, most bioequivalence studies, which compare the bioavailability of two or more dosage forms, usually employ only single-dose administration for each product, under fasting conditions. One major exception is bioequivalence studies of controlled-release products. The US Food and Drug Administration requires both single-and multiple-dose administration as well as a determination of the effect of food on the absorption of the drug from the dosage form. However, the requirement of multiple-dose studies in the assessing the bioequivalence of controlled-release products has received much attention recently and may be abandoned, with the thought that single-dose studies provide more sensitive information to assess the performance of these products.

Multiple-dose studies are more difficult to control and expose the subjects to more drug. However, multiple-dose study designs also have advantages. They are more representative of how drug products are usually used by patients, and they also require fewer blood samples and less-sensitive analytical methods. Such studies require a sufficient number of doses to permit the achievement of steady state, which may be defined as the point where the amount of drug being absorbed into the body is equal to the amount being eliminated from the body. A general rule is that dosing must continue for approximately five biologic half-lives to be within approximately 95% of steady state. Once steady state has been reached, the area under the blood concentration–time curve during a single dosing interval should be equal to the value of the AUC (0–∞) from a single dose (assuming dose-independent clearance of the drug). Thus, it is necessary to obtain blood samples over only a single dosing interval at steady state to determine the AUC. The dosing interval selected for sampling (e.g., 7 a.m. through 7 p.m. at steady state, if dosing occurs every 12 hr) should be identical for each study phase. Because the disposition of the drug could vary as a function of time of day, comparing an AUC determined during the period 7a.m. through 7p.m. for one product and the AUC determined from 7p.m. through 7 a.m. for a second product would not be valid.

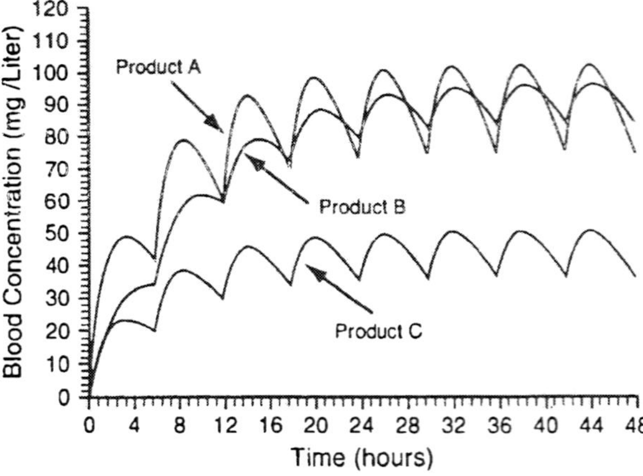

Fig. 1.3. Drug concentrations in blood vs. time after multiple doses of three products administered every six hours.

The results demonstrate the influence of the rate and extent of absorption on the steady-state plasma concentrations. The lower plasma concentrations shown for product C reflect the lower extent of absorption for this product. Products A and B have the same extent of absorption, but differ in rate of absorption. Product A is more rapidly absorbed than product B, and thus there is a greater fluctuation between the maximum and minimum concentrations at steady state.

Other study design considerations

In the design or evaluation of the results of a bioavailability or bioequivalence study, it is important to establish that adequate numbers of subjects were studied and that an adequate number of blood and/ or urine samples were collected. As in most scientific studies, the use of too few subjects precludes reaching meaningful conclusions regarding the significance of differences that may be observed. Moreover, values for T_{max}, C_{max}, or ER_{max} cannot be accurately determined if the time intervals between samples are too great. Further, accurate estimates of AUC and/or total urinary recovery of drug are not possible if blood and/ or urine collections are terminated prematurely.

As a general rule, collecting blood samples for at least two to three biologic half-lives is desirable, and urinary excretion studies should include urine collections for five to seven biologic half-lives. Some extension of these guidelines may be necessary if the study involves controlled-release dosage forms that may result in absorption for a prolonged period. If data are not available for the half-life of a drug, a reasonable guideline is to continue blood sampling until blood concentrations have declined to less than 10% of the peak concentrations. Similarly, urine collections should be continued until significant quantities of drug are no longer being excreted.

A typical bioavailability study utilizes from 12 to more than 24 healthy subjects who have no history of any disease that could affect the disposition of the test drug. The subjects are required to refrain from taking any drugs other than the test compound for a period (usually one week or more) prior to the study and throughout the course of the study. Certain drugs such as enzyme inducers could affect the disposition of the test drug. Further, depending on the specificity of the assay, other drugs may interfere in the quantitation of the drug of interest. Usually only subjects between the ages of 18 and 40 are employed unless there are specific reasons for employing other subject populations. Both male and female subjects should be included in the study, as well as subjects of differing race; realizing, of course, that the heterogeneity that one may accommodate in a study of 12 subjects is limited, if statistically meaningful comparisons are to be made between the groups. Finally, for typical single-dose studies, the subjects are required to fast from approximately 12 hr before the dose until 4 hr after the dose unless the objective of the study is to determine the influence of food on absorption of the drug.

Analytical methodology

One of the most important considerations in any bioavailability study is the validity of the analytical method. In addition to being reproducible, it must be sufficiently sensitive to permit the detection of low- drug concentrations in the biologic sample. After single-dose administration, drug concentrations in plasma are frequently in the low microgram or nano- gram per milliliter range. Further, the method must be specific for unmetabolized drug and be capable of accurately determining drug concentrations in the presence of metabolites of the drug and the constituents of blood and/or urine.

Most analytical methods involve some type of cleanup step such as solvent extraction, to separate the drug from the biologic fluid. In addition, most assays employ some type of chromatography, often using either gas chromatography or high- performance liquid chromatography. Assay validation is a critical component of any bioavailability or bioequivalence study and should consider the accuracy, precision, sensitivity, specificity, linearity, and reproducibility of the analytical method. The stability of the drug during storage in the biologic sample must also be given careful consideration.

Analysis and Interpretation of Data

Bioequivalence studies are usually intended to demonstrate that two or more formulations do not differ significantly (i.e., that the products are therapeutically equivalent and interchangeable). Once the data from a bioequivalence study is collected, statistical methods must be applied to determine the level of significance of any observed differences. Statistical comparisons of the C_{max} and AUC are performed after log transformation. Log transformation is appropriate because (i) many biologic and pharmacokinetic parameters are log-normally distributed and (ii) it is the ratio of C_{max} and AUC between drug products, and not the absolute difference between the mean values, that is most relevant for comparison. Two, one-sided statistical tests at a 0.05 level of significance are performed using the log-transformed data from the bioequivalence study.

It is important to note that 90% confidence intervals (CIs), and not the mean values, of C_{max} and AUC are employed to make this comparison and assure the bioequivalence of the drug products. In other words, the 90% CI for the mean C_{max} and mean AUC for the drug product must be between 80% and 125% of the respective mean values for the reference dosage form (e.g., a drug product with a mean Cmax of 83% of the reference product with a 90% CI of 79–87% would not be considered bioequivalent). In fact, if the mean C_{max} or mean AUC of the drug product differs by more than 10-15%, the CI is likely to fall outside the 80–125% range.

Typically an analysis of variance (ANOVA) method appropriate for the study design is applied to evaluate differences among dosage forms, subjects, and treatment periods. Mean T_{max} values are also computed, but unless large differences are observed, they are generally not used for the bioequivalence determination, largely owing to the fact that T_{max} values are highly dependent on study design and the time at which blood samples were collected.

The measurement of the bioavailability and bioequivalence of drug dosage forms is commonplace. The numerous reasons for the increased use of such studies include: rapid growth of the generic drug industry; an increased awareness of the effect of dosage form on the rate and extent of drug absorption;

the development of more sensitive and reliable analytic methods to quantitate drugs and metabolites in the body; and the need to have a means to evaluate the vivo performance of a dosage form by a means other than clinical trials in patients. Clearly bioavailability and bioequivalence studies have become a routine part of the drug product approval process by governmental agencies. Such studies provide valuable information regarding the disposition of a drug in humans and the factors that may influence the performance of a product. These data are useful in the development of new dosage forms and assist in the preparation of appropriate labeling for a drug product. Finally, bioequivalence studies have become an essential part of the comparison of pharmaceutically equivalent products manufactured by different pharmaceutical firms.

2

Drug Discovery and Development

Microarrays are grids of biomolecules (DNA, proteins, carbohydrates, small molecules) in which each element of the grid performs a specific assay such as identification of a specific binding molecule or measuring a particular enzymatic activity. A single sample is analyzed on each microarray providing simultaneous measurements for multiple parameters. Typically a complete experiment involves a large number of microarrays resulting in huge datasets. This deluge in data has led to approaches for integration of diverse datasets to enhance our understanding of both an individual molecular function and elaborate biological processes. This potential of microarrays to facilitate global analysis of genes and gene products has led to its adoption in nearly every area of biological science—from basic research to clinical diagnostics. They are being used to tackle one of the major challenges in the postgenomic era—to understand the regulation, expression, and function of entire sets of genes, transcripts, and proteins. This information will help in characterizing complex biological processes at the molecular level in various cell types, both in normal and in disease states.

Since their conception in the mid-1990s, microarrays have seen widespread use in almost all aspects of biological research and their range of applications continues to expand. These include (1) biomarker discovery, to find genes that can be used for measuring and following disease progression; (2) target selectivity, to identify genes that can distinguish one disease from another as well as subclasses of disease; (3) pharmacology and toxicogenomics, to help in identification of poor compounds and to optimize the selection of promising leads; and (4) drug screening, identification of protein activity modulators. As the cost of microarrays continues to drop, it is clear that microarrays are becoming a more integral part of the drug discovery process. In short, microarrays are redefining the drug discovery and development process by providing greater knowledge at each step and by helping to understand the complex workings of biological systems. This chapter provides a technical overview of microarrays, including information on array formats, production and use of microarrays for interrogating various molecular species—DNA, RNA, and proteins—and analysis of data. The challenges in experimental design to maximize microarray data quality, and the use of microarrays in understanding intracellular molecular networks as well as in drug discovery and development, are also discussed.

Array Formats

Planar Arrays

High-density microarrays

High-density arrays are ideally suited for analyzing a small number of samples against thousands of genes, proteins, or small molecules. Early transcript profiling studies used high-density arrays in the context of target discovery with the objective of obtaining a short list of high-priority candidates that showed interesting expression patterns in disease states. Arrays of oligonucleotides representing the entire human genome have been used for discovering polymorphic loci as well as the presence of thousands of alternative alleles. Other uses of high-density DNA arrays include determination of methylation patterns and identification of transcription factor binding sequences.

Manufacture of high-density protein arrays presents a greater challenge due to the inherent heterogeneity in the physicochemical properties and stability of proteins. However, arrays of recombinant proteins representing all yeast open reading frames (ORFs) have been manufactured and used for identification of novel binding activities. *Escherichia coli* transformed with cDNA libraries to express mammalian proteins have been arrayed to identify autoantibodies in serum from the mouse model of systemic lupus erythematosus.

Low-density microarrays

Low-density arrays can be used for simultaneously performing less complex analysis on many different samples. The ability to rapidly screen thousands of biological samples for multiple parameters in the same assay makes the process cost-effective and easy to perform. This format is based on either using slides with hydrophobic barriers to create wells or the 96- well microtiter plate formats, in which each well contains replicate mini-arrays of spots. Low-density arrays are becoming increasingly popular for cytokine measurements due to the relative ease with which preexisting conventional enzyme-linked immunosorbent assay (ELISA) assays can be adapted to a miniaturized format. In addition, low-density DNA arrays are being used for measuring polymorphisms to determine drug toxicity, and expression signatures obtained from high-density arrays are being used to guide the design of arrays with small sets of genes for use in cancer subclassification and prognosis. Over the last few years, several different types of microarrays of various probe densities and content—DNA or protein—have become commercially available. These provide microarray tools for analyzing samples derived not only from human tissues, but also from a wide spectrum of other species ranging from bacterial pathogens to Arabidopsis to mouse.

Solution Arrays

An alternative approach to planar arrays is three-dimensional arrays in solution. These have the advantage of parallel analysis and high throughput, in addition to better kinetics of binding in solution compared with planar arrays. Positional information in these arrays is retained by a variety of methods such as fluorescence-encoded beads (two dyes with varying ratios incorporated into the bead set) and bar-coded nanoparticles (self-encoded with submicron metal stripes). The independence of each element offers the flexibility to multiplex either a few or thousands of measurements without the need to customize each assay. The high degree of reliability and reproducibility has resulted in the development of fluorescence-encoded beads for multiplex diagnostic assays. This article will focus on technical issues, applications, and future directions in the use of planar arrays.

FACTORS FOR CONSIDERATION

Surfaces

Solid Supports

A wide variety of support materials have been used for manufacturing microarrays. Glass is the most commonly used support due to its low background fluorescence and amenability to automation. Polystyrene with fluorescence and binding properties similar to glass is beginning to be increasingly adapted for microarray use. These surfaces are usually modified by coating with one-, two-, or three-dimensional structures that provide either covalent attachment chemistry or enable binding of molecules through adsorption. Other microarray surfaces include membranes such as nitrocellulose and nylon and gold or silicon films. Synthesis of oligonucleotides has been performed *in situ* on fused silica wafers, and peptide arrays have been synthesized on cellulose and polypropylene membranes.

Chemistry

Microarray surfaces must maintain the stability and activity of attached biomolecules, while remaining surface-bound through all processing steps. Spot morphology and background noise, either due to nonspecific sample binding or from the detection system used, are important issues to be considered in choosing the right immobilization chemistry. A variety of surfaces have been derivatized to expose various active groups; these determine the type of attachment—ionic or covalent—of the biomolecule to the surface. Polylysine, which results in an amine surface carrying a positive charge, was among the early microarray surfaces used for binding to negatively charged biomolecules. Membranes such as nitrocellulose and nylon that have traditionally been used for a variety of blotting applications have been modified for microarrays by application onto glass backing.

Oligonulceotides modified to carry an amino group or proteins through their lysine residues can be covalently attached to aldehyde- and epoxy-derivatized surfaces. Other reactive surfaces used to covalently link both DNA and proteins include N-hydroxy succinimide and maleimide. Proteins expressed with polyhistidine and biotin tags have been attached to surfaces coated with nickel chelate and streptavidin, respectively. This strategy is likely to result in the proper orientation of the displayed molecules on the surface, thereby improving their functionality and stability.

Heterobifunctional cross-linkers have been used to attach activated biomolecules on surfaces functionalized with either aminosilane or mercaptopropylsilane. These strategies have resulted in up to fourfold higher signal-to-noise ratios compared with the polylysine surface for arrayed antibodies. Specific immobilization via interaction of surfaces functionalized with salicylhydroxamic acid derivatives and phenyldiboronic acid-labeled nucleic acids and proteins has also been demonstrated.

A new generation of chemistries has introduced poly(ethylene glycol)-functionalized surfaces that prevent nonspecific protein binding, thereby removing the need for a blocking step during processing. This commercially available chemistry also offers a wide variety of additional functional groups. A large spacer between the support and the biomolecule results in higher analyte binding by avoiding steric hindrance. Three-dimensional surfaces used for arraying biomolecules were shown to increase binding capacity and reduce denaturation of immobilized molecules, but they slowed down reaction kinetics due to reduction in diffusion rates. These same chemistries are applied for biomolecule attachment to beads in the manu facture of suspension arrays.

Probes

Printing

Printing refers to spotting arrays of presynthesized biomolecules directly onto a solid surface. This versatile approach can be applied to generate microarrays of almost any biomolecule in conjunction with a proper immobilization method. Printing can generate many copies of the same array more efficiently than *in situ* synthesis because the immobilized molecules need to be synthesized only once. Several kinds of microarray printing technologies have been developed, but the most commonly used method uses contact printing. In this method, pins are used to transfer samples from a source to the solid support by direct surface contact. Noncontact piezoelectric printers, which are also often used, can print more spots per unit time than contact printers by employing an electric current to accurately and rapidly dispense samples onto the solid support. Although the reproducibility of spot volumes delivered by contact printers typically has a coefficient of variation (*cv*) below 20%, piezoelectric printers have greater control over the volume dispensed resulting in *cv*s of under 5%. "*Dropouts*" or missing spots can be a problem, especially during high- throughput manufacture, and are primarily due to clogging of the dispensing components in the arrayer. To identify dropouts, microarrayers can be fitted with optical devices that can monitor dispensing and provide data on dropouts that can then be used to "fill in" missing spots. This system has vastly improved the quality of microarrays, reducing the need to print replicate spots of the same probe. Other less-common deposition methods include electrospraying in a stable cone- jet mode to generate highly reproducible spots of as little as 50-pL volumes and a laser transfer technique that allows the accurate deposition of picoliter volumes of proteins onto the solid surface.

In situ synthesis

Two typical *in situ* synthesis approaches are light-directed parallel synthesis and peptide synthesis on membrane (SPOT) synthesis. Although the former approach was initially developed for peptide synthesis, it has been adapted for the synthesis of DNA microarrays. This method uses a combination of photolithographic masks and combinatorial chemistry to synthesize oligonucleotides on fused silica wafers. High-density arrays have also been manufactured by maskless methods using either digitally controlled aluminium mirrors to fabricate oligonucleotides by photodeposition or by phosphoramidite chemistry in microfluidic chips with three-dimensional nano-chambers. The maskless method is also being used to create peptide arrays in microfluidic chips by parallel synthesis using digital photolithography and photogenerated acid during the deprotection step. Peptide arrays have also been manufactured by SPOT synthesis using a combination of novel polymeric surfaces, linker and cleavage chemistries, as well as robotic liquid-handling systems. These methods involve alternate synthesis and washing steps, increasing the possibility of contamination by reagents from adjacent spots, and thereby limiting array density.

Sample Processing

DNA analysis

Detection of single nucleotide polymorphisms (SNPs) was one of the early applications of high-density oligonucleotide arrays. More recently these arrays have also been used to assess DNA copy numbers. Each of these measurements requires the initial extraction of genomic DNA, which is then processed using several different methods each designed to incorporate labels for visualization of binding to specific probes on the array. Fragments from restriction digested genomic DNA were ligated with adaptors, amplified, and enzymatically end-labeled with biotin followed by hybridization to oligonucleotide arrays. Alternatively, labeling was done by incorporation of a biotin-tag during primer extension after hybridization of unlabeled amplified DNA fragments. The biotin was then detected using Streptavidin conjugated to a fluorescent dye. Genome-wide DNA–protein interactions have been mapped using intergenic oligonucleotide microarrays. In this approach, called chromatin immunoprecipitation (ChIP), epitope-tagged proteins of interest are allowed to bind specific regions in genomic DNA and then cross-linked. The DNA-bound epitope-tagged proteins are immunoprecipitated using a tag-specific antibody. The DNA is then delinked from the protein and, after fluorescent labeling, hybridized to arrays for identification of regions that bind to the protein of interest. A similar approach has been used for identification of methylation sites in genomic DNA. In this method, oligonucleotide primer adaptors are attached to restriction-digested DNA, followed by a secondary digestion with a methylation-sensitive enzyme, labeling with a fluorescent dye, and hybridization to arrays. These methods are providing a wealth of information on the factors that regulate gene expression and helping to understand these processes at a global level.

Transcript analysis

Microarrays permit the rapid analysis of complex gene expression changes in cells and tissues during development, both normal and disease. These changes give distinct patterns that can be used for discovering new disease-specific therapeutic targets, and molecular diagnostics, as well as for following treatment efficacy and disease prognosis. Typically for transcript profiling, a labeled nucleotide is incorporated during reverse transcription of the total cellular mRNA pools. Not only does this approach require a large amount of RNA (50 to 200 μg of total RNA) for hybridization, but RNA purity is also a critical factor in array performance due to potential nonspecific binding by other labeled macromolecules. Arrays have been widely used for obtaining relative mRNA concentrations between two samples, test and reference, in which each sample is labeled with a different dye (typically Cy3 and Cy5), followed by mixing of the samples before hybridization. An alternative method avoids incorporation of bulky dyes during reverse transcription by incorporating amino allyl labels to which N-hydroxyl succinimidyl dyes are chemically coupled in a later step. The use of a common reference RNA allows for the comparison of data between various array experiments. Typically a pool of RNA derived from a variety of tissues is used as a reference sample. Efforts are being made to implement common standards (MIAME, minimal information about a microarray experiment) for transcript profiling through the MGED Society to enable data sharing between different groups.

Methods in which the amount of mRNA has been amplified to produce labeled cRNA, by incorporating a T7 RNA polymerase promoter site into one end of the cDNA followed by *in vitro* transcription are also widely used. In this method, quantitative estimates of the amount of each transcript in a given sample can be calculated. In single-sample labeling experiments, a reference RNA may be spiked in during sample labeling and hybridization to facilitate quality control of the process as well as for comparison of data between different arrays. Despite its current widespread use and the drive toward ensuring high-quality microarray data by the implementation of MIAME guidelines, very little is known about the extent to which application of different technologies influences the outcome of transcriptional profiles and differential expression. However, microarray users should be aware of studies that have attempted to present a comprehensive evaluation encompassing different probe types (oligonucleotides and cDNAs), labeling techniques and hybridization protocols.

Protein analysis

The early adaptation of protein microarrays is the reformatting of already available ELISA. In these assays, which were first described by Roger Ekins, a protein antigen is identified and its quantity is measured using two antigen-specific antibodies—one surface-immobilized to capture the antigen, and the other chemically labeled to bind the captured antigen in the solution phase. The second antibody produces a detectable signal through the label. This method, in which the protein sample does not have to be labeled, has been widely used for measuring cytokine levels in a variety of samples such as serum and tissue culture supernatants. Protein expression profiles have also been measured by capturing dye-labeled protein lysates derived from cells and tissues on arrays of antibodies. These measurements have largely been ratiometric in which two samples each labeled with a different dye using protocols similar to those used for transcript analysis are mixed and incubated with arrays of antibodies. Single-sample analyses could be performed by spiking known amounts of control proteins into the samples before labeling.

Signal Detection

Detection chemistries

The most prevalent method for detecting binding of target to immobilized probes on microarrays are fluorescent dyes, of which Cy3 and Cy5 are the most widely used especially for differential transcript and protein profiling, whereas single-target hybridizations are commonly performed with fluorescein isothiocyanate. Although Alexa dyes allow use of more than two colors in a single experiment, they are less commonly used. Enzyme-labeled fluorescence (ELF), a phosphatase substrate that results in a precipitable product, has been used for both DNA and protein arrays. Chemiluminescent detection is also used, mainly to detect antigen capture on antibody arrays by sequential incubations with biotinylated secondary antibodies and Streptavidin-conjugated horse-radish peroxidase (HRP)]. Phosphorylation of arrayed kinase substrates in the presence of radiolabeled adenosine triphosphate (ATP) has been detected by autoradiography.

To increase sensitivity of detection, several signal amplification methods have been applied to the various types of molecular targets. Tyramide signal amplification (TSA) uses biotinyl-tyramide, an HRP substrate, to accumulate biotin at the reaction site. The "*amplified*" biotin is then detected using Streptavidin-HRP in conjunction with substrates that result in products detectable either by fluorescence, chemiluminescence, or colorimetry. Other signal amplification methods include rolling circle amplification (RCA) in which an oligonucleotide-conjugated antibody binds to biotin on the target, followed by hybridization of a circular DNA molecule to the oligonucleotide. The circular DNA is then replicated using a DNA polymerase in the presence of a fluorescently labeled nucleotide. Preformed branched DNA (dendrimers), each of which is attached to over 200 fluorescent dye molecules, have also been used for labeling array-bound targets.

Imaging systems

Assay format and cost are the primary determinants of the kind of devices used for imaging arrays. Fluorescence-based scanners that use lasers to excite fluorescent dyes attached to the target molecule (for transcript profiling) or to a specific secondary detection reagent (for ELISA assays) are the most widely used for signal detection and imaging. These instruments enable user-defined scanning resolutions and photomultiplier tube settings to adjust detection sensitivity. In addition, the availability of a wide range of fluorescent dyes makes this the most flexible system for use in microarray image detection. Chemiluminescence-based detection systems using a charge-coupled device (CCD) together with conventional camera optics are also commonly used. Although the latter systems are flexible for applications in a wide range of assay formats, fluorescence scanners provide a higher range of sensitivity and dynamic range. Label-independent methods such as surface plasmon resonance (SPR) can overcome variations caused by inconsistencies in labeling chemistries that are often seen in label-dependent detection systems. SPR has been used to measure affinities in binding reactions, especially between antigens and their cognate antibodies. These highly sensitive systems are beginning to be adapted for microarray-based measurements. Another recently described method relies on the change in fluorescence decay times of tryptophan and tyrosine residues in proteins to identify protein–protein interactions. In this method, a change in binding behavior of proteins in solution toward protein partners arrayed on a solid support is detected with regard to binding specificity and protein amount.

Data Analysis

Most commercial microarray imagers supply data extraction software that can accommodate the unique parameters of scanned images. In addition, printing precision has simplified the process of detecting spot boundaries and measurement of inter-spot distances. A useful consideration is the format for storage of primary scanned images (usually as tiff files) so as to be able to take advantage of future developments in image analysis software. Storage of raw image files retains maximum information, allowing the use of different normalization, image extraction, and quality metrics. Several commercially available software packages are available that interpret and transform an array image into a dataset. Software programs grid the elements of the array as a first step in processing the image. Background-corrected intensity values for each spots are obtained using one of several options: local (area around individual spots) or global (average signal in area outside of the grid) background corrections, or user-defined values such as those from negative control data points contained within the array. After background-corrected intensity values have been calculated for each spot, the data are normalized with respect to sources of systematic and biological variation. The choice of the normalization method is critical because it impacts precision of data comparison between arrays. Several methods for statistical analysis of microarray data are available depending on the experimental setup and the kind of biological question that needs to be addressed. Initial approaches to analyzing microarray data focused on unsupervised hierarchical clustering because these are simple ways in which data can be organized. It is still the most commonly used analysis tool especially if the experiment has been designed to obtain a bird's eye view of transcript or protein profiles during a particular process. Machine learning techniques such as neural networks and support vector machines should be used for more advanced analyses when preliminary information can be used to guide data interpretation. Most software packages have a user-friendly graphical user interface (GUI) that enables performing a number of simple analysis, including data normalization, various kinds of clustering, and principal component analysis.

Types of Arrays

DNA Arrays

Transcript profiling

Transcript profiling was one of the earliest applications of microarray technology. In this application, fluorescently labeled cellular transcripts are hybridized either to arrays of spotted cDNA or *in situ* synthesized oligonucleotides. The former have generally been used for hybridization of a mixture of two transcript pools, each of which are derived from a different biological sample (such as diseased and normal tissue), and labeled with a different fluorescent dye (Cy3 and Cy5) before mixing. A ratiometric analysis of fluorescence then helps to determine the relative expression levels of each transcript in the two samples. cDNA arrays have received wide acceptance within the academic community due to their low cost and ease of manufacture, as well as the ability to customize rapidly as new genomic sequence information becomes available. Customization of array content also easily accommodates the research interests of individual laboratories.

Oligonucleotide arrays, used for measuring transcript amounts from single samples, have the advantage of displaying a much larger number of very small spots (5μ), enabling the interrogation of multiple probes for each transcript, including mismatch probes for determination of hybridization specificity. Currently, oligonucleotide arrays that display probes covering all predicted genes in the human genome are commercially available from several vendors. The ability to obtain global transcript profiles has accelerated the process of discovery in all areas of biology ranging from basic discovery to drug development and diagnostics. Correlations between gene-expression patterns and disease states have led to the selection of the best drug targets for pharmaceutical development as well as for monitoring therapeutic outcomes. One area in which DNA arrays are making a critical impact is cancer, where expression profiles from hundreds of cancer tissue samples have allowed subclassification of cancers based on the identification of specific transcript expression signatures. These are likely to guide therapy and improve prognosis for cancer patients in the near future.

Physical characterization of genes

Oligonucleotide arrays have found use in the physical characterization of the genome by helping to map transcription factor binding sites and methylation sites. These arrays, with their ability to package hundreds of thousands of spots on each chip, have been widely used for SNP discovery. Clinically significant SNPs have then been rearrayed in a low-density format for analyzing large numbers of samples to determine clinical validity. A U.S. Food and Drug Administration (FDA)-approved SNP genotyping array for CYP450 has recently been used to identify patients with a decreased ability to metabolize risperidone. More recently, bacterial artificial chromosome (BAC) arrays have provided high-resolution maps of genetic changes, including gains and losses, as well as amplifications in chromosomal DNA by comparative genomic hybridization. Other applications of oligonucleotide arrays have been to analyze splice variants by hybridization of labeled transcripts with arrays that combine exon and junction-derived probes, which are either specific or nonspecific to a splice event.

Cell arrays

Immobilized arrays of plasmid DNA used to transfect cells in the presence of a transfection reagent are called cell arrays or reverse transfection arrays. These arrays are overlayed with cultured cells in medium and incubated so that cells superimposed on the DNA spot are transfected. The desired phenotypic change is visualized by staining the cells after a brief incubation period. This format allows a variety of readouts, including cytoskeletal changes, apoptosis, and DNA replication, which can be either visualized with a laser scanner or a fluorescence microscope. Similar approaches have been used for increasing the throughput of loss-of-function studies using RNAi to monitor effects on cell phenotype. These studies enable functional whole genome screens without the need for expensive screening facilities.

Protein Arrays

Protein profiling

Antibody Arrays. Antibodies are the most commonly arrayed protein class due to their structural similarity and stability. Many monoclonal antibodies generated over the years for binding to various epitopes on proteins offer a diverse source of capture and detection antibodies. These are being used in antibody arrays, especially for determination of growth factor and cytokine levels from a variety of biological samples. Arrays have been multiplexed with antibodies that were developed and used for conventional ELISAs to measure levels of more than 50 cytokines with a high degree of sensitivity (pg/mL) from low sample volumes (less than 50 μL). However, each set of arrayed antibodies needs to be characterized for specificity of binding to the target molecule to ensure data quality. Recent studies have shown significant cross-reactivity of arrayed antibodies to proteins other than their intended targets. Identification of disease biomarkers is a rapidly growing area of proteomic research. These biomarkers can enable better predictive capabilities in disease diagnosis and prognosis, as well as in drug development by identifying potential drug toxicities and side-effects. Although it has been suggested that antibody arrays can be used to profile serum and cell lysates, these measurements are complicated by the fact that protein concentrations in these samples cover 10 to 14 orders of magnitude, requiring systems that can simultaneously detect both low- and high-abundance proteins within a single array. The sample complexity issue may be alleviated by reduction in sample complexity before profiling. This can be accomplished using either liquid phase protein separation systems or by profiling the protein complement of various cell organelles separately. Samples can be labeled with either fluorescent tags followed by direct detection after capture or with other haptens such as biotin followed by detection with Streptavidin conjugated to a reporter molecule.

As well-characterized antibodies are available to only a small subset of total cellular proteins, profiling complex protein samples could be performed using arrays of *in vitro* synthesized antibody libraries. This format has the advantage of being able to directly array bacterial cells rather than purified recombinant antibodies. Once disease-relevant proteins have been identified through screening for global protein changes, arrays containing the "*diagnostic*" subset of antibodies that recognize disease-specific proteins can be used for high-throughput, large-sample analysis.

Antigen arrays

Several studies have been performed to demonstrate disease identification by analysis of serum antibodies to clinically relevant proteins. One study used arrays of autoantigen diagnostic markers to measure autoantibody titers in serum of patients with autoimmune disease. In an extension of this study, autoimmune patient sera screened for binding to arrayed antigens identified specificity of autoantibody responses defining autoantigens relevant in human disease. More recently, the diversity of B-cell response as a function of disease severity was measured using an array of over 225 distinct epitopes derived from several myelin-associated proteins. These arrays could identify distinct sets of epitopes and could demonstrate a correlation between reduced epitope spreading and improved disease outcome. This information is now being used to guide the development of a tolerizing DNA vaccine, which could potentially limit epitope spreading and improve disease outcome. These antigen arrays have been shown to have a much higher sensitivity than conventional ELISAs with a three-log linear dynamic range.

Protein function arrays

The development of high-throughput expression and purification methods have made a large number of proteins available for arraying. A small amount of material (pg to ng) is sufficient for printing numerous arrays that can then be used to perform rapid, functional screens. The first genome-wide protein display, an array of all yeast ORFs, was used to screen for binders to calmodulin and phospholipids. In this study, 5800 different yeast proteins with hexahistidine tags were arrayed on nickel-coated glass slides. The immobilized proteins were then probed with various labeled phospholipids resulting in the identification of more than 150 proteins that were shown to bind phospholipids for the first time. Other protein binding measurements include identification of protein–protein and protein–DNA interactions. In addition to binding assays, functional properties are also being measured on arrays. Protein kinase activity has been determined either by immobilizing fluorogenic substrates followed by the addition of specific kinases or on kinase arrays incubated with peptide substrates in the presence of radiolabeled ATP. Protein kinase arrays have also been used for identification of inhibitors by incubating small-molecule binders in the presence of substrates demonstrating the ability of arrays to screen for kinase inhibitors.

G-protein-coupled receptors (GPCRs) currently make up the largest class of therapeutic drug targets and are an obvious choice for microarray-based drug screening. An early study demonstrating the capability of microarrayed GPCRs for agonist and antagonist screening showed retention of activity through several activation/ deactivation cycles after ligand binding on arrayed rhodopsin. Competitive binding assays in which mixtures of fluorescently labeled ligands and unlabeled inhibitors were used to demonstrate binding selectivity to different receptor subtypes have also been described.

Other types of protein arrays

Peptides, arrayed either by deposition on the surface or by *in situ* synthesis, have been used for epitope-mapping, measuring enzyme activity, and cell capture. They have also been used for identification of peptide antagonists to proteins that are likely drug targets. In addition, protease specificities were identified using peptidyl coumarin substrate arrays created by immobilizing the fluorescent coumarin leaving group via the C-terminus to the solid support, enabling synthesis of a high-diversity peptide library at the N-terminal end.

Arrays of peptide–major histocompatibility complex (MHC) complexes have been created on acrylamide gel-coated glass surfaces and used for ligand-specific capture of CD4(+) and CD8(+) lymphocytes. This approach should be useful to characterize multiple epitope-specific T-cell populations during immune responses associated with infection, cancer, autoimmunity, and vaccination.

Covalent mRNA–protein fusions were displayed on single-stranded DNA arrays through nucleic acid hybridization of the mRNA in the fusion molecule. Similarly, capture agents such as nucleic acid aptamers have also been proposed for use in protein binding.

Tissue Arrays

Tissue microarrays (TMAs) are displays of several tens to hundreds of tissue specimens on a single slide for parallel analysis. Paraffin embedded tissue are generally used for arraying; however, arrays have also been constructed from frozen tissue. The ability to array archival paraffin embedded tissue opens up vast archives of patient samples for medical research. Arrayed tissue sections processed either for cytological staining or *in situ* hybridization, combined with automated image analysis systems, provides a powerful molecular profiling tool. TMAs are commonly used to confirm results obtained from expression microarrays, as well as in the development of diagnostic and prognostic markers for clinical applications.

Other Arrays

Although DNA and protein arrays continue to be widely used, other types of molecules are being arrayed and used for a variety of applications. These include small-molecule arrays in which individual members of a chemical library are deposited on a surface and used for performing binding assays with target proteins. Several strategies are being applied for displaying small molecules on surfaces. The simplest strategy is to spot molecules on glass after mixing with glycerol to maintain "wetness' after deposition. This strategy was used to create and screen arrays by spraying the target protein, human caspase 6, along with its fluorigenic substrate and screening for dark spots of enzyme inhibitors against noninhibitor fluorescent spots. An elegant method that takes advantage of DNA hybridization specificities to provide an address for arrays of *protein nucleic acid* (PNA)-tagged small molecules has been described. More sophisticated libraries of molecules that selectively modulate activities of mutated kinases have been used to identify chemical inhibitors that switch off individual kinases.

Carbohydrate arrays have been developed and used as novel high-throughput analytical tools for monitoring carbohydrate–protein interactions such as profiling protein binding to various sugars and to measure enzymatic activity on sugar substrates. These microarrays have also been used to discover anti-adhesion therapeutics by identifying carbohydrate binding specificities of pathogenic bacteria. The display of carbohydrate ligands on a surface in a manner that mimics interactions at the cell–cell interface is ideal for whole-cell applications. Similarly, monosaccharide-based arrays of N-acetyl galactosamine and N-acetylneuraminic acid derivatives were used to identify binders to cholera and tetanus toxins.

Implications of Array Technology

Experimental Design

Microarrays are observed as tools for "*descriptive*" research and not for "*hypothesis-driven*" research, which is primarily driven to answer specific questions related to a known set of molecules. However, most microarray-based studies do have clear objectives and are designed to answer well-defined questions. The plan for specimen selection should follow from the objectives of the microarray study. Studies may either be exploratory, whose results should be confirmed, or designed to test various models; in which case, the experiments have to be designed in a focused manner. Appropriate design of microarray studies is critical to draw valid and useful conclusions from the large amount of data that are invariably obtained from each experiment. Criteria for design will vary depending on the type of array used—DNA, protein, and small molecule—as well as the experimental objectives, and sources of variability within the system. Issues such as selection of samples, number of replicates needed, allocation of samples to dyes for ratiometric profiling, and sample size are important considerations in these studies.

Three sources of variation should be considered in the design of a micro array experiment: (1) biological, at the level of setting up of the cells, cell lines or animals, and sample treatment; (2) technical, which is introduced during sample processing; and (3) analytical, which highlights signal bias and readout. To minimize each of these variations, the experiment should be set up such that the biological material to be used for analysis should be handled separately from the initiation of the experiment providing biological replicates. If this results in an unwieldy experimental setup, pooling the samples at some stage of processing may still allow a reduction in biological variance. This approach is risky in the event of the presence of an extreme outlier in the pool, because this can unduly influence the expression values obtained from the pool. Samples from every stage of the experiment with a likelihood of introduction of variation should be treated separately. Replicate measurements from the same biological sample helps to reduce technical variation.

Ratiometric analysis of signal by comparing signal intensities between two samples from the same spot reduces errors due to printing differences. This has led to the use of a reference sample in transcript profiling experiments, and it is an integral part of differential profiling, making the choice of the reference sample critical. The most important considerations in choosing the appropriate standard are that it is readily available, homogeneous, and stable over a period of time. The reference sample does not need to have any biological relevance, because it merely serves to compare expression profiles between different experiments performed in different laboratories. Among the standards that have been used are mRNA populations obtained from a wide variety of cells or tissues with the aim of lighting up every element on the array. Alternatively, a reference sample is prepared from the samples that will be assayed in the experiment to ensure that every transcript present in the test samples will be represented in the reference standard. Care has to be taken, however, that no transcript in the reference sample saturates the signal in the detection system.

If a direct comparison needs to be made between two samples, for example, samples from pooled healthy tissue with samples from disease tissue, it would be necessary to perform forward and reverse labeling to remove any dye bias that may alter the results. Swapping dyes between samples reduces systematic bias in the data that can be corrected during the normalization step. Alternative design strategies that have been suggested are the balanced block design and the loop design. The same considerations can be applied to two-color antibody array-based protein profiling.

Molecular Network Analysis

Computational analysis is essential to transform the large amount of data generated by microarrays into a mechanistic understanding of various modules connecting at hubs and nodes to form molecular networks. Methods that identify the regulatory mechanisms underlying these modules and processes by an integrative analyses in the context of other data sources are often capable of extracting deeper biological insight from the data. Such integrative computational approaches include meta-analysis, functional enrichment analysis, interactome analysis, transcriptional network analysis, and integrative model system analysis. In addition, comparative analysis, combining human data with model organisms, can lead to more robust findings. Such methods that analyze biological processes in terms of higher level modules can identify robust signatures of disease mechanisms. Application of these methods to understand human cancers have delineated molecular subtypes of cancer associated with disease progression and treatment response.

A closely integrated data warehouse has been constructed to link different kinds and numbers of biological networks to experimental results such as those coming from microarrays. The basic idea is to consider and store biological networks as graphs in which the nodes represent promoters, proteins, genes, and transcripts, and the edges specify the relationship between the various nodes. Direct links to underlying sequences (exons, introns, promoters, amino acid sequences) in a systematic way enable close interoperability to sequence analysis methods. This approach allows us to store, query, and update a wide variety of biological information in a way that is semantically compact without requiring changes at the database schema level when new kinds of biological information are added. Such a system can be set up using software available from the public domain.

Drug Discovery and Development

Target discovery

Microarrays are increasingly being used in drug discovery for a wide range of applications, including target discovery and selection, pharmacology, and toxicogenomics. The objective of using transcript profiling in target discovery is to identify a short list of candidate genes with distinct expression patterns during disease. Typical selection criteria include disease-specific changes in expression levels and tissue or cell-type selectivity. A secondary screen is then typically used to examine the role(s) of short-listed genes by analyzing additional samples, and identifying correlations with disease progression. Validation experiments are performed to follow up the candidate genes using animal disease models or mice in which the target gene has been knocked out. Network analysis is especially relevant to antimicrobial drug discovery. The relatively small size of microbial genomes enables data from profiling experiments to be used for modeling gene networks because these would be several orders of magnitude lower in complexity compared with human cellular networks. In addition, the availability of whole-genome nucleotide sequence data from a growing list of microbial genomes allows designing of probes for DNA arrays. Such microarrays are already being used to obtain a global perspective of host–pathogen interactions. This is beginning to make an impact on our understanding of pathogenesis and the strategies taken to combat infectious diseases, including the identification of novel drug targets.

Target validation

Several approaches, including those that involve the use of arrays, can be taken to validate short-listed therapeutic candidates. Genes whose transcript profiles suggest additional analysis can be profiled using TMAs in tens to hundreds of tissues by immunohistochemistry. TMAs can be used to identify heterogeneities between primary tumors and their metastases, as demonstrated in the analyses of erbB2 in primary and metastatic breast cancers. The expression of a target gene in normal tissue from various vital organs can also be assessed using TMA panels. It is well known that mRNA levels do not reflect protein quantities and function. so proteomic analysis may help in making better decisions on targets to be developed for therapeutics. Cell-based gene knockouts can closely mimic the actions of potential drugs to identify phenotypic changes and potential side effects. The successful adaptation of RNA interference in a microarray format to facilitate efficient suppression of gene expression has enabled high-throughput target validation for a wide variety of cell types.

Pharmacology

A study that monitored the expression patterns of the entire complement of yeast genes under a variety of experimental conditions and genetic backgrounds was used to categorize drugs into various classes based on the expression pattern changes they induced. This database is being used to stratify novel drugs based on their mechanism of action by monitoring the changes in expression induced by them. Drug safety in animals is tested by monitoring a diverse spectrum of events, most commonly liver and kidney toxicity, and fatty liver. Transcriptional activation of drug metabolizing enzymes in livers of drug-treated animals or primary human hepatocytes has been widely used to identify drug metabolizing pathways. This helps to identify drugs early in development that might have toxicity issues due to inadequate metabolism. In human populations, certain polymorphisms in the cytochrome P450 genes result in slow drug metabolism leading to toxicity. Additionally, the identification of SNPs in the cytochrome P450 genes of patients during clinical trials can help to stratify patients in whom the treatment is likely to be effective.

3

INDIVIDUALIZED THERAPY

The rapid progress in molecular medicine has sought to understand the molecular basis of human disease with an ultimate goal of developing rationally designed therapies. The *gene discovery phase* has been largely driven by key technological advances including polymerase chain reaction (PCR) and other strategies and methods, high-throughput sequencing, and bioinformatics. Now that the genome is sequenced, there are ongoing efforts to identify genetic polymorphisms (e.g., single nucleotide polymorphisms, SNPs) that may point to disease predisposition or unique responses to therapy such as untoward drug side effects. Presently, physicians have to optimize a dosage regimen for an individual patient by a trail-and-error method. This kind of blind approach may cause adverse drug reactions (ADRs) in some patients. In fact, ADRs are found to occur in more than 2 million hospitalizations including approximate 100,000 deaths per year in the United States. Similarly, according to a German study, about 6% of ADRs are attributed to new hospital admissions, and these ADRs were found to be preventable.

This interindividual variability in drug response could be caused by multiple factors such as disease determinants, genetic and environmental factors, and variability in drug target response (pharmacodynamic response) or idiosyncratic response. These factors affect drug absorption, distribution, metabolism, and excretion. Drug concentrations in plasma can vary more than 600-fold between two individuals of the same weight on the same drug dosage. An understanding of the variability in efficacy and toxicity of the same doses of medications in the human population, therefore, may provide safer and efficient drug therapy. In general, genetic factors are estimated to account for 15–30% of interindividual differences in drug metabolism and response; but for certain drugs or classes of drugs, genetic factors are of the utmost importance and can account for up to 95% of interindividual variability in drug disposition and effects. The idea that drug response is determined by genetic factors that alter pharmacokinetics and pharmacodynamics of compounds evolved in the late 1950s, when an inherited deficiency of glucose-6-phosphate dehydrogenase was shown to cause the severe hemolysis observed in some patients exposed to the antimalarial primaquine. This discovery explained why hemolysis was observed mainly in African- Americans, in whom the deficiency is common, and rarely in Caucasians of northern, western, and eastern descent. In 1959, Vogel coined the term pharmacogenetics to describe inherited differences in drug responses.

Later in 1962, W. Kalow defined *pharmacogenetics* as "... the study of heredity and the response to drugs". It is a well-recognized fact that individuals respond differently to drug therapy; some drugs that are effective or well-tolerated by some people may be ineffective or toxic to others. This variability can often be traced by SNPs in genes encoding drug-metabolizing enzymes, transporters, ion channels, and drug receptors, all of which have been known to be associated with interindividual variation in drug response and have aroused considerable interest in recent years. Taken together, pharmacogenetics is the study of genetic polymorphisms in drug-metabolizing enzymes and the translation of inherited differences to the variability in drug effects. Genes are described as "*polymorphic*" when allelic variants exist in the population, one or more of which alters the activity of the encoded protein compared with the wild-type sequence. Typically, the polymorphism leads to reduced activity of the encoded protein. Although the focus of pharmacogenetics is the study of drug-metabolizing enzymes like the CYP family, polymorphisms in drug transporters (such as P-glycoprotein) band drug targets (such as receptors) have also received attention.

The original task of pharmacogenetic research is to aid physicians in the prescription of the appropriate medicine in the right dosage in an attempt to attain maximum efficacy and minimum toxicity based on a genetic test, performed before the initiation of the therapy. The new paradigm moves toward the approach of screening for polymorphisms associated with a drug response and tailoring clinical and therapeutic decisions for an individual patient. This strategy of targeting drugs according to the patient's genetic constitution is termed "*personalized medicine*". Toward the goal of personalized medicine, after completion of the human genome project, a haplotype map (HapMap) has been developed by the International HapMap Consortium with an intention of profiling DNA sequence variations across the human genome, which should provide a powerful tool to understand the genetic variants and drug responses (biomarkers). This knowledge may ultimately allow the development of personalized medications based on the genotype of each patient. The term "*pharmacogenomics*" was introduced to reflect the transition from genetics to genomics and the use of genome-wide approaches to identify genes that contribute to a specific disease or drug response. A pharmacogenomics approach could allow a specific drug therapy to be targeted to genetically defined subsets of patients and could lead to a new disease and treatment classification on the molecular level.

Although the "*blueprints*" of human disease and for the drug action may be genetically encoded, the execution of the disease process and the pharmacodynamics of a given drug occurs through altered protein function. Researchers in molecular medicine are currently going from genomics to proteomics. One goal for clinical proteomics will be to characterize the information flow within single cells, tissues, or entire organisms under normal or disease conditions. Therefore, identifying the genetic or epigenetic events leading to wanted or unwanted effects of drugs requires subsequent understanding of the proteomic consequences of these events. Therefore, *pharmacoproteomics* are focused on the influence of drugs on protein–protein interactions, their localization, or whether the encoded proteins are stable expressed, phosphorylated, cleaved, acetylated, glycosylated, or functionally "active." Mounting evidence confirms that the low-molecular-weight (LMW) range of circulatory proteome contains a rich source of information that may be able to detect or better characterize drug–protein interactions and stratify toxicological risk. Current mass spectrometry (MS) platforms can generate a rapid and high-resolution portrait of the LMW proteome. Emerging novel nanotechnology strategies to amplify and harvest these LMW biomarkers *in vivo* or *ex vivo* will greatly enhance our knowledge about pharmacoproteomics. As an example for an pharmacoproteomic approach, it was found that in comparison with tamoxifen-sensitive breast tumor cells, in an tamoxifen-resistant line, 12 proteins were found upregulated, whereas nine were downregulated. Three of the identified proteins (AGL-2 interacting protein and two GDP-dissociation inhibitors) could be directly involved in the resistance phenomenon. Curiously enough, the erythrocyte sedimentation reaction (ESR), which could be defined as a primitive forerunner of functional proteomics, has been used for a long time for clinical diagnostics and for monitoring of pharmacological therapy.

Although genetic variation is clearly important, it seems unlikely that personalized drug therapy will be enabled for a wide range of major diseases using genomic knowledge alone. Therefore, a third modern possibility for enabling personalized pharmacological therapy is the phenotyping by *pharmacometabonomics*. A major factor underlying interindividual variation in drug effects is variation in metabolic phenotype, which is influenced not only by genotype but also by different factors such as *in utero* effects, lifestyle, nutritional status, the gut microbiota, age, disease, environment, and the co- or pre-administration of other drugs. A new approach to personalized drug treatment is the examination of the metabolic profile. The profile, which is a measurement of small molecules such as sugars and amino acids, could be used to predict the pharmacodynamic or toxic response to drugs.

Pharmacometabonomics use a combination of pre-dose metabolite profiling and chemometrics to model and predict the responses of individual subjects. ^{1}H nuclear magnetic resonance (NMR) spectroscopy has been applied as a metabolite profiling tool for metabonomic studies, as it enables many endogenous metabolites to be quantified rapidly and reproducibly in biological fluids without derivatization or separation. Pharmacometabonomics has an important theoretical advantage over pharmacogenomics in that it can potentially take account of both genomic and environmental factors affecting drug-induced responses. However, because the time of practical use of pharmacoproteomics and pharmacometabonomics is obviously more distant from today as such for the genetic approaches, we will focus this chapter more on pharmacogenetics and pharmacogenomics. The present knowledge certainly does not allow or recommend individualized therapy on the basis of pharmacoproteomics as well as pharmacometabonomics. They are not ready for profound optimization of clinical drug application or rationale drug development to become a reality in the near future. Intensification of research capacities is assumed, providing optimism for personalized medicine. In the following sections, depending on the target respective, selected examples for the influence of genetic variability on the drug response are discussed. In most of the cases, we will cite publications from the first half of the year 2006, indicating the enormous progress in this field in the last months.

Drug Metabolizing Enzymes

A considerable body of evidence suggests that SNP in genes encoding drug- metabolizing enzymes might determine drug efficacy and toxicity. The cytochrome P450 (CYP) enzymes consist of a superfamily of haem-containing monooxygenases, and multiple forms of CYP exist in all mammals. CYPs are responsible for the oxidation of many drugs, environmental chemicals, and endogenous substrates. They exist in the liver and in extrahepatic tissues such as the intestine, lung, and kidney. In humans, xenobiotics are metabolized primarily by three CYP subfamilies: CYP1, CYP2, and CYP3. Genetic polymorphisms of the genes for CYP2C9, CYP2C19, and CYP2D6 affect the metabolism of 20–30% of clinically used drugs. The frequency of variant alleles of CYP families varies among populations according to the race and ethnic background. For instance, there are 78 reported variants of CYP 2D6 that associated with adverse drug reactions. Many of these polymorphic genes encode inactive enzymes. However, these inactive enzymes may produce adverse drug reactions among patients because of their poor metabolic activity (e.g., the adverse effects of the neuroleptic risperidone).

Similarly, several inactivating genetic polymorphisms have been reported in another member of the CYP family, namely CYP2C19 (CYP2C19*2 and CYP2C19*3), which is also associated with adverse drug reactions. This enzyme is responsible for the metabolism of proton pump inhibitors (e.g., omeprazole and lansoprazole) used for the treatment of gastric acid-related disorders such as peptic ulcer and gastroesophageal reflux disease. Approximately 2–4% of Caucasians and 4% of African-Americans have poor metabolism of these drugs. Poor metabolizing patients of proton pump inhibitors carry two nonfunctional alleles, heterozygous extensive metabolizers have one nonfunctional and one wild-type allele, and extensive metabolizers are homozygous for the wild-type allele. Another example is the coumarin warfarin, which is widely used for oral anticoagulation. Major side effects include bleeding complications. It was found that CYP2C9*2 and CYP2C9*3 alleles reduce the clearance of war farin and increase the risk of bleeding. The data indicate that patients carrying at least one variant CYP2C9 allele require lower maintenance doses and have a significantly higher risk of bleeding. However, SNPs in vitamin K epoxide reductase (VKORC1) may be more important. Recent studies have identified haplotype-dependent predictions for warfarin dosing. VKORC1 haplotype A predicted 21–25% of the required warfarin dose, and the inclusion of CYP2C9 genotypes reduced the required warfarin dose up to 31% in Caucasians. Combining nongenetic factors such as age, sex, body surface area, and drug interactions with the genotype information predicts up to 60% of warfarin dose. The remaining 40% of warfarin dosing variability remains unexplained. CYP2C9*13 allele is associated with reduced metabolism of lornoxicam. Similarly, CYP2C8 plays a role in the disposition of some therapeutic drugs.

The intestinal epithelium and liver contain the most abundant member of the CYP family, namely CAP3A, and these enzymes are responsible for the metabolism of more than half of the therapeutic drugs. Its activity also varies among members of a given population. In addition, this enzyme may undergo induction (rifamycins) and inhibition (calcium channel blockers) depending on the drug administration, which may account for its poor or higher metabolic activity. The interindividual variation in the immunosuppressive drugs cyclosporine and tacrolimus could be caused by interindividual differences in the expression of CYP 3A4 and 3A5 and the drug transporter P-glycoprotein. The most frequent allelic variant of CYP3A5 is CYP3A5*3, with a frequency of 87% of all alleles in a French population. An important P450 database in terms of genetic polymorphisms is the CYP alleles database. However, genetic variants identified in the CYP3A4 and CYP3A5 genes have only a limited impact on the CYP3A-mediated drug metabolism, and hence the identification of the genotype for the ABCB1 transporter gene may provide further clues for the individualization of therapy with certain drugs. Apart from CYPs, some other enzymes involved in the biotransformation of drugs include *N*-acetyltransferase (NAT), glutathione-*S*-transferase, and uridine diphosphate-glucuronosyl transferase 1A1 (UGT1A1). One of the earlier discoveries of pharmacogenetics is the attribution of the neurological side effects of the antituberculosis drug isoniazid to genetic variability of NAT2. A 98.1% correlation between genotyping of NAT2 and acetylation phenotype has been demonstrated using an allele-specific PCR. Gastric cancer patients treated with 5-FU and cisplatin and possessing the glutathione S-tranferase PI-105 Valine/Valine (GSTPI-105VV) genotype showed a response rate of 67% and medial survival time of 15 months compared with 21% and 6 months, respectively, in patients harboring one GSTPI-105 Isoleucine (GSTPI-1051) allele.

Pharmacogenetics of the UGT1A1 gene is known to influence irinotecan-induced diarrhea mediated via the glucuronidation of the active metabolite SN-38. Irinocetan is an inhibitor of topoisomerase used for the treatment of lung and colon cancer in adults and pediatric solid tumors such as rhabdomyosarcoma and neuroblastoma. The presence of seven repeats, instead of the wild-type number of six (UGT1A1*28) is associated with reduced UGT1A1 expression, leading to reduced SN-38 glucuronidation. It has been shown that the UGT1A1*28 allele leads to significantly increased amounts of SN-38 and a heightened risk of irinocetan-caused diarrhea and leukopenia. Patients homozygous or heterozygous for seven TA repeats have a sevenfold higher likelihood of diarrhea or leukopenia with irinocetan therapy than do patients with the wild-type genotype (six repeats). In a study conducted on Asians, UGT1A1*28 was found to be a common allele in Indians. Thus, it is possible that UGT1A1 genotyping can be used to predict toxicity to irinocetan therapy. The UGT database contains data on genetic polymorphisms of the various UGT alleles. A good example for clinical reality of pharmacogenetic methods is the very frequently performed test for pseudocholinesterase. Inherited deficiency in pseudo- cholinesterase activity results in prolonged respiratory paralysis when deficient patients receive standard doses of the neuromuscular blockers suxamethonium or mivacurium.

Drug Transporters

Genetic variability in drug transporters also plays an important role for individual drug response. For instance, polymorphism in the ABC-binding cassette (ABC) gene may affect the function and expression of proteins by inducing tumor cell resistance to anticancer therapy, altered disposition of chemotherapeutic agents, and associated chemotherapy toxicity, which may cause certain drug-induced side effects and uncertainty in treatment efficacy. ABCB1, also known as P-glycoprotein (Pgp) alias MDR1 for multidrug resistance, is a member of the ABC family that participates in the energy-dependent efflux of various substrates. A synonymous polymorphism in exon 26 (C345T) was found to influence drug response and exhibit interethnic variability. The importance of haplotype analysis was shown by a meta-analysis of the influence of this SNP on digoxin pharmacokinetics and Pgp gene expression.

The ABCB1 genotype of the donor, but not of the recipient, may be a major risk factor for cyclosporine-related chronic nephrotoxicity in recipients of renal transplants. The ABCB1 3435TT genotype, which is associated with lower Pgp expression in renal parenchymal cells, is strongly associated with cyclosporine nephrotoxicity (odds ratio 13.4). On the other hand, the cyclosporin disposition in heart transplant patients may be influenced by Pgp haplotypes rather than genotypes. Genetic polymorphisms in ABCB1 and ABCg2 may be important also in influencing the pharmacokinetics of irinotecan and its metabolites.

Another notable example is that in certain patients the reduced rate of methotrexate metabolism produced a severe methotrexate overdosing and nephrotoxicity. This defect is attributed to the heterozygous mutation (R412G) in the highly conserved amino acid arginine of the ABCC2 gene, which encodes the human multidrug resistant protein-2 (MRP-2). Interestingly, this mutated region is associated with substrate affinity and hence the mutant protein has a reduced rate of methotrexate elimination. In some other cases, a long-term use of methotrexate induces pancytopenia, which is determined by white blood cells and platelet counts. However, it is also known that polymorphisms always need not have to produce functionally defective proteins. For example, in the multidrug resistant gene (MDR1), certain polymorphisms may not have any effect on the drug response. However, this could be caused by nonsignificant statistical power. Gwee et al. have devised a rapid and robust assay to simultaneously screen SNPs of the MDR1 gene using a single-tube multiplex minisequencing strategy. Finally, there are several web-based transporter databases.

Ion Channels

Organic anion transporting polypeptides (OATPs) mediate the uptake of a broad range of compounds into cells. Substrates for members of the OATP family include bile salts, hormones, and steroid conjugates as well as drugs like the HMG-CoA-reductase inhibitors (statins), cardiac glycosides, anticancer agents like methotrexate, and antibiotics like rifampicin. The identification and functional characterization of naturally occurring variations in genes encoding human OATP family members is in the focus of transporter research. There is a high degree of functional heterogeneity among OAT3 variants, with three variants (p.Arg149Ser, o. Gln239Stop, and p.Ile260 Arg) that results in complete loss of transporter function, and several other variants with significantly reduced function. Common variation in the gene SCN1A affects the maximum dose of phenytoin and carbamazepine, which act on the sodium channel subunit encoded by this gene.

The etiology of drug-induced long QT syndrome (LQTS) could also be based on gene variability. A life-threatening form of cardiac arrhythmia has been associated with mutations in the ion channel genes. Therefore, screening of LQTS-associated genes before the initiation of therapy with known QT-prolonging drugs could serve as a precautionary measure against life-threatening adverse effects by avoiding such drugs.

Drug Receptors

Genetic polymorphisms in drug receptors may alter pharmacological response. For example, variations in β-adrenoceptors, angiotensin-converting enzyme (ACE), and 5-hydroxytryptamine (5-HT) receptors alter drug response to β-adrenoceptor agonists and blockers, ACE inhibitors, and antipsychotic agents, respectively. Genetic polymorphisms affecting amino acids at positions 16 and 27 within the β_2-adrenoceptor gene have been implicated in the asthma phenotypes and influence on the variability observed in response to use bronchodilator agents. It was found that Arg16 allele was slightly more frequent within the group with the unwanted tachyphylaxis phenomenon, whereas Gly16 allele carriers were overrepresented within the group of good responders (59.7%, $P = 0.0028$). On the other hand, the allele frequency of Gln27 and the proportion of Gln27 carriers was higher within the group with tachyphylaxis and Glu27 allele carriers were overrepresented within the group of good responders ($P = 0.026$).

Cancer Drugs

Cancer chemotherapy is an area that requires continual monitoring and adjustment of antineoplastic agents to achieve optimal therapeutic outcome, which makes pharmacogenetic approaches attractive in this field. Drugs such as azathioprines, mercaptopurines, and thioguanine have been used extensively to treat childhood acute lymphoblastic leukemia, rheumatic disease, inflammatory bowel disease, and used for solid organ transplantation. Thiopurine S-methyltransferase (TPMT) is a cytosolic enzyme that is involved in the metabolism of thiopurines. It has been shown that polymorphisms in TPMT result in severe toxicity for patients prescribed with normal doses of the cytotoxic agents mercaptopurine or azathioprine. The variant enzyme was shown to misfold and subsequently form aggresome. It has been reported that the TPMT genotype has a substantial impact on the mercaptopurine treatment response. Previous studies also have shown that patients with homozygous mutant TPMT alleles exhibit very low enzyme activity and develop a severe hematopoietic toxicity after treatment with standard doses of thiopurines. TPMT-deficient patients tend to accumulate excessive thioguanine nucleotide concentrations and are, therefore, at higher risk for hematological toxicity. TPMT deficiency can be largely attributed to three mutant alleles (TPMT*2, TPMT*3A, and TPMT*3C). Allele-specific PCR or PCR-restriction fragment length polymorphism strategies have been used to detect the three signature mutations, hence offering a rapid and affordable assay for identifying >90% of all mutant alleles. Today, one of the most frequently performed pharmacogenetic tests are for TPMT. Patients who inherit two nonfunctional variant alleles should be given 6–10% of the standard dose of thiopurines. TPMT deficiency has also been associated with a high risk of irradiation-induced brain tumors in patients given thiopurines concomitantly with radiation therapy.

Similarly, the response rate of 5-fluorouracil (5-FU)-based treatment of advanced colorectal cancer is significantly linked to 677 C → T polymorphism in the methylenetetrahydrofolate reductase gene. Additionally, polymorphisms in the thymidylate synthase gene promoter (TYMS enhancer region, TSER) has been linked to tumor downstaging in patients with rectal cancer who were treated preoperatively with 5-FU-based chemoradiation. In a study of 65 patients with stage T2–T4 rectal cancer, patients with at least one TSER*2 allele had a 38% increased frequency of tumor down staging at the time of surgical resection compared with TSER*3/TSER*3 patients.

The first genotype-guided clinical trial in North America is based on TYMS TSER genotype. Rectal cancer patients (stage T3 and T4) with the "good risk" TSER*2 allele are treated in a phase II study consisting of standard therapy (radiation and 5FU). The sample size was calculated to detect a downstaging rate of 60%, compared with the historical downstaging rate of 45%. Patients homozygous for TSER*3 ("bad risk" genotype) are also enrolled in a phase II study, in which they receive the standard radiation and 5-FU along with additional irinocetan. The sample size was calculated to detect an improvement from the previously reported TSER*3/TSER*3 downstaging rate of 22–45%. Preliminary data implied an improved response rate in both treatment groups, suggesting an enrichment for positive response.

Genetic polymorphisms in the epidermal growth factor receptors (EGFR) impact on pharmacological response to gefitinib and erlotinib, tyrosine kinase inhibitors used as monotherapy in the treatment of metastatic non-small cell lung cancer. The drugs are effective in only 10–15% of patients. Responders were found to harbor activating mutations in the gene coding for EGFR. The EGFR assay for tumor mutation analysis provides a platform in personalized therapy with the EGFR inhibitors gefitinib or erlotinib. The use of the other tyrosine kinase inhibitor imatinib, which blocks the enzymatic action of the BCR-ABL fusion protein, has represented a critical advance in chronic myeloid leukaemia (CML) treatment. However, a subset of patients initially fails to respond to this treatment. Use of complementary DNA (cDNA) microarray expression profiling, a set of 46 genes was differentially expressed in imatinib responders and non-responders. A six-gene prediction model was constructed, which was capable of distinguishing cyto genetic response with an accuracy of 80%. Another case of already practical use of pharmacogenetic methods is the test for mutations in tumors that overexpress the human EGFR, HER2. Trastuzumab, a humanized monoclonal antibody, is effective in only 10–15% of breast cancer patients whose tumors overexpress HER2. Therefore, the pretreatment detection of HER2 is essential for the trastuzumab therapy.

Cardiovascular Drugs

Variation in two genes encoding angiotensin-converting enzyme and endothelial nitric oxide synthase influence the effects of standard therapies. In addition, polymorphism in the sodium channel gamma-subunit promoter region is significantly associated with blood pressure response to hydrochlorothiazide. Similarly, SNPs in angiotensinogen (T1198C), apolipoprotein B (G10108A), and adrenoreceptor alpha 2A (A1817G) significantly predict the change in left ventricular mass during antihypertensive treatment. Although common variants may influence the blood pressure response to a given class of antihypertensive medication, studies of polymorphisms have generally provided conflicting results. For instance, polymorphisms in the alpha 2B adrenergic receptor does not show any association with azepexole hypertensive response. However, patients with Gly 389 variant and Ser 49 homozygous of the beta-adrenergic receptor require increases in heart failure medication. One study has reported that the effect of statins in lowering low-density lipoprotein (LDL) -cholesterol levels was slightly greater in -204AA homozygotes of CYP7A1.

Most of the studies to date have failed to demonstrate any link between polymorphism in tumor necrosis factor alpha and both cardiomyopathy and coronary artery disease. In the case of asthma that causes substantial economic burden, morbidity, and mortality, patients exhibit an extensive interindividual variation in the response to beta-agonists acting at beta 2 adrenergic receptors, which could be caused by one nonsynonymous polymorphism [1772M9 of adenylyl cyclase type 9 (AC 9)] gene. This variation results in decreased catalytic activity (M772) and, therefore, alters albuterol (bronchodilator) responsiveness in the presence of a corticosteroid. Additionally, in an Indian population, response to salbutamol treatment of asthmatic patients depends on polymorphism of the beta 2 adrenergic receptor.

Drug Acting on the CNS

A meta-analysis of the quantitative contribution of CYP2D6 polymorphism to the interindividual variation in dosage of antidepressants has shown that the metabolism and dosage of imipramine, doxepin, maprotiline, trimipramine, desipramine, nortryptiline, clomipramine, and, partially, paroxetine depend on the CYP2D6 genotype and phenotype. Pharmacokinetic data suggest dose adjustments for these drugs that range from 28% to 60% of the normal dose for poor metabolizers and from 180% to 14%

of the normal dose for ultrarapid metabolizers. In general, based on the impact of CYP2D6 on dosage adaption of antidepressants and antipsychotics, 40–50% of drugs may be subject to important pharmacokinetic alterations owing to CYP2D6 polymorphism. A considerable variability also exists in efficiency and toxicity of other antipsychotic drugs. For instance, in the case of mood disorder, approximately 30–40% of patients do not completely respond to pharmacological treatment. However, serotonin transporter gene promoter (5HTTLPR) length polymorphisms has been implicated in the pathogenesis of mood disorders as well as in the therapeutic response to serotonergic drugs. Reduction in the Liebowitz social anxiety scale and in the brief social phobia score during treatment with serotonin reuptake inhibitors (SSSRIs) was significantly associated with 5HTTLPR genotype. When patients were treated with serotonin-blocking antidepressants, a significantly higher occurrence of side effects was found in patients with the HTTVNTR2.10/2.10 genotype (52.6%) than in patients with the 2.10/2.12 (12.5%) and 2.12/2.12 (0%) genotypes.

In patients with schizophrenia, Taq I polymorphism in the dopamine D2 receptor is associated with greater improvement of symptoms after treatment. Similarly, Gly 9 allele (Ser 9 Gly) of the dopamine D3 receptor and His 452 Tyr polymorphism in the 5-hydroxytryptamine 2A receptor (5-HT2A) are associated with response to clozapine. The side effects (weight gain) induced by antipsychotics seems to be associated with the –759 C allele of the 5-HT2C receptor. Additionally, Gly 9- variant of dopamine D3, the 102C-variant of the 5-HT2A, and the Ser 23-variant of the 5-HT2C receptors (in females) seem to increase the susceptibility to tardive dyskinesia.

Epilepsy is a difficult disease to treat because different patients require different ranges of doses, and some patients may even experience side effects such as increase in seizures, depression, and double vision. To control epilepsy, drugs such as phenytoin and carbamazepine have been extensively prescribed throughout the world. At present, evaluation of the allelic variation between individuals relies on the prior identification of candidate genes and their therapeutic effects of antiepileptic drugs. Variants in the CYP2C9 and SCN1A (encodes a brain protein) genes are often found in patients treated with the highest doses of both phenytoin and carbamazepine. Additionally, in Han Chinese, the carbamazepine side effects like Stevens–Johnson syndrome and toxic epidermal necrolysis are strongly associated with the HLA-B* 1502 gene, which also means that genetic suscep tibility to carbamazepine-induced cutaneous adverse drug reactions is phenotype-specific. Pharmacoresistant epilepsy is still a major clinical problem in epilepsy, and it could be caused by multiple factors, but also multidrug transporters may play a key role in resistance phenotypes. However, studies on one variant in the ABCB1 gene provided inconclusive evidence so far. Long-term treatment of Parkinson patients with L-Dopa exhibits L-Dopa-induced dyskinesis in some patients, which could be caused by genetic polymorphisms among patients. Therefore, pharmacogenetic studies may provide an explanation of neuronal plasticity among Parkinson patients. Furthermore, drug addictions are major social and medical problems and therefore impose a significant burden on society. Epidemiological, linkage, and association studies have shown a significant contribution of genetic factors to the addictive diseases. Studies of polymorphisms in the mu-opioid receptors and transporter genes have contributed significantly to the knowledge of genetic influence on opioid and cocaine addiction and the efficacy of opioid therapy in pain management.

Endocrinology

At present, a lot of scientific efforts are being employed to use pharmacogenetics/ pharmacogenomics for protein/peptidergic hormone therapy as well as for treatment with steroids. The main topics are polymorphisms in the membranous and nuclear receptors, including their subtypes and isoforms, and the genetics of steroid transforming enzymes (aromatases, 5α-reductases, sulfotransferases). It seems that, in comparison with other fields of pharmacological approaches, the pharmacogenetics in endocrinology are relatively advanced and, in certain parts, ready for clinical use.

Growth hormone receptor (GHR) transcripts exist in several isoforms in humans, among which is the retention (GHRfl) or exclusion (GHRd3) of exon 3, which encodes a 22-residue sequence in the extracellular domain of the membrane- located receptor. In Western Europe an populations, it has been estimated that 68–75% of alleles are GHRfl, whereas 25–32% are GHRd3. In short children, the homozygous or heterozygous presence of GHRd3 resulted in a significantly greater growth response in both year 1 and year 2 of GH therapy. Logically, patients who are homozygous for GHRd3 were less responsive to short-term and long-term hGH therapy. Exogenous sexual hormones are used worldwide by women as oral contraceptives and hormonal replacement therapy. Some epidemiological studies have shown an increased risk of venous thromboembolism (VTE). It was found, that the risk/ benefit ratio could be, in part, mediated by the genetic predisposition of women. Genetic thrombophilia might be implicated in the risk of VTE patients who use exogenous hormones.The most common causes of genetic hypercoagulability known today are factor V Leiden, G20210A prothrombin polymorphisms, and the genetic variant C677T of the methylenetetrahydrofolate reductase (MTHFR) gene. Therefore, an increasing number of kits for these two thrombophilic mutations are becoming commercially available, and screening for inherited thrombotic risk before giving the "pill" is among the most requested genetic tests in molecular diagnostic laboratories.

It seems that use of oral contraceptives or postmenopausal hormone replacement in women with the germ line mutations in the two genes BRCA1 and BRCA2 are more at risk for breast cancer than women also carrying these mutations but without hormonal interventions. CYP1A2, CYP2C19, and CYP3A5 are responsible for estrone oxidation. These enzymes are all known to be genetically variant in the human population, and studies to asses the role of these CYP P450 enzymes in breast cancer risk are indicated. The estrogen receptor-subtype ERα mediates the hepatotoxicity of 17α-ethinylestradiol (EE2). Upon EE2 treatment, ERa represses the expression of bile acid and cholesterol transporters (bile salt export pump, BSEP), Na^+/taurocholate cotransporting polypeptide (NTCP), OATP1, OATP2, ABCG5, and ABCG8 in the liver. The genetic variability of some of these transporters is well known and could explain, at least in part, the interindividual differences for the tolerability of oral contraceptives.

Estrogen receptor α variations increase or decrease the action of estrogens; but, at present, no clinical studies are available that show that pharmacogenomic checking of ERα before estrogen-treatment (OCs or hormone replacement) can reduce the risk of adverse drug reactions. The progesterone receptor 660L allele (PGR-12(rs1042638)V660L) may be associated with a moderately increased risk of breast cancer. The polymorphism of UDP-glucuronosyl transferase (UGT2B17) is strongly associated with the bimodal distribution of the testosterone excretion. Interestingly enough, besides the encouraging findings of genetics in the field of clinical endocrinology, proteomic approaches on the effects of estrogens, progestins, and androgens on the mammary gland are advancing step-by-step. And what happens with diabetes mellitus? In 525 Caucasian type 2 diabetic patients, the common E23K variant of KCNJ11 encoding the pancreatic β-cell adenosine 5′-triphosphate-sensitive potassium channel subunit Kir6.2 was associated with increased risk for secondary failure to treatment with sulfonylurea-like glibenclamide.

Environmental Factors

Needless to say, the genetic background and the gene variability is only one aspect of pharmacodynamics. Apart from potential gene–gene interactions, drug actions are also deeply affected by gene-environment interactions such that a particular genetic marker may present a variable pharmacological response in individuals with different nutritional states, lifestyle habits, and general well-being. Thus, the genetic information is not a reliable predictor of drug response, and therapeutic drug monitoring, with several notable exceptions, remains generally empirical. The sum and substance is as follows: Prescription genotyping serves more a predictive rather than a diagnostic role.

Here, we give only two examples for the role of the environment. Interindividual variability has been seen in liver UDP-glucuronosyltransferase 1A6 (UGT1A6) enzyme activity that glucuronates various drugs and toxins. Its expression is associated with polymorphisms in the 5′-regulatory and exon 1 regions. The three most common non-synonymous polymorphisms are S7A, T181A, and R184S. However, it did not explain the inter individual variability in glucuronidation and alcohol consumption, which suggests that environmental factors may have a significant role in alcohol consumption. Similarly, alcohol dependence is not associated with single-nucleotide polymorphisms in the corticotrophin releasing hormone receptor 1 (CHRH 1) gene.

Ethnicity

To use genomic knowledge to develop drugs and to improve health, we need to consider ethnical differences in different populations. There exists inter- ethnical differences in polymorphisms of genes encoding drug metabolizing enzymes, transporters, and disease-associated proteins. Meanwhile, a population genetics-based method to calculate the probability value for a variation in the gene is proposed. Genetic differences are greater within socially defined racial groups than between other groups. Additionally, it has been found that genetic diversity decreases in noncoding regions, whereas diversity of coding non-synomous SNPs is lower in regions containing a known protein sequence motif in individuals of European origin. Drug treatment may be tailored for greater effect if important genetic variation exists between racial and ethnic groups. By knowing these variants, patients can be classified into low-, intermediate-, and high-dose groups. For instance, coumarins are characterized by a narrow therapeutic index and a wide interindividual variability in dose response; daily maintenance doses of warfarin range from less than 1 mg to over 20 mg and, additionally, warfarin therapy shows a wide variation among patients of different ancestries. This variation could be caused by polymorphisms in the gene encoding vitamin K epoxide reductase complex 1. Accordingly, Chinese patients require lower dosages of heparin and warfarin than those usually recommended for white patients. Additionally, the combination of isosorbide dinitrate and hydralazine for treatment of heart failure in African-American heart patients reduced mortality by 43%, claiming that African- Americans and Caucasians differentially respond to the treatment, which is claimed to be because of genetic differences in the pathophysiology of heart failure between the two groups. In other words, biological differences exist between the two racial groups. However, in this study, there is no comparison population and hence results should be interpreted cautiously. The distribution of haplotype profile of MDR1 (Pgp, ABCB1) has also been shown to exhibit inter-ethnic variabililty.

The ethical and moral concerns that develop in the midst of genetic testing are factors that hamper the development of personalized medicine. The deciphering of the genetic code may pose a threat to the protection of one's privacy. Moreover, some variants that predict drug response are also markers for disease predisposition. For example, the apolipoprotein E4 allele known to influence response to cholesterol-lowering (statin) is also associated with an increased risk of Alzheimer's disease, which may subsequently lead to medico-legal implications, such as the issue of data confidentiality and the possibility of stigmatization: whether employers and insurance companies should be given rights to asses the genetic data and the chance of the information falling into the hands of unauthorized parties. In addition, a positive result for a genetic determinant underlying therapeutic failure for a critical illness may inflict additional emotional trauma and dampen the willpower of the patient to combat the disease.

Nevertheless, the debate on the biological basis of race and ethnicity and pharmacogenetics may provide a useful understanding of ethnic and racial differences. Even in this case, however, we should not ignore several important parameters such as diet, economic, environmental, and psychosocial factors. However, pharmacogenetic studies on race and ethnicity are worthwhile because they are useful indicators of genetic variation. However, this kind of race and ethnicity classification for medical treatment could lead to discrimination.

Technological Aspects

Mutation screening technologies can generally be categorized into mass screening for novel variants and specific genotyping approaches. Although the former approach is more often adopted in academic research to uncover novel mutations and unravel functional consequences, the latter is more suited for practical diagnostic purposes. Rapid, precise, and cost-effective high-throughput technological platforms are essential for performing large-scale mutational analysis of genetic markers. However, genotyping techniques have generally been laborious in nature, rendering large-scale analysis time-consuming and inefficient from a cost perspective. However, SNP detection technologies have recently evolved to some of the most highly automated, robust, and affordable methods in biomedical research. Genotyping is often performed in conjunction with phenotyping (e.g., pharmacometabonomics).

It is not the task of this chapter to discuss the advantages or disadvantages of the different technological platforms and bioinformatics tools in detail. Only a short presentation is possible. Commercially provided services, such as Signature Genetics are based on the analysis of integrated results from a detailed genetic test and comprehensive questionnaire. The report addresses the efficacy and toxicity of medications, potential drug interactions, and customized information on nutrition and recommended lifestyle modifications. Another example of a personalized medicine company is focused on SNP testing, haplotyping, and clinical genotyping. DxS has applied the Amplification Refractory Mutation System and Scorpions (a homogenous fluorescent PCR detection system) technologies to the development of a highly sensitive oncology test panel.

The Roche AmpliChip CYP Genotyping test is FDA-approved and combines Roche's PCR amplification technology and Affymetrix high-density microarray technology to allow rapid, simultaneous analysis of multiple SNPs within the CYP family. This genotyping strategy relies on the hybridization of complementary fluorescent-tagged DNA sequences to an array of sequence-specific oligonucleotide probes. Drug MEt is another microarray-based pharmacogenetic test used for simultaneous detection of 29 SNPs of CYP and phase II enzymes involved in drug metabolism. Invader UGT1A1 Molecular Assay is an *in vitro* diagnostic test for genotyping UGT1A1 alleles and is FDA-approved. This assay appears to be an accurate method for the rapid detection of UGT1A1 polymorphisms.

The TRUGENE Human Immunodeficiency Virus (HIV-1) Genotyping Kit and OpenGene DNA Sequencing System is yet another example illustrating the use of genetic testing in personalized medicine. TRUGENE is a sequence-based assay designed for detecting HIV genomic mutations (in the protease and part of the reverse transcriptase regions of HIV) that confer resistance to certain antiretroviral drugs. The assay has been shown to be robust, reproducible, and accurate and is considered a significant advance in the treatment of HIV infection. New technologies like matrix-assisted laser desorption ionization-time-of-flight (MALDI-TOF) mass spectrometry (MS) and GOOD assay (requires no purification steps) have to bring in wider use. The next challenge is the demand for more accurate, economical, and large-scale technologies for SNP association studies. There are several review papers describing the technological platforms in pharmacogenetic research. The technological challenges for pharmacoproteomics are exceptional. Protein microarrays are an emerging class of nanotechnology for tracking many different proteins simultaneously. However, translation into the medical practice is very slow. On the other hand, proteomic changes in cultured cell lines might not fully reflect pharmacodynamic interactions because of the lack of the tissue microenvironment.

Although the molecular genotyping and phenotyping techniques are well established in major research institutes, the facilities for genetic testing and measurement of parent and metabolic concentrations are not always accessible in the diagnostic laboratory. Furthermore, mutational screening using the current state- of-the-art technology is still laborious and time-consuming. The hassle of having to courier samples to an external laboratory and the turn around time for sample processing diminish the feasibility of adopting the approach in the fast-paced healthcare setting.

Limitations

A big problem limiting the progress of the pharmacogenetic approach is the fidelity of genotyping results and the confidence in associating SNPs with altered drug response. The ambiguity that sometimes develops in classifying an individual's genotype based on the laboratory results is another important contributory factor. In addition, the phenotyping method may give rise to false-positive results because the metabolic ratio can be influenced by other factors, such as epigenomic signaling, concomitantly administered drugs, nutritional state, and general health, hence affecting the validity of genotype-phenotype correlations.

The exact association between many SNPs of the drug target genes with therapeutic outcome is still unclear. However, few mutations have been characterized to ascertain their potential functional severity and limited definitive functional correlates established. As such, the functionality of these SNPs and their causative role remain largely speculative. In cases of functionally characterized SNPs, care should be exercised when translating research findings into an investigative tool, particularly in the extrapolation of observations from *in vitro* studies to a physiological effect. Even if the pharmacokinetic parameters are altered by genetic variants, the impact on pharmacodynamic or therapeutic effects may not be apparent. No standard guidelines exist on how the dosages of a drug should be adjusted, as a specific drug target may affect its panel of substrates to different extents, which increases the com plexity of drug prescription because the dose adjustments differ among the various substrates in individuals carrying the same gene mutation.

Clinical use of pharmacogenetic testing has been severely limited by a lack of prospective clinical trials. Such trials are required to establish that pharmacogenetic testing benefits the selection of the appropriate drug and dose for the individual patient, thereby improving therapeutic responses or reducing ADRs. One key point that will affect the integration of pharmacogenetics into clinical practice will be the cost-effectiveness of these approaches, which may be influenced by several factors. Drugs with a narrow therapeutic index with more severer and expensive side effects are ideal candidates for phar macogenetic testing. Drugs for which there are no established methods for monitoring adverse events (e.g., methotrexate) are also best-suited for pharmacogenomic analyses. However, for such approaches to be cost-effective, a well-established association should exist between genotype and clinical phenotype, and the frequency of the variant gene should be high. For example, if the frequency of a vriant allele is only 0.5%, then ~200 patients will have to be tested to identify one patient with the variant allele. Similarly, the strength of association between genotype and clinical phenotype will be important.

Educational Aspects

The resistance in the medical community to switching from the "*trial-and-error*" treatment approach to the gene-based approach is still prominently evident. Physicians in clinical practice, trainee physicians, and medical undergraduates have not been adequately educated in the field; the concept of pharmacogenetics has not been incorporated in the curriculum of medical courses worldwide. They are, thus, neither well-versed in the selection of target genes for ordering a genetic test nor equipped with the knowledge to interpret and analyze the report. Thus, the bridging of the gap between basic science and medicine requires the collaborative efforts of researchers and clinicians.

Professionals in medicine and the life sciences must be prepared to adapt to this new approach. However, systems-based pharmacogenomics is unlikely to be ready for clinical application in the near future. To benefit patients today, the already available options of pharmacogenetics should be carefully implemented in clinical practice as soon as possible. Teaching the current, continuously updated knowledge of pharmacogenomics should not be postponed until the new paradigm arrives.

The well-known interindividual differences in drug response could be caused by genetic and environmental factors and by the dose-response curve of a given drug. Knowledge of the individual genetic variability in drug response is. therefore, clinically and economically very important. Pharmacogenetics (focus is on single genes) and pharmacogenomics (focus is on many genes) are the two recent developments to investigate interindividual variations of drug response. This type of genetic profiling of the population doubtless provides benefits for future medical care by predicting the individual drug response.

The field of pharmacogenetics/pharmacogenomics has seen exciting advances in the recent past. The Human Genome Project and International HapMap projects have uncovered a wealth of information for researchers. The discovery of clinically predictive genotypes (e.g., UGT1A1*28 for irinocetan therapy; TPMT alleles for avoiding severe ADRs if patients receive standard doses of mercaptopurine and azathiopurine; TYMS TSER for treatment of rectal cancer; HER2 for optimizing the trastuzumab treatment in mammary Ca patients; BCA1, BRCA2, and factor V Leiden for improvement of oral contraception as well as hormone replacement), haplotypes (e.g., VKORC1 haplotype A for individualization of warfarin therapy), and somatic mutations (e.g., epidermal growth factor receptor for tailoring of tyrosine kinase inhibitors), along with the introduction of FDA-approved pharmacogenetic tests (UGT1A1*28) and the initiation of a genotype-guided clinical trial for cancer therapy (TYMS TSER in rectal cancer) have provided the first steps toward the integration of pharmacogenomics into clinical practice.

The translation from population-based (one dose fits all) to personalized medicine in the clinical setting is progressing at an incredibly slow pace. But why?

Several issues and problems need to be considered and solved before pharmacogenetics can be fully integrated into clinical practice (and also into drug development in the pharmaceutical industry). The ideal pharmacogenetic assay would quickly, accurately, and inexpensively provide composite genotypes for an individual patient to allow selection of the most suitable drug for the patient. Today, some approaches including suitable assays are very successful and have reached the level of clinical routine methods. Most other approaches (some are presently under investigation) are not mature. However, ongoing research is sure to bring one of the promises of the human genome project to fruition soon, that being individualized drug therapy. We should always keep in mind that, although in some cases polymorphism in a gene is associated with poor efficacy and adverse drug reactions, in many cases the clinical relevance remains to be understood or is irrelevant. Therefore, pharmacogenetics/ pharmacogenomics may not be applicable to all diseases and all treatments. However, the many pharmacogenomic complexities, and particularly time-dependent changes of gene expression, will never allow personalized medicine to become an error-free entity.

The suggestion that individuals will be genotyped at birth and their "*HapMap genotype*" carried lifelong as an implantable identity may be too Orwellian for some. However, it may be close to the reality of clinical pharmacology practice in decades to come. By the way, we will have the data needed to extract the genetic risk from a genome and effectively model dosages and the risks of adverse reactions based on an individual's genotype, which is further than most imagined electronic prescription would go, but it is an attractive prospect. Pharmacogenomics has a long way to go to achieve this goal, but its potential is clear enough.

However, at present, pharmacogenomics' practical impact on medicine is more or less minimal, and the greatest challenge is to understand the genotype- environmental factor interactions, extensive geographic variations in genes (ethnicity) and to optimize study design for the accuracy, high level of quality, and consistency of technologies. In comparison with pharmacogenomics, the successful transition of proteomic technologies (including novel nanotechnology strategies) from research tools to integrated diagnostic platforms will require much more effort and much more time. After the great enthusiasm about mastering of the Human Genome Project, at present, we are in the post-genetics skepticism, which should not block our efforts for bringing pharmacogenomics and pharmacoproteomics into the clinical practice, which, however, is a long and interesting road. Like other methods in medicine, pharmacogenomics as well as pharmacoproteomics will optimize only certain parts of pharmacological therapy, not the whole field of clinical pharmacology. Taken together, prescription genotyping is only intended to aid the doctor in making individualized therapeutic decisions and is not a substitute for a physician's judgment and clinical experience.

4

Formulation Development

In the development of a formulation, the degradation of the protein is assessed under several conditions to determine under which conditions the active compound is most stable. Typically, variations in pH, ionic strength, buffer components, tonicifiers, and surfactants are investigated. Stressed conditions such as exposure to elevated temperatures, freezing, or harsh lighting are used to purposefully damage the protein. These conditions may not reflect the actual storage conditions, but can give insight into the mechanisms by which the protein may degrade.

In 1999, there were 96 biotechnology products approved by the Food and Drug Administration (FDA) for either the detection or treatment of human diseases. More than 350 biotechnology-produced drugs and vaccines are currently being tested in clinical trials, with hundreds more in earlier stages of development. The approved products treat a wide variety of conditions and diseases, including hemophilia, multiple sclerosis, acquired immune deficiency syndrome (AIDS)-related illnesses, growth failure, infertility, cancer, diabetes, hepatitis, anemia, Crohn's disease, diabetic ulcers, prevention of transplant rejection, stroke, and acute myocardial infarctions. The successful treatment of a disease state requires that the drug be delivered in an active form over a specific time frame to the location in the body where it is needed. This necessitates the development of a suitable formulation and drug delivery system that ensures the stability of the active compound, the delivery of the drug to the site of action, and its presence at the site of action over a desirable time frame.

The goal of a successful formulation is to minimize the degradation of the protein during storage as a formulated bulk (drug substance) and over the shelf life of the final drug product. Storage conditions for the purified drug substance must be determined to ensure minimal changes to the protein before the material is manufactured as the final drug product. It is in the manufacturer's best interest to have as much stability as possible for the drug substance for two reasons: (1) the ability to build adequate inventory of the drug substance frees the manufacturer to produce the bulks at will instead of trying to time the manufacture of the drug substance to meet the needs of the market and (2) degradation of the protein while stored as the drug substance minimizes the shelf life of the drug product. Typically, at least 2 years of shelf life is required to ensure suitable time for the manufacture, testing, and distribution of the drug product. Any degradation observed during storage of the drug substance would adversely impact the expiration dating for the drug product. The selection of the form of the drug product (e.g., liquid or solid state) and the final storage conditions are made with the goal of achieving the most cost-efficient and stable product possible.

In addition to developing a stable product, it is also necessary to determine the most desirable form for the administration and marketing of the product. Drug products administered in a hospital setting have different requirements for development compared with those administered by a patient (or parent of a patient) at home. Consideration must also be given to the formulation/delivery system for any competing products that are on the market. For example, if the competition sells a drug that is administered orally, it would not be prudent to sell a drug that must be administered by injection on a daily basis, unless it provided superior efficacy or safety benefits. Patients would not have the motivation to switch to a more painful and less convenient route of administration otherwise. Thus input from the field regarding user preferences and competitive products must be considered throughout product development.

This article will discuss the strategy used for the development of a therapeutic formulation for clinical trials that will eventually lead to a marketed product. What questions does the formulation scientist need to answer to develop a suitable drug product? First, the degradation and inactivation mechanisms for the protein are determined. After all, it is those reactions that the successful formulation scientist is attempting to prevent. How can the degradation be minimized? Next, consideration is given to the state and composition of the formulation. Will it be a liquid product? Is it better to have a lyophilized product that can be stored at ambient temperature rather than a liquid product that must be stored under refrigerated conditions? With the decision regarding state, the excipients that will comprise the formulation are selected. What should the pH of the formulation be? Is a bulking agent necessary to form a good lyophilized cake? Does the formulation need to be isotonic? With which excipients is the formulation most stable? Linked to both the selection of state and excipients is a decision regarding the route of administration and a prototype of the final product. Is delivery by injection the preferred route of administration for this product? Are there devices available that will enhance the product? Careful consideration of these questions may lead to the successful design of a drug product.

Degradation/Inactivation

Proteins may degrade via several routes. In some cases, denaturation of the protein may cause its inactivation. Some of the potential sites of degradation may be anticipated from the primary structure of the protein, such as the high probability of deamidation of Asn when followed by Gly. Other sources of instability are only discovered during the course of studies in which the stability of the protein is assessed.

These instabilities fall into two general classes: *physical instability*, in which the protein changes its tertiary or quaternary structure, and *chemical instability*, in which a chemical reaction causes a change in one or more of the amino acids in the protein. In the development of a protein formulation, the amount of degradation products of either type that are formed over the shelf life of the drug product must be minimized. The denatured protein may have altered activity, pharmacokinetics, or safety. There is concern that the denatured protein may cause an immunogenic response when administered to a patient, even if no response is observed with the native protein. For this reason, it is crucial for the formulation scientist to develop a drug product that minimizes any changes to the protein over its shelf life.

Physical Instability

Physical instability is caused by *aggregation* or *surface denaturation* of the protein. *Soluble aggregates* result from proteins that self-associate into discrete units such as dimers or trimers through ionic interactions, hydrophobic interactions, or changes in disulfide bonding of the native protein. Precipitation, which is the formation of *insoluble aggregates*, usually results from nonspecific protein interactions, although in some proteins, it may result from the formation of extremely large, ordered aggregates. Some disease states are the result of the formation of insoluble protein aggregates in vivo. Amyloidosis (AL) and light chain deposition disease (LCDD) are caused by aggregates of immunoglobulin light chain fragments either as ordered, fibrillar aggregates (AL) or as amorphous aggregates (LCDD). Alzheimer's disease has been associated with the presence of amyloid fibrils that form plaques.

In some cases, it is desirable to have a pharmaceutical protein in an aggregated state because it is the bioactive form of the protein. An example of this is surfactant protein B (SP-B), a pulmonary surfactant protein necessary for normal lung function in neonatal infants. The protein exists exclusively as a homodimer in which the monomers are linked by a disulfide bond. In studies investigating efficacy of the SP-B monomer compared with the dimer in transgenic mice, it was found that although the surfactant action was preserved in the monomeric form of the protein, altered lung hysteresis was noted. The authors concluded that SP-B dimerization is required for optimal lung function.

Aggregation of a protein may also be desired when the aggregate is a more stable form of the protein. For example, insulin is formulated in the presence of Zn^{2+}, which coordinates insulin dimers to form an ordered hexameric form of the protein. Zn^{2+} added to the formulation has been shown to increase the physical stability of an insulin solution.

However, most often, aggregation is not desired. The presence of a nonnative aggregate is a cause of concern to biopharmaceutical scientists because this aggregate may have altered activity, clearance, and toxicity compared with the native protein. Aggregates of ribonuclease A were found to be less active. Covalent aggregates of insulin resulted in the appearance of antibodies to the protein in the blood of insulin-using diabetic patients.

Because of the potential effects on safety and activity, it is necessary to minimize the aggregate content in the final formulation. In the formulation screen for the recombinant humanized monoclonal antibody to vascular endothelial growth factor (rhuMAb VEGF), a reversible self-association of the protein was observed, whose levels were found to be dependent on protein concentration, pH, and ionic strength of the formulation. It would be possible to minimize the aggregate content in the formulation by controlling these variables.

In addition to aggregation, *surface denaturation* causes physical instability of the protein. Surface denaturation occurs when the protein interacts with the container surface, or when it comes into contact with an interface (e.g., air/liquid interface). At these interfaces, the protein may partially unfold, leading to a nonnative structure. This unfolding can result in aggregation, precipitation, or adsorptive loss of the protein to the container surface. At relatively high protein concentrations ($>$10 mg/mL), adsorptive losses are rarely observed because the amount of protein lost to the surface is very small compared with the total amount of protein in solution. At low protein concentrations ($<$1 mg/mL), the adsorptive losses are often significant and must be considered during the selection of a formulation and a container/closure system for the product. The protein interaction with the container surface is usually nonspecific and is caused by hydrophobic interactions.

One study investigating protein adsorption examined the stability of factor VIII, a protein used to treat hemophilia B, in polyvinylchloride (PVC) minibags. These bags are commonly used in clinical settings for administration of drugs to patients because of the ease of administration. After 48 hr of storage at room temperature in these PVC minibags, the activity of factor VIII dropped to 2% of the expected concentration of 2 IU/mL, or 44% of the expected concentration of 10 IU/mL. These losses in activity were determined to be because of protein adsorption onto the PVC surface. Patients treated with factor VIII that had been stored in PVC bags would have received significantly lower doses of the protein than expected.

For liquid formulations, shaking the formulation increases the air/liquid interface in the formulation and often leads to protein denaturation. Several proteins are susceptible to denaturation by shaking, including human growth hormone (hGH) and recombinant factor XIII, both of which formed insoluble aggregates after shaking.

For lyophilized formulations, it is often critical to add a surfactant to the formulation to minimize aggregation. Denaturation of the protein may occur during the freezing or dehydration portion of the process. Interactions of the protein at the solid/air, liquid/air, or water/ice interface may result in aggregation, and it is these interactions that the addition of surfactant to the formulation may minimize.

Chemical Instability

Chemical degradation of proteins generally involves several common reactions in the protein. Some information regarding the chemical reactivity may be deduced from the primary sequence of the protein. Powell compiled hydropathy and flexibility information for 71 proteins and found that the hydropathy value, coupled with known "hotspot" sequences, predicted degradation with high certainty for deamidation and fragmentation. *Deamidation* primarily occurs through the hydrolysis of Asn or Gln residues, often from the formation of an intermediate cyclic imide. *Oxidation* may occur through several different mechanisms, including reactions with free radicals and metal ions. *Disulfide exchange* results from either the reduction or β-elimination of existing disulfide bonds, which in turn form new bonds, or from the creation of new disulfide bonds from free thiol groups. Isomerization may result from several pathways. For example, proline isomerization may be caused by peptidyl prolyl isomerase that exists in trace amounts in the purified bulk. *Fragmentation* may result from enzymatic cleavage or from hydrolysis of the peptide bond. Each of these sources of chemical instability is detailed below.

Deamidation and succinimide formation

Deamidation of proteins at Asn or Gln residues proceeds through one of two pathways. Direct hydrolysis of the amide bond occurs under both basic and acidic conditions and results in cleavage of the peptide bond, thus forming fragments. This reaction will be discussed further under "*Fragmentation.*" The second route for deamidation in proteins occurs through the formation of a succinimide intermediate. This pathway involves a unimolecular interaction in which a deprotonated amide nitrogen undergoes nucleophilic attack on a carbonyl side chain of Asn to form the succinimide. Loss of an ammonia molecule from this structure results in the formation of a carboxylic acid. Figure 4.1 shows the deamidation reaction for Asn. Asn residues typically are much more susceptible to deamidation compared

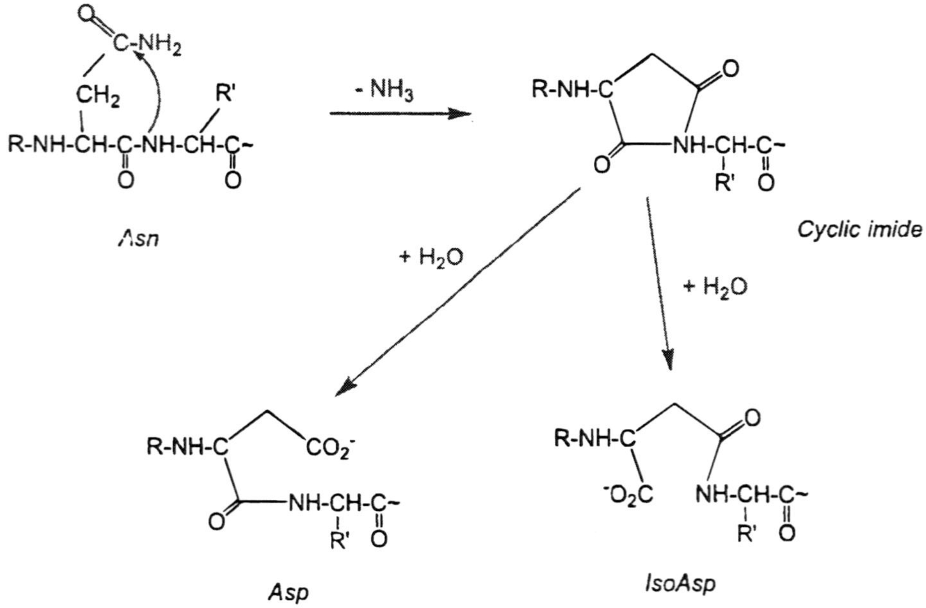

Fig. 4.1. Deamidation of aspargine.

with glutamine. Both the succinimide and the deamidated form are considered to be degradation products. The susceptibility of Asn to deamidation has been studied by Robinson and Rudd, who found that an Asn followed in sequence by Gly deamidated at a much faster rate compared with an Asn adjacent to bulkier residues. This is presumably because the smaller amino acid allowed greater flexibility in the peptide chain, facilitating the formation of the cyclic imide. Because water is a reactant in this mechanism, the deamidation reactions occur much more readily in solution than in solid phase. Deamidation is one of the key routes of degradation for insulin and DNase.

Succinimide formation may also result from the degradation of Asp or Glu. This reaction may occur under either basic or acidic conditions. As mentioned previously, the presence of succinimide is considered a degradation product of the protein. Conversion of Asp to the succinimide product was observed to be optimal at pH 4–5 in basic fibroblast growth factor (bFGF).

Oxidation

Oxidation of proteins and peptides is extremely common, and there are several reviews that cover this topic in depth. Many amino acids are susceptible to oxidation. Methionine, cysteine, histidine, tryptophan, and tyrosine all undergo oxidation under specific conditions. Oxidation may be photolytic, metal-catalyzed, or through the presence of reactive oxygen species in the system that have been introduced as contaminants during the manufacturing process (e.g., peroxide). Even trace amounts of an oxidizing agent may wreak havoc with a protein because the oxidizing agent serves as the initiator for a propagation reaction. Photolysis occurs when light causes the formation of reactive oxygen species that in turn attack the protein. Molecular oxygen may be activated by converting it to an excited singlet state ($^1O_2$) , or by reducing it to species such as the superoxide radical ($^{\bullet}O_2^-$), hydrogen peroxide (H_2O_2), or hydroxyl radical ($^{\bullet}OH$).

Metal ions lead to protein oxidation either by reacting directly with an amino acid to form a radical, or by generating reactive oxygen species in solution. Amino acids that chelate transition metal ions (e.g., histidine) are most prone to metal-catalyzed oxidation because the complex generates the reactive oxygen species that lead to oxidation. The proximity of the nascent reactive oxygen species to the chelated amino acid makes that amino acid most susceptible to attack.

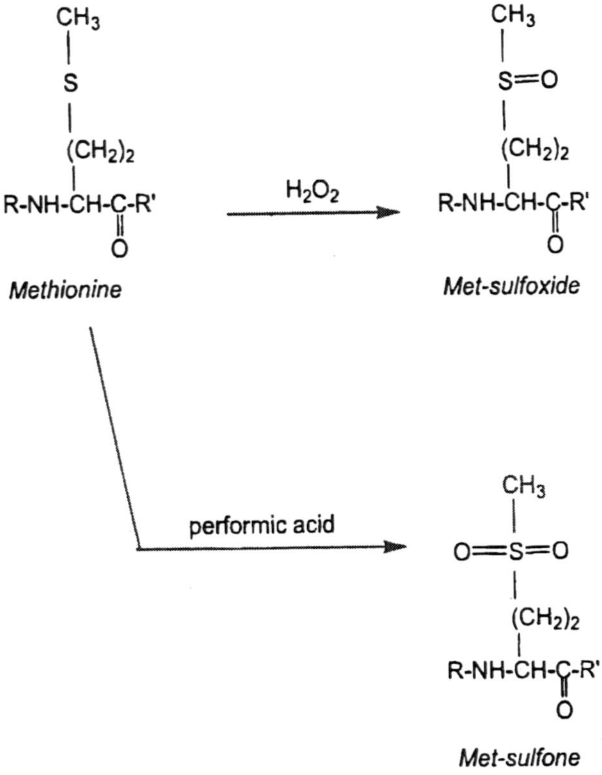

Several commonly used solvents and/or excipients may contain trace levels or reactive oxygen species that could cause oxidation in proteins. Bleach, a commonly used cleaning agent, may leave trace levels of hypochlorite on storage containers and processing equipment. Polysorbate 20 and polysorbate 80 are widely used excipients in protein formulations that help prevent aggregation and surface denaturation. During the manufacture of polysorbates, a bleaching step is sometimes used, which results in the presence of trace levels of alkyl-hydroperoxide and hydrogen peroxide in the final polysorbate product. The polysorbates generate

Fig. 4.2. Oxidation of methionine.

peroxides on storage. Oxidizing agents have been introduced as contaminants with mannitol. To examine the effects of oxidation on proteins, one must understand which amino acids are most susceptible to oxidation and what the resulting products of oxidation are. Methionine is one of the most readily oxidized amino acid in proteins. Under mild oxidation conditions, Met-sulfoxide is formed. This is the primary oxidation mechanism under acidic conditions. The reaction to form Met-sulfoxide is reversible chemically or enzymatically. If oxidation occurs under harsher conditions, then the sulfone is formed The reactions for the formation of these two products are displayed Figure 4.2.

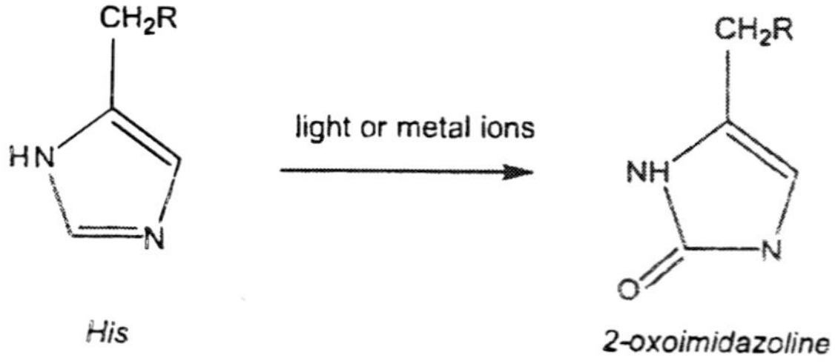

CH_2R ... HN ... N — light or metal ions → CH_2R ... NH ... N ... O

His → 2-oxoimidazoline

Fig. 4.3. Oxidation of histidine.

Histidine may undergo either photo-catalyzed or metal-catalyzed oxidation. Photolytic oxidation results in the formation of 2-oxohistidine, also known as 2-oxoimidazoline. Because His is an effective chelating agent, it is highly sensitive to metal-catalyzed oxidation. Additional oxidation products may be observed through metal-catalyzed oxidation of His, including the formation of Asp or Asn, but the mechanism for the formation of these products is not understood.

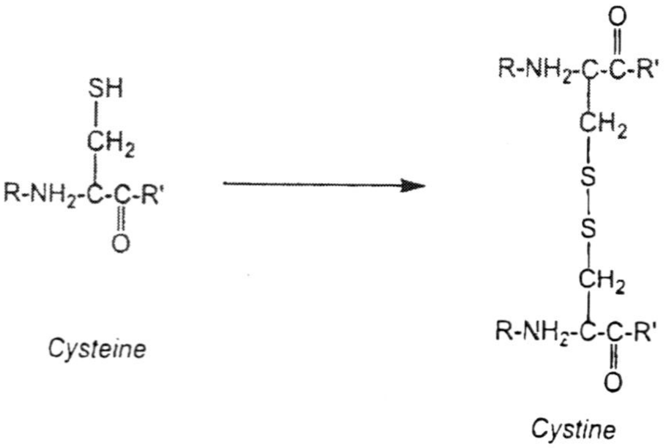

SH, CH_2, R-NH_2-C-C-R', O → O, R-NH_2-C-C-R', CH_2, S, S, CH_2, R-NH_2-C-C-R', O

Cysteine → Cystine

Fig. 4.4. Oxidation of cysteine.

Cysteine has a free thiol group that may oxidize to form a disulfide bond (cystine). This reaction is favored at higher pH values, where the thiol is deprotonated. The oxidation of Cys may be spontaneous (resulting from the presence of O_2) or metal-catalyzed. Spontaneous oxidation of free thiols in bFGF was promoted in the presence of heparin and led to aggregation of the protein.

Tryptophan oxidizes primarily via reactive oxygen species, although it may occur as a result of photo- oxidation in the presence of dyes. Trp and Met are the only amino acids that are capable of being oxidized below pH 4. The primary oxidation products of Trp are *N*-formylkynurenine and kynurenine, with many other products observed including Gly and Ala. As with His, the detailed mechanism for understanding the oxidation of Trp is poorly understood.

Tyrosine is oxidized via a photolytic mechanism to produce 3,4-dihydroxyphenylalanine and bityrosine. Because bityrosine formation may be intermolecular, the product of oxidation is often the formation of aggregates.

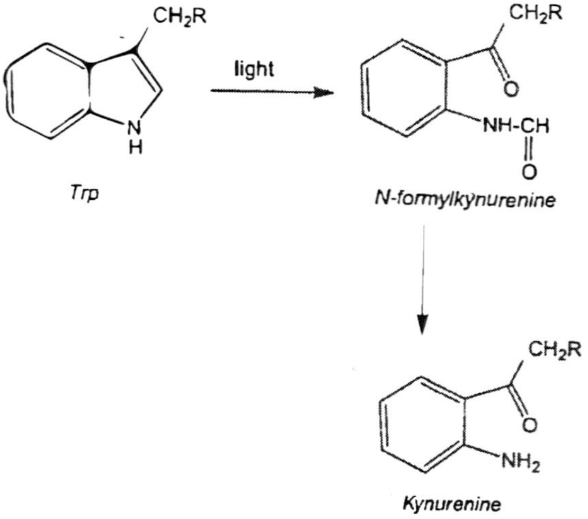

CH_2R ... N H — light → CH_2R ... O ... NH-CH ... O → CH_2R ... O ... NH_2

Trp → N-formylkynurenine → Kynurenine

Fig. 4.5. Oxidation of tryptophan.

Because protein oxidation may occur at any stage of the manufacture of the product, it is necessary to assess the susceptibility of the protein to oxidation through several mechanisms. Hydrogen peroxide, tert-butyl hydroperoxide (TBHP), and light are often used to promote oxidation in protein samples.

Metal ions such as Cu^{2+} and Fe^{3+} have been added to protein formulations to purposefully assess whether a protein is susceptible to metal-catalyzed oxidation.

The oxidation of recombinant interferon-γ (IFN-γ) and recombinant tissue plasminogen activator (t-PA) was investigated by Keck. Two of five Met in IFN-γ and three of five Met in t-PA were oxidized to the sulfoxide state with TBHP. In each case, the Met was located on the surface of the protein. No other amino acids were oxidized in this experiment. Additionally, oxidation of IFN-γ by H_2O_2 resulted in the conversion of all five Met to Met-sulfoxide, again with no other oxidation products observed. DalleDonne, Milzani, and colombo probed the oxidation of actin with TBHP and found that although none of the Met oxidized, one of five Cys did undergo modification, which caused a marked decrease in the rate of actin polymerization. Oxidation of human epidermal growth factor 1-48 (hEGF1-48) was achieved using light exposure. In this protein, the lone Met converts to Met-sulfoxide on exposure to light when the protein solution is stored in glass. The rate of oxidation was observed to be greatest in colorless glass. Storage in amber glass afforded some protection, whereas storage in foil-wrapped glass showed the slowest rate of oxidation. Metal-catalyzed photooxidation of hGH was found to specifically oxidize His21, one of three residues involved in a cation-binding site. Other potential sites of oxidation, including three Met and two additional His, were found to be unaffected by photooxidation of hGH.

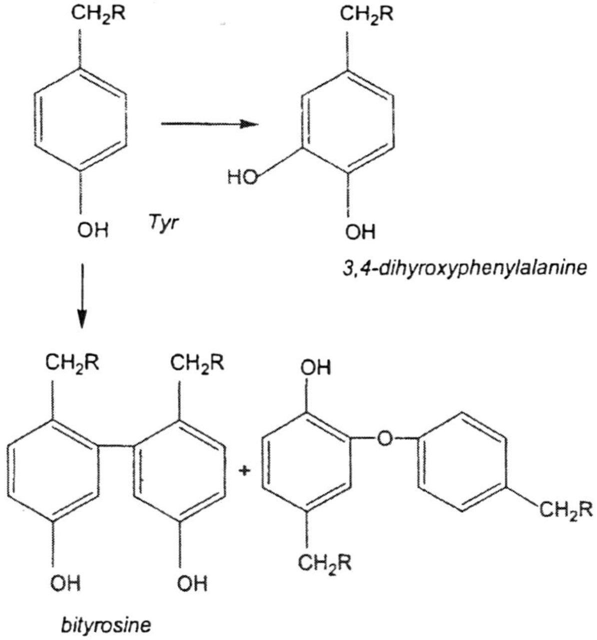

Fig. 4.6. Oxidation of tyrosine.

Oxidation of relaxin has been extensively studied and serves as a useful example of how oxidation may be achieved through different mechanisms. Relaxin is a two-chain, disulfide-linked hormone with a molecular mass of ~6 kDa. Early formulation screens by Cipolla and Shire demonstrated that oxidation of relaxin was enhanced by light or in the presence of methylcellulose—a carbohydrate used to make a topical formulation. Under these conditions, Met4 and Met25 on the B-chain formed sulfoxides. Oxidation of relaxin by hydrogen peroxide gave similar results, with only the sulfoxide form of the two Met observed. No other amino acids displayed oxidation. Li et al. demonstrated that metal-catalyzed oxidation achieved by a combination of ascorbate/ cupric chloride/oxygen resulted in modification of His12 on the A-chain in addition to the previously mentioned Met, as well as physical instability of the protein at pH >6.0. The physical instability was postulated to be an indirect result of His modification, and this hypothesis was supported in later studies by comparing the protein to the porcine version that does not contain His12. These examples demonstrate that oxidation products of proteins depend highly on the mechanism used to achieve oxidation.

Disulfide exchange

Disulfide exchange occurs when a disulfide bond undergoes β-elimination to form free thiols, and the free thiols reoxidize with incorrect pairings. When disulfide exchange occurs, a change in secondary, tertiary, or quaternary structure may be observed. Lyophilized insulin was shown to undergo β-elimination followed by formation of mixed disulfides when stored at high temperature and/or high humidity. β-Elimination has been proposed as the mechanism for degradation of recombinant human macrophage colony-stimulating factor (rM-CSF) stored under alkaline conditions.

Isomerization/racemization

All amino acids except Gly are susceptible to isomerization or racemization. Enzymes such as peptidyl prolyl isomerases exist solely to isomerize specific amino acids. The cyclic imide pathway of degradation for both Asn and Asp can result in a racemic mixture of products. Isomerization has been observed in Asp residues of bFGF and Asn residues of insulin.

Fragmentation

Fragmentation result, from multiple pathways including deamidation, Asp–Pro cleavage, and protease activity. Direct hydrolysis of Asn-containing peptide bond could occur, causing fragmentation and deamidation. Cleavage after Asn101 in aging α-crystalline was determined to occur through a deamidation pathway. Asp, because of the electronegative carbon center in the carbonyl group, is particularly susceptible to cleavage of the peptide bond when followed by Pro in the protein sequence. Recombinant human interleukin-11 and rM-CSF both degrade primarily via cleavage at Asp–Pro sites in acidic solution. Finally, fragmentation may occur because of protease activity. Although the final protein bulk obtained from manufacturing is highly pure, it is sometimes possible for trace amounts of proteases or other enzymes to copurify with the protein of interest. The quantities of the proteases may be too small to observe analytically—even a trace amount of a protease can result in significant fragmentation in the protein during storage. Fragmentation at locations on a protein other than those described above may be the only evidence for the presence of a protease in the formulation.

Glycation

Glycation occurs when a sugar molecule chemically reacts with one of the amino acid side chains to form a carbohydrate adduct on the protein. This occurs via a Maillard reaction in which the carbonyl of a reducing sugar undergoes a condensation reaction with the amino group on Arg, Lys, or N-terminal amino acid. The product of this reaction has a Schiff's base. This reaction is accelerated in the solid state and is favored when the formulation pH is less than neutral. Amadori rearrangement of the Schiff's base product may lead to browning of the solution. Glycation has been observed in a lyophilized formulation of relaxin in which a glucose adduct was identified. Formulation of recombinant human DNase with lactose in a spray-dried state resulted in the addition of lactose molecules to five of the six Lys in the protein. A similar reaction was observed in a lyophilized formulation of hGH in lactose. Because of the tendency of reducing sugars to undergo the Maillard reaction with proteins, they are not the carbohydrates of choice for use in formulations. With the information from an assessment of the primary structure of the protein, the formulation scientist now begins the task of developing a suitable system for storage of the protein.

FORMULATION DEVELOPMENT

The first stage of formulation development is called preformulation. During the preformulation stage, short studies are conducted to assess the relative types and rates of degradation observed as a function of pH, protein concentration, and temperature. It is from these early studies that the formulation scientist first gains information regarding which specific degradation mechanisms may be important to the protein of interest.

With the results of the preformulation studies, the formulation scientist can begin to address some of the specific questions pertaining to the development of the final formulation. The *state* of the dosage form is selected. The inactive ingredients in the formulation, *excipients*, which promote stability of the final product, are screened. Finally, supportive *accelerated stability studies* are conducted to aid in the selection of the final formulation.

Selection of State

The purified bulk that is obtained from the manufacturing process of proteins typically arrives as a liquid solution. A decision is made by the formulation scientist regarding the state of the final drug formulation (i.e., liquid or solid state) to be produced from the liquid bulk. The selection of state for the final product involves balancing several criteria, including cost, stability, route of administration, dose, and intended storage conditions for the final product.

Many different routes are employed to achieve solid-state formulations, including crystallization, lyophilization, spray drying (SD), and spray–freeze drying (SFD). *Crystallization* is the only one of these techniques to form a purposefully ordered solid. Formulations of crystallized glucose oxidase and crystallized lipase have been reported to be more stable than their amorphous counterparts, presumably because the crystal packing structure does not allow reactions that require flexibility of the peptide chain to occur. However, Pikal and Rigsbee noted that amorphous insulin exhibited greater stability compared with the crystalline form of the protein. The authors postulated that the decreased stability of the crystalline form was because of local configurational differences around Asp21, the primary site of degradation. The crystallized forms of three monoclonal antibodies were found to be efficacious when delivered subcutaneously. The investigation of crystallized protein formulations is expected to be a hot topic in the next decade. Because little information is available regarding actual examples of crystalline protein formulation production and stability, the remaining portion of this section will focus on amorphous solid-state formulations obtained by one of the drying processes.

The most common method to achieve a solid-state formulation is *lyophilization*, or freeze drying, in which the formulation is frozen and the bulk water is removed by sublimation. The resulting cake is composed of the protein, any nonvolatile excipients, and a small amount of residual water tightly associated with the protein. Excipients such as sucrose, mannitol, or glycine are often added to formulations to be lyophilized to serve as bulking agents and to protect the protein during the freezing and drying processes. There is a wealth of literature available that examines the lyophilization process and its effects on protein integrity.

SD uses atomization to form microdispersed droplets. The water in these droplets quickly evaporates when passed through a stream of hot gas, resulting in the formation of a fine powder of microparticles containing protein and excipients. Although the protein solution passes quickly through the hot gas stream and evaporation provides some cooling, the potential for thermal degradation of the protein is a concern using this technique. This technique was successfully applied to the preparation of powders of hGH and t-PA.

SFD is a combination of the two previously described drying techniques in which the microdispersed liquid particles are generated through the jet nozzle in the absence of heat, then collected and frozen in liquid nitrogen before sublimation occurs. The frozen particles are then lyophilized. SFD is used in place of SD when the protein cannot withstand the temperatures in the SD process. Preparation of SFD powders of DNase and an anti-IgE monoclonal antibody were found to be superior to those prepared by SD.

How does one decide which state to pursue for a dosage form? Production of a liquid formulation is cheaper than any of the solid-state forms because it takes fewer steps to manufacture, thus requiring a shorter time. At most, a formulated liquid bulk may need to be diluted before a liquid fill is performed, although often the bulk is filled directly into the final container. For a lyophilized product, the filled containers must undergo the freeze-drying process that can take up to 1 week. For spray-dried formulations, the bulk must be further processed to achieve the powder formulation that then must be filled into the appropriate final containers. SFD formulations have the added cost of both powder production and lyophilization prior to filling. These added manufacturing steps result in a higher production cost for the solid state. In addition, losses in protein yield are observed for SD and SFD processes. Thus the cost in terms of time, money, and sometimes product yield for the liquid formulation is smaller than that for solid-state formulations.

If the cost is higher, why would one pursue a solid- state formulation? One critical issue is stability. Generally, solid-state formulations degrade much more slowly than liquid-state formulations because water plays a key role in several of the degradation mechanisms (e.g., deamidation) for proteins. The decreased rate of degradation in a solid-state formulation potentially enables storage of the drug product at higher temperatures than would be allowed for liquid products, which are generally stored under refrigerated conditions. However, it should be noted that some mechanisms of degradation are accelerated in the solid state (e.g., glycation), and simply switching to a solid- state formulation does not ensure that no degradation will be observed.

The ability to store a drug product under non- refrigerated conditions is particularly critical for products, such as vaccines, intended for export to developing countries. Although sometimes inconvenient, it is easy to find refrigerators for storage of drugs in the United States and other industrialized countries. In developing countries, access to refrigeration may be quite limited. It is critical that drugs manufactured for use in developing areas have sufficient stability under local ambient conditions to enable their use. Solid-state formulations may allow one to achieve that goal.

The need for a multidose formulation may also dictate the use of a solid-state formulation. As the name implies, multidose products are intended to provide the patient with a product that contains several doses of the therapeutic within one container. Multidose formulations contain preservatives to kill any bacteria and prevent mold growth that may result from repeated entry into the drug product. Phenol and benzyl alcohol are two widely used preservatives in protein-based parenteral pharmaceuticals. Frequently, the addition of a preservative to the formulation compromises the long-term stability of the drug product, typically because the protein becomes physically unstable and/or exhibits oxidation. If the formulation scientist can obtain sufficient short-term stability (e.g., 2 weeks) for a formulation containing a preservative, then the use of a solid-state product may enable production of a multiuse formulation. In this case, the preservative is NOT added to the liquid bulk used to prepare the solid state. Instead, when the solid-state formulation is reconstituted prior to use, a preservative is included in the water for reconstitution. Thus the final product to be used is a multidose formulation that will experience only short-term exposure to the preservative.

The desired protein concentration may also dictate the use of a solid-state formulation. At large scale, protein solutions are concentrated using ultrafiltration. During ultrafiltration, the protein concentration at the membrane can become several fold higher than the concentration of the bulk solution. The result of this high-protein concentration is limited diffusion of the solvent through the protein layer, which in turn limits the bulk protein concentration that may be achieved using this process. Depending on the protein, the maximum concentration that may be reached using ultrafiltration varies between 40 and 200 mg/mL. This concentration limitation is very important when one is developing a formulation intended for administration subcutaneously or intramuscularly. Both of these routes of administration require that 1 mL or less total volume be given per injection. For proteins that require high concentrations for efficacy, the concentration achievable through ultrafiltration may be insufficient to meet the dose necessary for subcutaneous (SC) or intramuscular (IM) administration.

To work around this concentration limitation, formulation scientists often use a solid-state formulation as a means to achieving a higher protein concentration for the final drug product. By reconstituting the solid formulation with less water than was used to initially formulate the drug, one gets an increased protein concentration in the reconstituted product. It is important for the formulation scientist to remember that, in addition to the protein, the excipients in the formulation are also increased in concentration when the solid formulation is reconstituted to a lower final volume. Care should be taken to maintain a suitable final product osmolality for injection. The ability to achieve a higher concentration on reconstitution of the solid-state product also may allow the formulation scientist to side-step potential stability-limiting aggregation that may result in a liquid formulation of high-concentration protein.

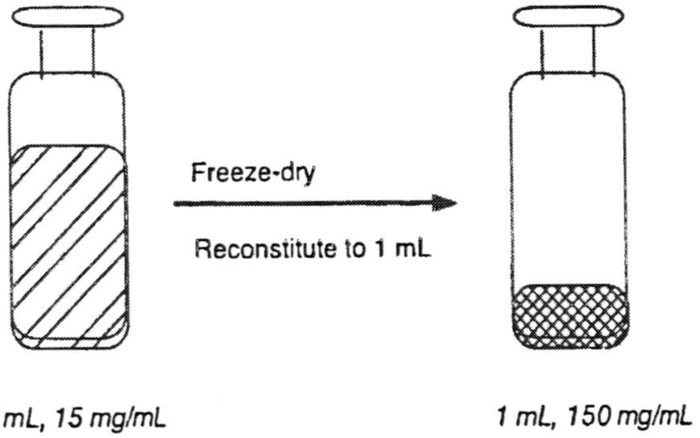

Freeze-dry

Reconstitute to 1 mL

10 mL, 15 mg/mL

1 mL, 150 mg/mL

Fig. 4.7. Using reconstitution to achieve high protein concentrations.

Excipient Selection

Excipients are the inactive ingredients added to stabilize the drug substance and the final drug product. The excipients may serve many purposes, including maintaining solution pH, adjusting solution osmolality, antioxidants, preservatives, and bulking agents; and minimizing surface denaturation. Although it might be tempting to add a little bit of each type of additive to the formulation, the desire is to add only what is necessary for stabilization of the drug. This is because the added excipients may interact with the protein or with each other, thus compromising the desired activity. In addition, an increased complexity of the formulation because of the number of excipients used also increases the risk of errors in the manufacture of the formulation that can result in product failure.

Formulation scientists tend to only use excipients that have been previously incorporated in other formulations. The reason for this is very clear--the demonstrated safety of the excipients in humans. For a new excipient to be used for a particular route of administration, the FDA requires that safety of that excipient is demonstrated in a human clinical trial. This may be an additional trial to that used to study the safety of the active drug product; therefore it is a significant added expense to the development of the drug product. If an excipient that has been used previously accomplishes the same goal in a formulation as one that has not been previously tested, it is prudent for the formulation scientist to proceed with the previously tested excipient. For a list of previously used excipients, one is often referred to the GRAS list, additives that are Generally Regarded As Safe by the FDA. Caution should be used when consulting this list as it refers to compounds that have been administered orally and specifically to food additives. The safety of excipients administered by other delivery routes may be quite different than those administered orally. The FDA publishes the Inactive Ingredients Guide, which lists all inactive ingredients in approved drugs with the route of administration, the number of drugs approved containing the ingredient, and the range of concentrations used. The Physician's Desk Reference (PDR) includes formulation information for specific prescription and over-the-counter drugs. Information from the PDR has been compiled by Powell, Nguyen, and Baloian to provide the formulation scientist easier access to this information.

Buffer and pH

The first variable typically specified for a formulation will be the pH. Several factors will aid the selection of pH. stability of the protein, solubility of the protein, and acceptability of the pH for the route of administration. The pH at which the drug undergoes minimal degradation is usually the preferred pH of the formulation. However, proteins reach minimal solubility when the solution pH approaches the isoeletric point (pI) of the protein. At the pI, the net charge on the protein is minimized and as the solution pH reaches the pI, precipitation is often observed. Generally, one must be greater than one pH unit away from the pI to achieve meaningful solubility. The final consideration is the pH that will be acceptable for administration. For drugs that are administered via the IM or SC routes, and especially to the lungs and eyes, it is desirable to be as close as possible to the tissue fluid pH of 7.4.

Administration of a drug at a pH that differs significantly from neutral could result in pain on administration, possibly because of cellular damage at the site of administration.

Using the desired pH and the list of buffers that have been previously used for drugs, the formulation scientist quickly narrows the buffers available for testing that meet both criteria. It is notable that there are actually very few choices at any pH. This list is typically decreased further if one is planning to formulate a solid-state product because some of the buffering components (e.g., acetic acid) are volatile. A reconstituted formulation that originally contained sodium acetate/acetic acid would no longer have a buffering species or pH control. Tris and other amine buffers are known to have a strong temperature dependency on pH. For this reason, analysis of protein stability as a function of pH under elevated temperature conditions is often difficult to interpret because the pH varies with the temperature.

Table 4.1. Approximate pK_a for commonly used buffers for parenteral administration

Buffer salt	*pK_a at 25°C*
Acetate	4.76
Citrate	3.13
	4.76
	6.40
Glycine	2.35
	9.78
Histidine	6.04
Phosphate	2.15
	6.82
	12.38
Succinate	4.21
	5.64
Tris	8.30

The concentration of the buffering species to be used also needs to be assessed. As with excipients in general, the rule of thumb is to use only the concentration of buffering species necessary to maintain pH or solubility of the formulation. One of the reasons to minimize the concentration of buffer components in the formulation is to prevent pain on administration. Products that are formulated at pH values that are not equivalent to that of the human tissue fluids are somewhat painful when administered subcutaneously, intramuscularly, topically to open wounds, or in the eye. The use of a buffer that maintains the pH of the formulation delays the equilibration of the administered drug's pH to that of the body. Thus, higher concentrations of the buffering species prolong this equilibration and result in pain on use. As anyone who has been on the receiving end of administration of a painful formulation can attest, the development of a drug product should minimize the potential for pain because of the excipients added. A second reason to minimize the buffer concentration is to limit the extent of buffer-catalyzed reactions. It has been observed with the peptide, gonadorelin, that an increase in the concentration of phosphate buffer led to an increase in the degradation rate of the peptide, and this increase in degradation rate was independent of the ionic strength of the buffer.

A preformulation screen performed for hybrid (BDBB) interferon-α (IFN-α) provides an interesting study in the balance of factors that must be considered on the selection of pH and buffering species used for a formulation. The authors compared the degradation of IFN-α in liquid solutions ranging in pH from 1.0 to 7.6 using citrate, acetate, glycine–HCl, or phosphate as the buffering species.

Formulations prepared with glycine–HCl at pH 5.0 and 6.0 did not allow sufficient solubility of the protein, presumably because of the proximity of the bulk pH to the pI of the protein (5.5). Formulations in acetate (pH 3.4–5.0) and glycine–HCl (pH 1.0 and 2.0) were found to degrade the fastest, as assessed by reversed-phase high- performance liquid chromatography (RP-HPLC), a technique used to monitor oxidation and fragmentation for this protein. Citrate formulations ranging in pH from 2.0 to 4.5 showed the next highest rates of degradation. Glycine–HCl (pH 3.0–4.5) and phosphate (pH 7.6) formulations displayed the slowest rates of degradation. These results demonstrate that for IFN-α: (1) formulation at low pH (e.g., 4.0) and near neutral pH (7.6) provides the most stability according to this method; and (2) glycine–HCl is the preferred buffering species at pH 4.5 compared with acetate and citrate. No difference in the rate of degradation was observed when the concentration of phosphate in the pH 7.6 formulation was changed twofold.

Although the relative rates of degradation for the pH 7.6 and 4.0 formulations of IFN-α were almost equivalent, the mechanisms of degradation were found to be very different. The pH 7.6 formulations exhibited higher levels of aggregation with concurrent decreased solubility as compared with the pH 4.0 samples. Oxidation was observed at pH 7.6, whereas none was observed at pH 4.0. Lower-molecular-weight species were formed at pH 4.0. Thus the next stage of formulation development for this protein for the pH 7.6 solution would require the use of excipients to minimize aggregation and oxidation, whereas stabilization of the pH 4.0 solution would require determination of the mechanism for fragmentation and the steps that could be taken to minimize degradation by this route.

Salts, sugars, and polyols

After selection of pH and buffer, the osmolality of the solution is adjusted using salts, sugars, or polyols. The osmolality of the blood is ~290 mmol/kg, and this is typically the target osmolality used for formulations that will be administered subcutaneously, intramuscularly, or to the eye. Solutions that are more than twofold or threefold hypoosmolar or hyperosmolar may result in cell lysis, an undesirable side effect of dose administration. Solutions that are administered via the intravenous (IV) route do not necessarily have to be isoosmolar because the dilution into the large volume of blood quickly normalizes the osmolality of the drug. For liquid formulations, the choice of using either a salt or a carbohydrate to adjust the osmolality of the solution is made by the impact on protein stability. Sodium chloride is one of the most commonly used salts in the formulation of both traditional pharmaceutics as well as biological pharmaceutics. It is extremely safe, well tolerated, and inexpensive. However, the presence of sodium chloride in a formulation of rhuMAb HER2 was found to increase oxidation when the formulation was stored in stainless steel containers, presumably because the sodium chloride promoted corrosion of the stainless steel. Interactions of salts with the proteins must be investigated on an individual basis because the type and concentration of salt may lead to protein aggregation. Sugars and polyols have often been used in formulations as well, particularly those that are in solid state. Commonly used carbohydrates include mannitol, sucrose, and trehalose. As previously described, the formulation scientist is strongly advised to steer clear of incorporation of reducing sugars (e.g., glucose and lactose) in formulations to avoid glycation and browning of the solution.

In lyophilized, SD, and SFD formulations, carbohydrates are employed as both bulking agents and as lyoprotectants. A bulking agent is necessary for these solid-state formulations because the physical amount of protein is very small. The addition of a bulking agent makes the sample amount more adequate for handling and generally improves the appearance of the final product. More importantly, the carbohydrate additives usually impart physical stability to the protein during the drying process. Specific ratios of carbohydrate to protein were found to be important to the stabilization of the protein structure in the solid state for two recombinant humanized antibodies and for recombinant human interleukin-1.

Surfactants

Surfactants are added to formulations to minimize denaturation of the protein at interfaces, typically liquid/air, solid/air, and liquid/container interfaces. Surfactants bind to hydrophobic areas of proteins. By minimizing the accessibility of the hydrophobic contacts in a protein solution, the surfactant reduces the protein–protein interactions that lead to aggregation. Furthermore, surfactants compete with the protein for binding at hydrophobic surfaces and are added to minimize protein losses because of surface denaturation. The concentration of surfactants required in these formulations generally is above the critical micelle concentration (CMC) for the particular surfactant. Polysorbate 20, polysorbate 80, and pluronic F68 are commonly used surfactants in protein therapeutics.

Several studies have demonstrated the need for surfactants in protein formulations. A formulation of recombinant factor VIII SQ required either polysorbate 80 or polysorbate 20 to prevent losses because of surface adsorption. Another study examining the stability of factor VIII SQ found that polysorbate 80 prevented losses of protein activity on filtration and freeze–thaw process. Polysorbate 20 was added to a formulation of recombinant factor XIII to stabilize the protein against both agitation and freeze–thaw-induced aggregation. Polysorbate 80 was added to a freeze-dried formulation of recombinant hemoglobin and found to protect the protein from aggregation resulting from the freeze–thaw process, although long-term stability of the protein against aggregation was not achieved. Pluronic F68, Brij 35, and polysorbate 80 all prevented aggregation of recombinant hGH that was induced by vortexing the solution. As described previously, care should be taken when using polysorbate 80 in formulations because of low levels of peroxides that may be present as a result of manufacturing or form during storage.

Antioxidants

Antioxidants are incorporated into formulations in which oxidation is a degradation mechanism for the protein. Typically, the antioxidant is a compound that is highly susceptible to oxidation and serves to scavenge any oxidative species in the solution before the oxidants can attack the protein. Addition of Met and thiosulfate to a formulation of rhuMAb HER2 effectively inhibited oxidation of the protein. In cases where metal-catalyzed oxidation is observed, the incorporation of a chelating agent such as ethylenediamine-tetraacetic acid (EDTA) may reduce the rate of oxidation of the protein by effectively scavenging free metal ions in solution before they have a chance to oxidize the protein. An alternative approach to reducing metal-catalyzed oxidation is to include Zn^{2+} in the formulation to bind to residues that may be susceptible to oxidation. Because Zn^{2+} does not promote oxidation, it protects the amino acid to which it chelates.

Preservatives

The next class of excipients that may be added to formulations is that of preservatives. These usually are not added to enhance stability to the formulation, but rather to give flexibility in the use of the drug product. With single-use formulations (those lacking a preservative), there is a requirement that each drug- filled container be entered only once. This is a safety precaution because exposure of the drug product in the container/closure system to air may result in the introduction of bacteria to the drug product. This is not a problem if the drug is used immediately because there is not sufficient time for the bacteria to colonize. However, on storage, it is possible for a significant number of bacteria to grow, particularly in formulations that are produced at neutral pH and that contain carbon and nitrogen sources on which the bacteria may feed. It would be unwise to inject a patient with a drug full of bacteria.

For this reason, a drug product that is to be used multiple times (multidose) must contain a preservative to prevent bacterial growth. However, most of these are not usually compatible with protein formulations. Some, such as the parabens, are not active in the presence of nonionic surfactants—

excipients that are typically required in protein formulations. Others may not be acceptable for a particular route of administration. Benzalkonium chloride, a commonly used preservative in topical formulations, causes ototoxicity when applied to the ear. As with buffering species, the list of preservatives available to the formulation scientist quickly narrows to just a few compounds including benzyl alcohol, phenol, m-cresol, and benzethonium chloride. A benzyl alcohol-containing formulation of epoetin alfa has been shown to be stable, even when dispensed in plastic syringes.

In screening preservatives for use in formulations, it is necessary to determine what levels of preservatives are efficacious at preventing bacterial growth in the particular formulation. Preservative challenge tests are conducted in which the protein formulation is spiked with different organisms such as *Pseudomonas aeruginosa*. The levels of each organism are monitored over time to determine if the preservative acted to kill or prevent growth of the particular organism. The United States Pharmacopeia (USP) and the European Pharmacopeia (EP) have prescribed levels of efficacy that a preserved formulation must pass to be used. Because the efficacy of the preservative is dependent on other excipients in the formulation, the formulation scientist must be careful to assess the final formulation conditions in the preservative challenge test. Even a change in protein concentration can affect the efficacy of the preservative.

Proteins are generally not exceedingly stable in the presence of preservatives. Preservatives are typically small hydrophobic compounds that may interact with hydrophobic regions of the protein, leading to a disruption in protein structure. Lam, Patapoff, and Nguyen found that addition of benzyl alcohol to a formulation of IFN-γ resulted in a loss of tertiary structure as determined by CD spectroscopy. Aggregation of interleukin-1 receptor was found to be the predominant pathway for degradation in the presence of phenol, *m*-cresol, and benzyl alcohol.

Others

There are numerous other excipients that may be required for use in formulating proteins. Amino acids such as His, Arg, and Gly have been used as bulking and solubilizing agents. Metal ions such as Ca^{2+} and Zn^{2+} are sometimes added for maintaining structure or activity of the protein. Other additives may be required to meet the needs of a specific route of administration, such as the necessity of including a gelling agent for topical formulations. To minimize losses because of protein adsorption, additives may be incorporated in the formulation to prevent or reduce surface denaturation of the active protein. Previously unpublished dilution studies were performed using trans-forming growth factor-β1 (TGF-β1) to determine the lowest concentration feasible at which the protein could be reasonably formulated. TGF-β1 is a potent cytokine, and very small amounts are required for biological action. In the absence of an additive to the formulation, the recovery of TGF-β1 from either a glass container or from a polypropylene tube was 80–90% at 10 μg/mL. At 10 ng/mL, the recovery dropped to 20–30% of the expected concentration. In the presence of a 0.5% (wt/vol) 100 bloom gelatin solution, the recovery increased to 100% at concentrations of 100 ng/mL or greater, and almost 70% at 10 ng/mL. Thus to achieve consistent protein dosages, gelatin addition to the formulation was required to minimize the losses of the TGF-β1 to the container surfaces used for storage of the drug and for analysis of the formulation.

In the last 10 years, there has been great concern regarding the use of animal-derived excipients in pharmaceutical formulations. There is a possibility of contamination of an excipient by either an undetected virus [e.g., hepatitis C, human immunodeficiency virus (HIV)] or prion that may cause transmissible spongiform encephalitis (TSE). For this reason, formulators have moved away from plasma-derived additives (e.g., human serum albumin, gelatin) and animal- sourced excipients (e.g., polysorbate 80) to either recombinant or vegetable-derived sources for these excipients. For example, the lyophilized formulation of recombinant factor VIII SQ was modified to remove human albumin (present to minimize surface adsorption and to function as a bulking agent and stabilizer) and to replace it with a combination of polysorbate 80, histidine, sucrose, and sodium chloride to achieve a stable product that would not have the potential of containing human viral particles.

Accelerated Stability Studies

Once the formulation scientist has narrowed the list of excipients to test in a formulation, an accelerated stability study is initiated. In this study, potential formulations are exposed to conditions such as elevated temperature, harsh light, mechanical stress, and freezing to assess which formulation provides the most stability to the active protein.

Accelerated temperature studies are conducted to assist the formulation scientist in the selection of the optimal formulation for a particular protein. Degradation is often accelerated at higher temperatures, allowing a faster assessment regarding formulation parameters. The temperatures selected for use in the accelerated temperature studies in part depend on the melting temperature (T_m) for the protein. Generally, protein formulations are assessed under refrigerated temperatures, at room temperature, and at least one higher temperature at which protein degradation is forced. Care must be taken to avoid temperatures that are too high; degradation at extremely high temperatures (e.g., 60°C) may not be representative of that which would occur under normal storage conditions. Using an Arrhenius plot of the data collected from several temperatures, it may be possible to estimate the shelf life for a product under the recommended storage conditions.

In addition to exposure to elevated temperatures, an assessment is made of the protein degradation under exposure to freezing conditions. Protein solutions may be stored in the bulk form at -20°C to -40°C for long-term storage. Data from several proteins, including hGH and hemoglobin, show that the freezing process may result in aggregation or denatura-tion. This damage may be because of formation of ice, a change in pH caused by freezing, or cold denaturation of the protein. As ice forms in the solution, the remaining components of the formulation are concentrated into the liquid phase. The resulting concentrate may be conducive to protein denaturation. Furthermore, a shift in pH of the solution during freezing may occur when one of the buffer salts (e.g., disodium phosphate) has limited solubility in this concentrated solution.

Exposure to harsh lighting is used to support handling of the drug product during the filling, finishing, and inspection of the protein. Excessive degradation on exposure to light may necessitate the use of colored glass to limit the amount of light exposure for vialed proteins. The previously mentioned study of hEGF1-48 demonstrated that the rate of photooxidation decreased when the product was stored in amber glass compared with the rate observed on storage in colorless glass. However, use of colored glass or other types of packaging made to limit light exposure of the product makes visual inspection of the product more difficult.

The susceptibility of the protein to degradation as a result of mechanical stress is conducted to support the manufacture and distribution of the protein. Protein solutions are often shaken mildly for 24–48 hr to provide information on mechanical stress-induced degradation. With shaking, the protein formulation's exposure to the air/liquid and liquid/container interfaces is maximized. Under these conditions, protein solutions may exhibit physical instability or oxidation. Stirring may also provide information on degradation induced by mechanical stress on a protein. Unlike shaking, stirring a protein solution generally does not significantly change the exposure of the protein solution to the interfaces. Rather, stirring results in an increase in the shear stress experienced by proteins. Physical instability is the main route of degradation from shear stress.

However, still to be considered are the route of administration and the use of a delivery device for the drug product. These impact the final selection of the formulation and will be covered in "*Drug Delivery Systems.*"

Drug Delivery Systems

A drug product can only be successful if it is delivered in a timely manner to the site of action in a way that will be amenable to the patient and in a way to ensure product quality. Different *routes of administration* may be used to achieve either systemic or local delivery of the protein. *Devices* such as needle-free injectors and nebulizers may be used to deliver the protein and to enhance patient compliance with use of the drug. Both the route of administration and the decision to use a device are optimally determined early in clinical development of the protein so that there is plenty of clinical experience with the final product. Some considerations regarding the selection of route and device are given below.

Route of Administration

One of the key pieces to development of a successful drug product is the ability to deliver the drug to the site of action with minimal discomfort or inconvenience to the patient. For small molecule therapeutics, there is a wide range of options available for drug administration. Delivery via injection (IV, IM, and SC), oral, nasal, ocular, transmucosal (buccal, vaginal, and rectal), and transdermal routes is possible with small molecule drugs. However, the size of proteins and the complexity of their structures severely limit the routes of administration available to proteins.

Injection

Parenteral injections of proteins often provide the fastest route of development for protein-based formulations. For systemic delivery of proteins, IV administration is considered to be the most efficient approach. Because of the efficiency of IV administration, the bioavailability of drugs is determined by comparing the blood levels achieved with the route of interest to that obtained via IV administration. For drugs administered through a route that has poor bioavailability, larger doses must be given to achieve the same serum levels of the drug compared with those achieved by IV administration. This additional amount of drug required would then lead to higher manufacturing costs associated with each dose.

Administration by injection is not without its drawbacks: It is considered to be painful, inconvenient, and invasive. For proteins in competition with traditional therapeutics that can be delivered via noninvasive methods, this is considered to present a significant marketing disadvantage. For SC and IM delivery, there is a volume limitation for injection. Typically, a maximum of 1.2 mL may be injected to a single SC site (~3 mL for IM), with larger volume doses necessitating the use of additional injection sites. For this reason, formulations intended for SC or IM delivery usually contain higher protein concentrations than those intended for IV delivery. The achievable protein concentration in the formulation may prove to limit the ability to deliver proteins by SC or IM routes.

Oral

Oral delivery of proteins has been the lofty goal of many formulation scientists and is the topic of several review articles. It is a traditional route of delivery for small molecules. However, the ability to deliver proteins orally presents several challenges to the biotechnological formulation scientist. First and foremost, the purpose of the gastrointestinal tract is to aid in the digestion and absorption of dietary proteins. The low pH and high enzymatic content of the gastric fluid make the environment highly unfavorable for protein therapeutics. This environment could be circumvented by designing a formulation with an enteric coating that allows the protein to escape unscathed from the stomach into the small intestine, where the pH is closer to neutral and the enzymatic content is lower. A formulation comprised of enterosoluble microparticles was developed for Enzeco lactase to facilitate oral delivery of this acid-labile enzyme to the small intestines for treatment of lactose intolerance. Polyethylene glycol-coated liposomes containing recombinant human epidermal growth factor were found to be efficacious in a rat model for gastric ulcer healing when delivered orally.

Although oral administration may allow for local delivery of protein therapeutics, the permeability of intact proteins through the stomach and intestinal membranes is extremely low, thus limiting systemic delivery of protein via the oral route. These are membranes that, by design, allow passage of small molecules and amino acids from the gut into the bloodstream. Protein therapeutics, in general, are too large and too hydrophilic to pass through these membranes. The low permeability, which may be extremely variable, translates to low bioavailability. For example, the bioavailability of an oral formulation of insulin, a small therapeutic protein, was found to be less than 0.5%. For a successful oral formulation to be developed for protein-based pharmaceutics that need to reach the bloodstream, it would most likely require the addition of a permeation enhancer to facilitate absorption of the drug. Only proteins requiring either a low dose for efficacy with a large therapeutic window, or requiring only local delivery to the gastrointestinal tract are viable candidates for oral delivery.

Pulmonary

Although routine oral delivery of proteins has not been realized, some protein formulations have been developed for pulmonary delivery. Pulmonary delivery can result in either parenteral or local administration of the drug and, like oral delivery, is considered noninvasive. As with other routes of delivery, the size of the protein may limit its ability to be delivered systemically via the pulmonary route of administration. Pulmozyme, a DNase-based formulation approved for the treatment of cystic fibrosis (CF), is delivered to the lungs by a nebulizer to clear blockage of the airways in the CF patient. Formulations for insulin to be administered by inhalation for systemic delivery of the protein have been developed, including a formulation comprised of microencapsulated insulin in particles formed from 3,6-bis[N-fumaryl-N-(n-butyl) amino]-2,5-diketopiperazine.

Topical

Topical delivery of small molecule drugs has been used to deliver therapeutics transdermally and transmucosally. Again, because of the size of the protein, it is often not feasible to deliver enough protein to achieve systemic levels of the drug. It is possible to deliver protein-based therapeutics locally by a topical formulation. Regranex, a platelet-derived growth factor-based topical formulation, has been approved by the FDA for the treatment of diabetic ulcers. Clinical trials are planned to investigate the efficacy of Oralin, a liquid aerosol preparation of insulin that is applied to the buccal mucosa.

Delivery Devices

Traditional parenteral delivery of biotechnological products has been accomplished through the use of a syringe equipped with a needle. Using this, it is possible to deliver proteins intravenously, intramuscularly, or subcutaneously. Devices have been developed to make this method of administration either less painful or more user-friendly. Robertson, Glazer, and Campbell have written a review of available devices for delivery of insulin. Devices have been manufactured to shield the needle to prevent accidental needle sticks. Prefilled cartridges coupled with a pen-type device reduce the need for the patient/nurse to withdraw drug into the syringe, thereby reducing the steps necessary for delivering the drug. Needle-free injectors that use a propellant to drive the drug solution through the dermis to deliver proteins subcutaneously or intramuscularly have been developed. This type of device would not be suitable for use with protein formulations that are susceptible to denaturation by shear stress.

Implantable pumps have been developed to administer drugs continuously, and there has been renewed interest in these devices for delivery of insulin. A small palm-sized pump is surgically placed subcutaneously in the abdomen of the patient with a catheter extending from the pump to the desired site of administration. The battery-operated pump is controlled externally with a device that adjusts delivery rate and volume. The pump may be refilled using a long needle. When the battery dies, the pump must be replaced. A clinical trial comparing delivery of insulin from an implantable pump to

SC injection demonstrated several advantages of the pump, including lower levels of antibodies to insulin, improved lipid metabolism, and no weight gain. Another study demonstrated reduced glycemic variability and hypoglycemic incidences with pump therapy.

There are several formulation concerns related to delivery of proteins from an implantable pump. Because this pump is placed within the body, it requires a formulation that is stable at body temperature (37°C) over the length of time the pump will deliver the protein until it is refilled. Motion of the body results in agitation of the solution contained within the pump; therefore it is necessary to ensure that the formulation is stable to shaking. The high surface-to-volume ratio of the catheter used for delivery may result in losses of protein because of surface adsorption. Each of these potential pitfalls may be overcome with the appropriate selection of excipients for most proteins.

Depot delivery systems offer an alternative for continuous delivery of protein therapeutics. Cleland, Daugherty, and Mrsny have written a review that covers the current technologies for depot delivery. With depot delivery, a formulation is injected or implanted, which provides sustained release of the therapeutic. The delivery may be for either local or systemic administration of the drug. Typically, the formulation contains a biodegradable matrix such as hyaluronate or poly(lactide-co-glycolide) (PLG), which entraps the therapeutic drug and slowly degrades in the presence of enzymes. During degradation of the gel or polymer, the drug incorporated in the matrix is released. Careful selection of the matrix may yield delivery times that release drug over several days or weeks. As with the implantable pump, depot formulations require sufficient stability at body temperature to ensure delivery of active protein. Nutropin Depot is a formulation of hGH in PLG microspheres that has been shown in clinical trials to release active hGH for 1 month after injection.

For pulmonary delivery of proteins, there are three broad categories of devices available: nebulizers, metered dose inhalers (MDIs), and dry particle inhalers (DPIs). Each of these must meet specific criteria for successful use, such as generation of appropriately sized particles for inhalation, chemical and physical compatibility of the device with the drug formulation, and consistency of dose delivery. Jet nebulizers use a pump to pressurize a liquid solution held in a reservoir through a nozzle, forcing the creation of tiny droplets that are deposited in the lung airways when the droplet stream is inhaled. The efficiency of delivery with this device is typically low because there is a large hold-up volume in the reservoir. Because the larger droplets that are formed do not leave the reservoir, the protein may experience several trips through the jet. The shear stress that the protein encounters during these repeated trips may lead to protein denaturation.

Additionally, milliliters of dosing solution are required per administration, and the length of time required for drug administration is not convenient (15–20 min). Ultrasonic nebulizers, which generate the droplet stream by ultrasound, require much smaller volumes (25–50 μL) and delivery times. However, the small volume necessitates a high concentration formulation that is able to withstand the ultrasonic exposure without degrading the protein. Formulations of aviscumine were compared to determine which formulations were able to protect the protein from shear-induced degradation caused by nebulization.

MDIs have not been used extensively with protein therapeutics. With an MDI, a small amount of drug is aerosolized using a propellant, typically a hydrofluoroalkane. Poor delivery efficiency and reproducibility, coupled with concern regarding the stability of proteins in the presence of the hydrofluoroalkanes, have led to a lack of interest in pursuing the use of this type of device for pulmonary delivery of proteins.

Dry powder inhalers that are currently marketed use the patient's inspiration to move the powder from the device to the lungs, although powered DPIs are also under development. Fine powders of the protein formulation are stored either in a large reservoir in the DPI (for multidose administration), or in individual blister packs (for single-dose administration.) As the patient inhales, the DPI is activated to release powder into the airstream. For this method of delivery to be successful, the protein formulation must retain the fine, dry powder consistency necessary for delivery. Exposure to high humidity may cause the particles to clump, which may lead to clogging of the device and a decrease in delivery efficiency. For the multidose formulation, a preservative is required in the powdered formulation.

Future Prospects

With the development of biotechnology-derived products for clinical indications that are not life-threatening, there will be an increased drive to move away from drugs that must be given by injection, particularly by IV administration. The ability to formulate proteins at high concentrations will allow more to be administered subcutaneously. Crystalline forms of proteins are now being investigated as potential formulations and with the possibility that these could be given as depots to allow extended delivery of the protein. Devices to increase the convenience of delivery will continue to be attractive for protein therapeutics. Development of formulations for pulmonary delivery should increase significantly within the next decade. Pulmonary delivery is non-invasive, and the advent of formulations that may be administered by dry powder inhalers makes this route extremely attractive to patients.

In the development of a formulation, the potential degradation mechanisms for the protein must be considered. From the primary structure, one may anticipate some of the potential degradation pathways for a given protein (e.g., deamidation at Asn–Gly; fragmentation at Asp–Pro). Other types of degradation (e.g., surface denaturation) cannot be predicted as easily and must be determined experimentally.

Information from preformulation and formulation studies allows the formulation scientist to determine the state and composition of the drug substance and drug product. Using accelerated stress conditions such as exposure to elevated temperature, harsh lighting, freezing, and shaking helps the scientist to elucidate the likely degradation products for the protein of interest. Data from these studies are instrumental in determining storage conditions for the drug substance and drug product.

Selection of the appropriate route of administration and delivery device is critical for the commercial success of a drug product. Although injections are the most efficient delivery method for proteins, they are not always the most suitable from the patient's perspective. Few routes of administration (IV, IM, SC, pulmonary, and topical for local delivery) have been successful to date with protein therapeutics because of the size and complexity of the protein structure. Consideration of the bioavailability via a given route must be made when determining the dose required. Use of a delivery device such as an implantable pump, needle-free injector, or dry-powder inhaler may yield a product with a commercial advantage over a competitor's product.

Testing, Filling, and Packaging

The present article will continue the discussion of the development of the formulation, with a focus on the requirements for stability testing and manufacturing to be able to successfully deliver the final formulated product to patients.

Once the selection of delivery route, excipients, and physical state is made during formulation development, studies to examine the stability of the product under recommended and stressed storage conditions must be performed to ensure product quality and safety. Does the product require refrigeration? Should the bulk be stored frozen? Is there sufficient stability for a viable product? These studies utilize analytical methodologies to evaluate the stability of the protein. What does each of the assays tell the scientist about the degradation of the protein? Are the assays stability indicating? Additionally, the manufacturability of the product must be considered. Is the formulation compatible with the manufacturing equipment? Does the protein degrade due to shear stress experienced during the filling operation? What steps must be taken to maintain sterility of the product? It is through this process that an active protein drug may be formulated into a viable drug product.

Stability Studies

In an earlier study, a discussion of the factors that must be considered during formulation development of a protein therapeutic was presented, including the selection of state, solution conditions (e.g., pH, buffer type, and concentration), and route of delivery. Once the formulation has been selected, stability studies of the drug substance and drug product are required to support expiration dating by the FDA and other regulatory agencies in submissions for product approval. If a device is being used to administer the drug, studies must also be conducted to demonstrate the compatibility of the formulation with the device.

These stability studies are typically conducted in a GMP environment using established protocols and analytical methods. The International Conference on Harmonisation (ICH) has recommended for adoption by the regulatory bodies of the U.S.A., Europe, and Japan guidelines for conducting stability testing for biotechnological products. The guidelines for biotechnological products are different from those used for traditional small molecule drugs due to the complexity of the protein structure. Three areas that are covered in this guideline are selection of batches, the stability indicating profile, and storage conditions.

Selection of Batches

The selection of batches refers to the specific drug substance and drug product batches that will be tested to support expiration dating. At the time of regulatory submission for approval (e.g., BLA), a minimum of six months of stability data is needed on at least three batches of drug substance and final drug product for which the manufacture, container, and storage are representative of the manufacturing scale of production. The quality and process used to manufacture each must be representative of material used in preclinical and clinical trials. Expiration dating is based upon real time/real temperature storage data.

Stability-Indicating Profile

The stability-indicating profile for a biotechnological product generally comprises information from a battery of assays, not from a single stability-indicating assay. To support the expiration dating, the stability of the drug product and drug substance must be assessed by methods that have been validated and are detailed in a protocol specific to that product. This protocol includes the testing intervals and the specifications that the product must meet. Some of the methodologies that could be used for this purpose are described in a later portion of this article.

Storage Conditions

The storage conditions for biotechnological products need to be clearly defined because protein stability is generally temperature dependent. Unlike small molecule drugs, accelerated temperature studies are not used to determine expiration dating for biotechnological products. However, accelerated temperature studies may be used to provide supporting data and to determine the pathway(s) of degradation for the protein. Humidity control is generally not a concern for biotechnological products because most are packaged in containers that protect against humidity.

For those products that are not, stability data gathered at different humidities must be provided. Studies should be conducted to support shipping and handling of the product. These may include exposure to light and to a wider range of temperatures that would be tested for recommended storage temperatures. Interactions, or lack of thereof, of the product with the container/ closure must be assessed. For products that are further prepared for administration in the field (e.g., reconstitution of a lyophilized product followed by dilution into an IV bag containing saline), data must be provided that supports expiration dating and recommended storage conditions of the diluted product that will be administered to a patient.

Methodology for Assessing Protein Stability

As stated throughout this entry, one goal of the formulation scientist is to understand and minimize degradation of the protein in the formulation during storage. Additionally, the FDA and other regulatory agencies require that the purity and potency of pharmaceuticals are monitored during the shelf life of the products. Achieving these requirements involves using a combination of analytical techniques such as chromatography, electrophoresis, and spectroscopy among others. Because proteins are capable of denaturing via several mechanisms, it is necessary to use more than one technique to demonstrate stability. Jones has written an in-depth review of analytical methodologies used to assess protein stability.

Liquid Chromatography

High performance liquid chromatography (HPLC) is the workhorse for many of the analytical technologies used to assess protein stability. It relies on protein separation by interaction of the protein with a resin, called the stationary phase. The protein is removed (eluted) from the resin using a solution called the *mobile phase*. Differences in the interactions between protein variants (e.g., aggregates, deamidated products) and the stationary phase are exploited to achieve separation. The length of time that the protein variants are retained by the resin, the retention time, is determined to gain understanding of the nature of the variants. There are four basic types of chromatographic separations used by formulation scientists: size exclusion chromatography (SEC), ion exchange chromatography (IEC), hydrophobic interaction chromatography (HIC), and reversed phase chromatography (RPC).

In SEC, also referred to as gel filtration or gel permeation chromatography, the protein variants are separated according to differences in hydrodynamic radius. The stationary phase for SEC employs porous microparticles while the mobile phase is typically an aqueous salt solution. When the protein and its variants enter the SEC column containing the stationary phase, they are greeted with a tortuous path to reach the end of the column. The smaller variants (e.g., fragments) have access to a greater number of paths through the porous material that results in a larger accessible volume for these variants and therefore a longer retention time on the column. Larger variants (e.g., aggregates) have fewer paths (detours) available, and therefore elute first from the SEC column. The smallest particles are those that elute with the longest retention time. Molecular weight is usually estimated by a comparison of the retention time of a variant to those of molecular weight standards. However, because the retention time is determined by the hydrodynamic radius rather than molecular weight alone, it is often important to confirm estimated molecular weights using a second technique such as static light scattering or mass spectrometry.

One advantage that SEC has for the formulation scientist is the ability to study protein aggregation/fragmentation in the environment of different formulations. Also, it is possible to add denaturants such as sodium dodecyl sulfate (SDS) to the mobile phase to gain a greater understanding of the sources of molecular weight heterogeneity.

Ion exchange chromatography exploits charge differences between protein variants to achieve separation. The resin used in the IEC stationary phase is either for cation exchange or anion exchange. For protein with basic pI, cation exchange chromatography is typically used. The protein is injected onto the stationary phase where it interacts with the resin. Using a gradient of salt and/or pH, the protein is eluted from the column when the pH or ionic strength of the mobile phase is sufficient to overcome the protein's ionic interaction with the column. The products of deamidation are typically resolved using IEC chromatography.

With HIC, the protein variants are separated by differences in hydrophobicity. In this technique, the stationary phase is comprised of a resin with a hydrophobic backbone. The protein is injected onto this column under high ionic strength conditions. This promotes hydrophobic interactions. A mobile phase gradient is used in which the ionic strength decreases with time. Less hydrophobic variants elute with an earlier retention time than those with higher hydro phobicity. Products of oxidation may often be resolved by HIC.

Reversed phase chromatography is used to separate protein variants by hydrophobicity as well. The stationary phase is also comprised of particles containing hydrophobic backbones. However, separation is achieved using a gradient that employs an increasing content of an organic solvent such as acetonitrile or methanol. Trifluoroacetic acid (TFA) is typically added to the mobile phase to improve the interactions of the protein with the resin through ion pairing with charged residues on the protein. Unlike the other chromatographies described, this technique often results in denaturation of the protein during chromatography due to exposure of the protein to both low pH (TFA) and the organic solvent. As with HIC, products of oxidation may be separated by RPC. Reversed phase chromatography generally offers much better resolution than HIC, but has limitations on the size of protein that may be separated.

With all of the HPLC techniques, it is often possible to gain more information by modifying the protein prior to injection either by reduction or through mild enzymatic treatment. By purposefully fragmenting the protein, it may be possible to identify the site of degradation or to at least increase the resolution achieved in the chromatographic separation. Peptide maps generated from complete enzymatic digests, together with mass spectrometry, have proven extremely useful for determining sites of degradation in many proteins, including recombinant human macrophage-colony stimulating factor (rhM-CSF) and relaxin.

Electrophoresis

In electrophoresis, protein variants are separated due to differences in their mobility in the presence of an electrical field. Traditionally, electrophoresis has been performed using a stationary slab gel. The most common electrophoretic technique is sodium dodecyl sulfate-polyacrylamide gel electrophoresis (SD S-PAGE). In this technique, a polyacrylamide gel provides a sieving matrix for the protein solution. The protein is mixed with an SDS solution prior to loading onto the gel. By coating the protein with SDS, the charge to mass ratio becomes uniform between proteins. This allows proteins to be separated solely on molecular weight in the presence of the electrical field. The protein/SDS solution is loaded onto the gel which is continually bathed in an SDS-containing buffer. A voltage is applied across the gel, and the protein is mobilized. Smaller proteins travel through the gel faster than larger ones. Protein visualization occurs through the staining of the gel, usually with either established silver staining or Coomassie staining techniques. Molecular weights are estimated by comparison of mobilization distance to molecular weight standards.

Native PAGE is conducted in the same manner as SDS-PAGE, with the exception that SDS is added neither to the protein solution nor to the bathing solution surrounding the gel during electrophoresis. In the absence of SDS, protein separation results from a combination of the charge and mass of the protein. For this reason, analysis of a native gel is more difficult than that of traditional SDS-PAGE. However, native gels can provide information on protein interactions under very specific conditions (buffer, pH) that could not be studied using SDS-PAGE.

Isoelectric focusing (IEF) separates proteins on a gel by exploiting differences in the isoelectric point (*pl*) of the protein variants. At the *pl*, the sum of all of the charges on the protein is zero. Degradation that results in a charge in the *pl* (e.g., deamidation, fragmentation) may be detected using IEF. Separation by IEF occurs in the presence of ampholytes that maintain a pH gradient in the presence of an electrical field. The protein variants migrate on the gel until they reach the pH in which they are neutral. The *pl* of a variant is determined by comparison to the location of *pl* standards.

During the 1990s technological advances were achieved in the field of capillary electrophoresis (CE), resulting in its emergence as one of the primary tools in assessing protein degradation. In CE, an electric field is applied across a capillary containing a separation medium and the protein solution to achieve separation of the protein variants. Once the separation occurs, the solution in the capillary is mobilized and passes in front of a detector to assess the separation. UV and fluorescence detectors are commonly used to assess protein separations. Capillary electrophoresis has the ability to separate proteins based on size (SEC, SDS-PAGE), charge (IEC), *pl* (IEF), and hydrophobicity (HIC, RPC). The amount of protein required for CE analysis is substantially smaller than that required for traditional HPLC or gel electrophoretic techniques. This makes CE attractive when only small amounts of protein are available. It is not feasible, however, to use CE as a separation technique when one wishes to collect the fractionated proteins for use in another assay because the amount of protein is too small.

The separation medium used in the capillary dictates the type of separation that will be observed. In capillary zone electrophoresis (CZE), an aqueous buffered solution at a specific pH is used. Protein variants are separated according to their charge to mass ratio at that specific pH. In capillary isoelectric focusing (CIEF), ampholytes are used in the separation medium. Proteins are separated by *pl* in CIEF. Micellar electrokinetic capillary electrophoresis (MEKC) employs micelle forming surfactant solutions to achieve separations that resemble RPC. Various sieving matrices may be used in the capillary in conjunction with SDS to achieve separations based on molecular weight.

Spectroscopy

Spectroscopy measures the interactions of the protein chromophores with light. Information regarding the concentration and conformation of the protein may be obtained through different types of spectroscopy.

Using ultraviolet/visible (UV/Vis) absorption spectroscopy, it is possible to measure the protein concentration using Beer's Law: $A = \varepsilon | c$, where A is the measured absorbance of a solution, ε is the absorptivity of the protein, | is the pathlength of the cell used to determine the absorbance, and c is the protein concentration. Proteins typically exhibit two strong, broad absorption bands in the UV/Vis part of the spectrum. The first and most intense band is centered at 214 nm and arises from absorption of light by the peptide backbone. The second absorption band is typically found at ~280 nm. This band arises from absorbance from the aromatic side chains of Trp, Tyr, and Phe. Disulfide bonds may exhibit weak absorption in this range as well.

During stability studies, the concentration of the protein is monitored to ensure that there is no loss due to physical instability of the protein. Most typical routes of chemical degradation do not result in a change of absorbance. A change in color of the solution may occur as a result of degradation of some excipients, (notably His) or in the presence of a reducing sugar.

The UV/Vis absorption spectrum has the capability of providing important information regarding the stability of the formulation by using the spectrum to ascertain the level of light scattering that the solution exhibits. The intensity of light scattering by particulates depends on the fourth power of the frequency of light and on the size of the particulates. As one progresses to bluer (shorter) wavelengths, the intensity of light scattering dramatically increases. The formulation scientist can exploit this to monitor formulations for low levels of particulates, particularly before the particulates are large enough to be observed by visual inspection. Dynamic laser light scattering may also be employed for this purpose, although the equipment for this is usually more costly than the average spectrophotometer.

Circular dichroism (CD) is often used by the formulation scientist to monitor the secondary and tertiary structures of the protein of interest. Circular dichroism results from the preferential absorption of left vs. right circularly polarized light. In the far UV region of the spectrum (190–250 nm), the circular dichroism absorption of proteins arises from peptide bonds. Each type of secondary structural elements (e.g., alpha helix, beta sheet) has a unique circular dichroism spectrum. Using algorithms which compare the spectrum of the protein of interest to libraries of spectra from proteins with known secondary structural elements allows the formulation scientist to estimate the contribution of each secondary structure element to the total structure of the protein. This ability may aid the formulation scientist in the selection of a suitable formulation for a protein. A combination of excipients which results in an increase in the content of random coiled structure within the protein would not provide a suitable formulation for long term stability of the protein. Signals in the near UV region (250–400 nm) of the CD spectrum of a protein predominantly arise from absorption of the aromatic side chains of Trp, Tyr, and Phe. The dichroism in this region is highly dependent on the tertiary structure of the protein. For this reason, the near UV CD spectrum is often used to monitor changes in the native environment of proteins that result from instability. For example, Lam, Patapoff, and Nguyen used the near UV CD spectrum of IFN-γ to determine that there was an incompatibility of the protein with a combination of excipients (succinate, benzyl alcohol) that resulted in a loss of structure.

The secondary structure of proteins may also be assessed using vibrational spectroscopy, fourier transform infrared spectroscopy (FTIR), and Raman spectroscopy both provide information on the secondary structure of proteins. The bulk of the literature using vibrational spectroscopy to study protein structure has involved the use of FTIR. Water produces vibrational bands that interfere with the bands associated with proteins. For this reason, most of the FTIR literature focuses on the use of this technique to assess structure in the solid state or in the presence of non-aqueous environments. Recently, differential FTIR has been used in which a water background is subtracted from the FTIR spectrum. This work-around is limited to solutions containing relatively high protein concentrations.

Raman spectroscopy offers the advantage of being able to collect spectra in aqueous environments, because the vibrational frequencies arising from water are almost invisible in the Raman spectrum. However, this technique has not been used as extensively as FTIR because the technique was more time consuming and the equipment more costly. The recent development of FT-Raman systems has allowed this technique to be used more readily than in the past.

Appearance Assays

In addition to the various physical techniques, a simple visual inspection of the formulation is conducted to determine if there are changes to the formulation. The human eye is extremely sensitive to many changes observed in protein formulations, and for this reason visual inspection is a valuable tool in the bag of techniques used to assess stability. For liquid formulations, the appearance of precipitates or a change in color of the formulation signifies trouble. For lyophilized formulations, the visual appearance of the lyophilized cake is an important characteristic of the formulation. Collapse or discoloration of the cake could indicate a compromised formulation.

Potency/Activity Assays

The most important assessment during stability studies is analysis of the protein by an activity assay. Degradation of a protein that results in compromised activity is of great concern because this affects the potency of the drug product. Expiration dating of the drug product is made to minimize the loss of potency. Potency of drug candidates is typically assessed in vitro. An appropriate potency assay must be biologically relevant to the clinical indication for which the drug is targeted. For example, the potency of a growth factor whose action is believed to induce proliferation of epithelial cells in vivo would need to be assessed by an in vitro epithelial cell-based proliferation assay.

Thermal Techniques

Thermal techniques such as isothermal calorimetry (ITC) and differential scanning calorimetry (DSC) have been used in formulation screens to predict the formulation with the greatest stability based on the assumption that excipients that increase the T_m of the protein will stabilize the molecule at the recommended storage temperature. For example, a screen of preservatives performed during formulation development for interleukin-1 receptor found that the T_m for the formulation correlated with the extent of aggregation observed on storage at 37°C. Such thermal analysis may be useful to rank order formulations.

Other

Other methodologies may be employed for specific drug products. For microencapsulated, spray-dried, and spray-freeze-dried formulations, an assessment of the particle size may be critical. Lyophilized, spray-dried, and spray-freeze-dried formulations must be monitored for moisture content. Gel-based formulations typically require monitoring the viscosity of the semi solid formulation.

Filling, Finishing, and Packaging

Filling, finishing, and packaging are the processes by which the drug substance is turned into the final product and are performed according to current Good Manufacturing Practices (cGMPs). These steps in the manufacturing process are tightly regulated to ensure patient safety. A thorough review of the cGMPs related to filling, finishing, and labeling of drug products is given by Willig and Stoker.

Filling

Filling refers to the operation in which the drug substance is placed into the container that will be sold to the consumer. The filling operation involves transferring the drug substance from its storage tank to the filler, accurately pumping the drug substance through the filling machine into the final container, and then closing the container. In the case of lyophilized products, the filled vials are transferred to a lyophilizer and freeze-dried prior to closing the container. A recent review gives detailed information on this process.

Prior to filling, care should be taken to examine the compatibility of the product with the equipment used in the filling process and with the shear that may be experienced by the protein during the filling operation. For example, the protein is sterile-filtered to ensure sterility. The effects of the rate of the filtration on the protein quality and the compatibility of the protein with the type of membrane used for the filtration should be explored prior to filling. Fill speeds should be adjusted to minimize foaming of the protein product during the filling process. Compatibility of the product with the materials of construction for the filling and storage equipment should be assessed to ensure product quality.

The most typical filling operation for a biotechnology-derived product involves filling a liquid into a glass vial that is then closed with a stopper and sealed with a cap. The vial/stopper combination is referred as the "container/closure system" and provides the barrier to microbial contamination for the drug product during its shelf life. Several container/closure systems are used in the biotechnology industry, including vials/stopper, ampoules, and pre-filled syringes. The vial/stopper combination has been the most widely used based on the relative flexibility that this system provides. The stopper (typically made of a type of rubber) is inserted at the top of the vial. The depth of penetration into the vial and the shape of the stopper affect how well the container/closure system works. Typically, an aluminum crimp cap is used to achieve a better seal with the stopper and to provide a barrier against accidental removal of the stopper from the vial. Ampoules, made of glass or plastic, are manufactured by forming the shape of the container from softened glass or plastic, cooling slightly, filling the product, and then using heat to seal the container. Because the container is a single piece, contamination may only occur if the container is improperly formed, cracked, or broken. Prefilled syringes are similar to vials/ stoppers in the type of components to which the product is exposed. In the case of the syringe, a glass or plastic-barreled container is filled with the drug. A stopper is placed near the plunger end of the syringe to prevent leakage from the bottom, while a rubber cap is typically used to protect from leakage at the needle-end of the syringe. As with vials/stoppers, the quality of the seals will be affected by the shape and depth of penetration of the stopper and cap.

The container/closure system used for the product must be validated to ensure that the system is effective in maintaining a boundary to microbial contamination during the shelf life of the product. This validation begins in the manufacturing area to ensure that appropriate components and parameters are used during the fill. First, compatibility of the components with the manufacturing fill line must be ascertained so that appropriate equipment are used. Factors such as the pressure required to insert the stopper into the vial are determined. The ability of the filling process and the container/closure system to prevent microbial contamination is validated by several methods, including media fills and dye leak tests. Filling the container/closure system with growth-promoting media is performed to demonstrate that the filling operation does not introduce colony-forming organisms to the final product. With this method, the sealed vial containing media is monitored for several days to ensure that no growth is observed. A dye-leak test is typically performed to demonstrate that the container/closure system provides an adequate seal. In this method, the container/closure system is immersed into a water solution containing dye, and the system is monitored for ingress of the dye into the container. This test is often performed at the end of shelf-life to demonstrate that the container/closure system maintained integrity under the recommended storage conditions for the drug product.

The FDA "Guidelines for Sterile Drug Products Produced by Aseptic Processing" describes the critical points that must be considered when filling the final product. Biotechnological products cannot be terminally sterilized, because the heat or radiation used for sterilization of the final product damages the protein. Therefore, the filling operation is performed in an aseptic environment to minimize the risk of introduction of bacteria to the product. At this stage in manufacture, the presence of bacteria in the product could present a serious safety risk for patients who use the drug.

To minimize the potential for introducing microbes and other foreign particles to the final product, several precautions are used in the filling area. All components used for the filling operation, including the components for the final package (e.g., vial, stopper, blister-pack) and filling equipment, are washed and pre-sterilized. For a liquid drug substance, a sterile filtration is performed into a pre sterilized filling vessel to ensure that the drug substance is bacteria-free. Any area in which the sterilized product or the open container/closure systems are exposed to the environment must meet special requirements. Class 100 rooms are used in which the air is high efficiency particulate air (HEPA)-filtered at the point of delivery and contains less than 100 particles sized $\leq 0.5\ \mu m$ per cubic foot of air. The airflow is unidirectional in this room. The microbial load should be no higher than 0.1 colony forming unit (CFU) per cubic foot of air. Operators working in class 100 rooms are required to be completely gowned in sterile garb. They must minimize movements and talking within the room so as not to disturb the airflow. Validation of the filling environment and operations is accomplished by performing media fills periodically and by testing the sterility of the media- filled units. At least 3000 units should be filled in order to be able to detect a contamination rate of one in 1000 units with a 95% confidence interval. For lyophilized products, the vials are filled with the liquid drug substance and partially stoppered before being placed into a lyophilizer contained within the class 100 area. Lyophilization occurs in three steps: freezing, in which the temperature inside the lyophilizer is decreased to freeze the product; primary drying, in which the resulting ice is removed by sublimation that is facilitated by pulling a vacuum on the lyophilization chamber; and secondary drying, in which the temperature is raised to remove any water molecules that are not tightly bound to the protein. The rate of freezing, primary drying, and secondary drying can profoundly affect the overall lyophilization time. Careful selection of the temperatures, pressures, and rates for each of these processes must be made to ensure good product quality.

Filling and packaging by blow/fill/seal technology has gained wider acceptance for use in the biotechnology industry in the past decade. The blow/fill/seal process is one continual, integrated operation in which the container is formed by "*blowing*" a molten plastic such as low density polyethylene (LDPE) into a mold, filled using a nozzle provided with a class 100 HEPA airflow, and then sealed by molding of the still molten plastic at the neck. The result is a plastic ampoule. Due to the highly automated procedure used, minimal personnel are required for the filling operation. This reduces the sources of potential viable and nonviable particulate contamination in the final product.

Finishing and Packaging

Once the protein formulation has been filled into the final container, several packaging and finishing steps are performed before the product may be shipped for use. For vialed formulations, the final vial must be capped to ensure that the stopper does not inadvertently come off of the vial. This protects potential leakage from the vial or the introduction of contaminants to the vial. The product is inspected and representative samples are tested to ensure consistency, safety, and potency. The final container is labeled with product information such as the name of the drug, the manufacturer, the amount of the drug in the container, the lot number, and the expiration date. Once the labeling has been done, a second inspection is performed on a representative sample of units to ensure that the correct label has been used. Outer packaging is selected (e.g., a carton) in which all of the components for the final product are assembled for sale. This packaging may be as simple as one vial in a carton or as elaborate as one containing a lyophilized product packaged with a vial of diluent and a syringe to enable easy access to the tools necessary for reconstitution of the product. This package is appropriately labeled to include the name of the drug, the manufacturer, the amount of drug per unit, the number of units, and the expiration date among other information. Included in the final package is a "*package insert*," a very detailed description of the composition of the drug product, its intended use, and any side effects noted with use of the drug. Once packaged, the product is ready for distribution.

The successful development of a biotechnology-derived product relies on several factors, including the appropriate selection of dosage form. In the application to the FDA for product approval, the section describing drug product and drug substance stability information is one of the critical sections related to manufacturing as it will define the expiration dating for the drug substance and the drug product. Relatively short expiration dating for either the drug substance or drug product would result in increased frequency of manufacturing and a higher level of complexity in product distribution.

The use of appropriate analytical techniques during formulation development aids the formulation scientist in determining the degradation products and the rate of formation of those products. Since proteins are complex structures, a combination of techniques must be used to ensure that the formulation scientist is able to assess potential degradation of the protein. This information is critical for the successful development of a therapeutic formulation.

The protein formulation must be filled and packaged prior to delivering to the patient for use. Compatibility of the protein formulation with the filling equipment and filling process should be assessed to confirm that product quality is not compromised during these operations. After filling, the product is labeled for distribution and packaged into its final container. Tight regulations around the filling, finishing, and packaging operations are in place to ensure patient safety.

5

Dosage Form

Over the past several years, the fraction of new drug products that are new chemical entities has steadily decreased, reflecting the tremendous cost required to bring new chemical entities to the marketplace. Increased understanding of drug metabolic and toxicologic factors, such as the effect of the patient age on drug distribution, the genetic factors that may result in dramatic intersubject variability in metabolism, short-term versus long-term exposure toxicities, and the potential for teratogenic, mutagenic, and embryo- toxic effects, has increased the scrutiny under which governmental agencies view the new chemical entity. This careful inspection is intended to minimize the possibility of toxic reaction(s) and to demonstrate the safety and efficacy of new drug products. The regulatory process has also resulted in significantly more costly and time-consuming testing prior to commercialization.

Physicochemical Approach

This increased emphasis on safety has placed an additional burden on those who are involved in the development of new drugs, while increasing financial pressures have led to the need for decreased development time. The investigation of approved drugs has resulted in enhanced patient safety and therapeutic efficacy by directing research efforts toward the more efficacious delivery of known pharmacologically active agents to the appropriate physiologic site. This trend has caused pharmaceutical researchers to seek the most suitable methods to deliver both new and existing compounds in the most pharmacologically appropriate manner. The methods may be designed to optimize bioavailability, minimize toxicity and side effects, and improve stability. The objective of this article is to present approaches that have been employed to improve bioavailability and/or minimize the toxicity and side effects of various drugs. A rational approach to dosage form design requires a complete understanding of the physicochemical and biopharmaceutical properties of the drug substance. For example, the successful design of an efficacious oral dosage form requires an understanding of the pathways of physiologic disposition of the drug. On oral administration of an immediate release dosage form (the most common delivery system), the dosage form must disintegrate, the drug must dissolve in the gastrointestinal (GI) fluids, cross the GI mucosa, enter the mesenteric blood system, and pass through the liver prior to reaching the systemic circulation and the site of action. The drug may be metabolized by GI fluids, by enzymes in the gut wall, or by hepatic metabolism prior to reaching the systemic circulation. The net result is incomplete bioavailability due to first-pass metabolism (inactivation), and/or metabolic formation of a pharmacologically active species.

The physicochemical and biopharmaceutical properties of the drug can have a tremendous impact on its bioavailability and, hence, on its efficacy and toxicity profile. Thus, understanding these parameters is often tantamount to the selection and development of the optimum dosage form.

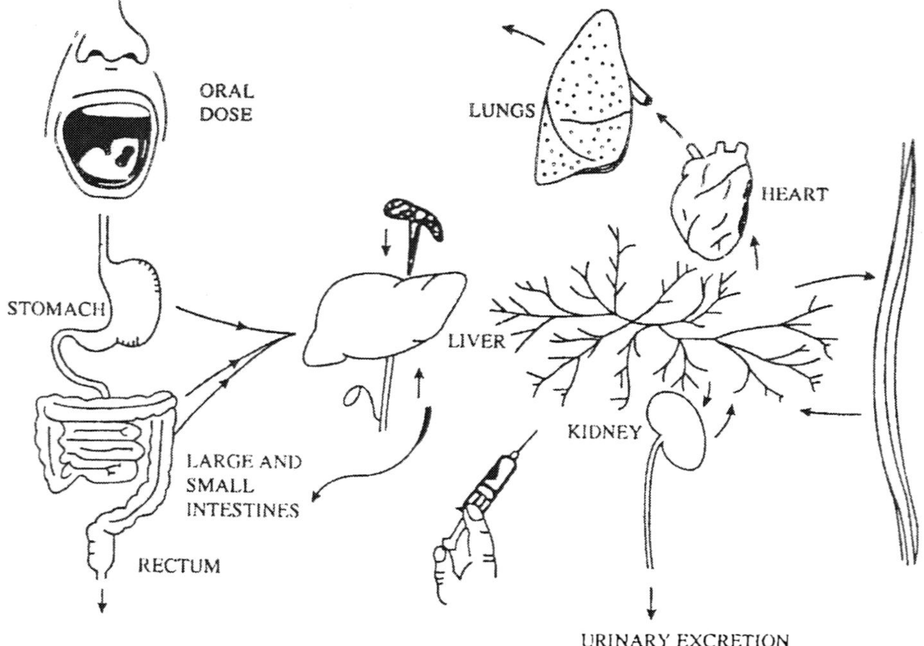

Fig. 5.1. Physiological factors associated with bioavailability.

These properties of the drug are its:

1. pH solubility profile and dissolution rate
2. Partition coefficient between lipoidal barriers and aqueous physiologic media
3. Stability and/or degradation rate in the physiologic fluids
4. Susceptibility to metabolic inactivation
5. Mechanism of transport through biologic membranes.

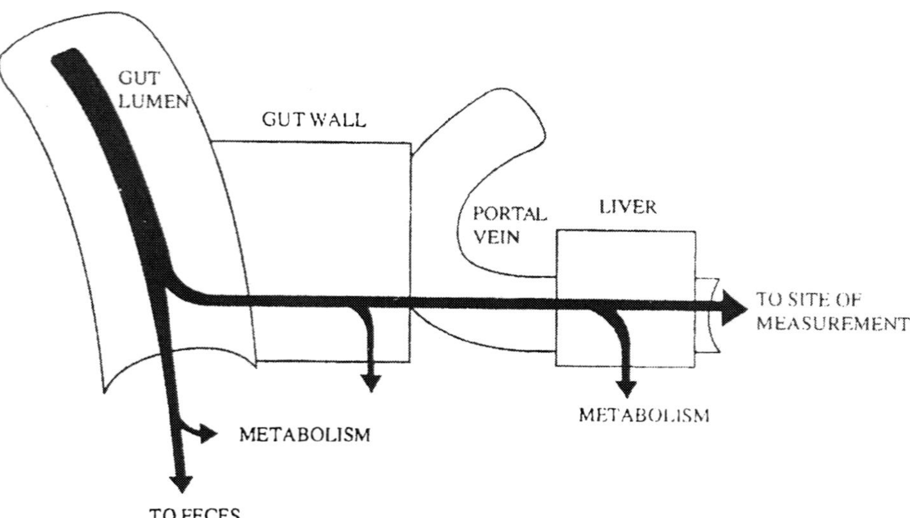

Fig. 5.2. A drug, given as a solid encounters several barriers and sites of loss in its sequential movement during gastrointestinal absorption.

The aqueous solubility of a drug in the 2–8 pH range has a direct influence on its oral and parenteral formulations. A drug with poor solubility (i.e., less than 0.1 mg/ml) in acidic media may show poor and erratic oral bioavailability due to the dependency of absorption processes in GI fluids. Intravenous dosing requires that the drug be administered in a soluble form. The adjustment of pH, the addition of a cosolvent or a ligand for complexation, or the formation of an emulsion may permit solubilization, but each of these techniques has limitations. Rapid intravenous administration of a solubilized drug can result in rapid dilution in an environment in which the drug is insoluble, resulting in incomplete availability and a delayed response due to the formation of particulate matter within the vascular system.

Poor aqueous solubility is not always a limitation; in fact, it may be a desirable feature for a sustained effect after oral or parenteral administration. Oral sustained release may be achieved if the drug combines poor aqueous solubility with the ability to be adsorbed throughout the GI tract. Parenteral sustained release can be achieved after intramuscular administration of a suspension of a drug with low solubility under physiologic conditions or from a drug that precipitates from an aqueous vehicle or that forms a reservoir or depot from an oil-containing dosage form.

The lipid-aqueous partition coefficient of a drug molecule affects its absorption by passive diffusion. In general, octanol/pH 7.4 buffer partition coefficients in the 1–2 pH range are sufficient for absorption across lipoidal membranes. However, the absence of a strict relationship between the partition coefficient of a molecule and its ability to be absorbed is due to the complex nature of the absorption process. Absorption across membranes can be affected by several diverse factors that may include the ionic and/or polar characteristics of the drug and/or membrane as well as the site and capacity of carrier-mediated absorption or efflux systems.

Compounds that are intended for oral administration and can undergo rapid degradation at low pH may require protection from the acidic environment of the stomach. Protection can often be afforded by administering the drug in the form of an acid-insoluble chemical species or in a dosage form with an acid- resistant coating. The insoluble chemical species must remain insoluble and unavailable for solution degradation as it passes through the stomach and must dissolve upon reaching the chemically more stable environment of the intestine at a higher pH. To be effective, an acid-resistant coating must remain intact and protect its contents until it reaches the required pH to dissolve the coating and release the contents in the intestine where the drug may be more stable.

Metabolic inactivation of a compound following oral administration can occur in the GI lumen, the GI mucosa, or the liver. The site of metabolism and the susceptibility of the metabolic processes to saturation are factors that may influence oral bioavailability. Occasionally, some of these factors may be altered to optimize oral bioavailability. For example, segment specific metabolic sites within the GI tract may be avoided through the use of pH-dependent coating materials that rely on the local pH environment of the GI tract to release the drug. Absorption from the lower colon and rectum can reduce exposure to the portal circulation and the first-pass inactivation that can occur in the liver and, thus, provide the opportunity to improve systemic availability following oral administration. Enzyme systems may be saturated by the rapid release of the contents of the dosage form at a local site or by coadministration within the dosage form of a competitive inhibitor.

Once the physicochemical and biopharmaceutical properties of the drug are determined and the desired plasma concentration profile is defined, the pharmaceutical scientist can select and develop an efficacious dosage form by utilizing a formulation approach, a prodrug approach, a device approach, or an alternative administration route approach.

Formulation Approach

Use of formulation techniques can improve the bioavailability and/or minimize the toxicity and side effects of drugs. Factors to consider include those that impact on solubility and dissolution rates.

chemical and enzymatic stability, and absorption capability. Several parameters, including particle size, crystalline habit, and salt form, can affect the solubility and dissolution rates of the drug. The effect of particle size on the dissolution rate of relatively insoluble compounds becomes significant when the drug is administered as a suspension or solid dosage form and the material is well dispersed within the GI tract. However, caution must be exercised when compressing the material into a final dosage form because excessive force can result in particle agglomeration and an actual increase in the effective particle size.

Polymorphism is the ability of a chemical species to crystallize in more than one distinct crystal habit. The pharmaceutical applications of polymorphism have been reviewed by several authors. The differences in dissolution rate and solubility that polymorphs can produce may have a dramatic impact on bioavailability when dissolution is the rate-limiting step in the absorption process. Tawashii investigated the GI absorption of two polymorphs of aspirin, the stable and metastable forms, forms I and II, respectively. He found that the metastable form produced a 70% higher total serum salicylate levels than the stable form I.

The selection of a salt form directly influences the physicochemical and biopharmaceutical properties of a compound. The impact of salt selection has been reviewed. Nelson examined the dissolution of theophylline salts and commented on their impact on oral administration. The dissolution rates of the theophylline salts proceeded independently of the pH of the medium but was governed by the diffusion layer pH. The choline and isopropanolamine salts dissolved three to four times faster than the ethylenediamine salt and produced higher and prolonged blood levels.

For highly insoluble amine bases, such as ergotamine and certain antimalarials, the drug may precipitate in the small intestine as soon as the pH rises following stomach emptying. The authors' experience has been that committing the effort and expense required to develop a new, more soluble salt form of this type of drug may be futile, especially if the new salt is only two to three times more soluble than existing salts. Thus, the selection of the most appropriate salt form should be made early in the development process to optimize bioavailability.

The stability of a drug in the gut is influenced by both chemical and enzymatic factors. Protection from chemical degradation may be accomplished via coating techniques, and enzymatic protection may be achieved with enzymatic inhibitors.

An enteric coating protects the drug during transit through the acidic medium of the stomach. Upon entering the higher pH environment of the duodenum, the coating is dissolved, and the drug becomes available for absorption. Such a coating also provides protection for the gut mucosa when the drug is capable of producing GI irritation. This method has been employed for a number of drugs, including potassium chloride, ammonium chloride, aspirin, diethylstilbestrol, erythromycin, and divalproex. Nishimura et al. employed enteric coating of levodopa to improve its bioavailability. Levodopa is absorbed from the upper portion of the small intestine but undergoes rapid degradation in the intestinal mucosa by levodopa decarboxylase. The authors developed an enteric-coated dosage form with an effervescent core. The dosage form remains intact through the stomach, dissolves upon reaching the small intestine, and bursts open due to the effervescence of the incorporated sodium bicarbonate. The rapid release in the duodenum results in concentrations of levodopa sufficient to saturate the enzyme at the absorption site.

The limitations of enteric-coated dosage forms include the possibility of duodenal irritation from caustic drugs and an increase in intersubject variability due to the presentation to the small intestine of a dosage form that needs to undergo disintegration and dissolution versus a disintegrated and partially dissolved drug substance. Enzyme inhibitors compete with the active drug for the enzyme and, thereby, reduce the degradation of the drug and deliver it more efficiently to the systemic circulation. An example is the carbidopa–levodopa combination. Carbidopa competes for levodopa decarboxylase, thereby reducing the levodopa degradation and improving the low bioavailability of levodopa.

Alternatively, the enzyme in the gut can be utilized to control the release of the active drug in the gut. For example, sulfasalazine, which is employed in the treatment of ulcerative colitis, is a combination of sulfapyridine and 5-aminosalicylate chemically linked via an azo bond. It remains absorbed and intact throughout the GI tract until it reaches the large intestine, where bacterial azoreductase enzymes degrade the azo bond and release sulfapyridine and 5-aminosalicylate to act locally on the lesions.

Altering the availability for absorption permits tailoring of the concentration-time profile for a drug. In the case of synthetic contraceptive steroids and theophylline dosage forms, the approach should be to slow the release rate so that undesirable spikes in the plasma levels are minimized. This effect can be accomplished with a sustained-release formulation. Informulating a drug in a sustained-release dosage form, the following must be taken into consideration: the effective drug plasma level, the rate of absorption of the compound, the rate of elimination of the compound, and the site(s) of absorption. Having established these parameters, calculating the required release rate from the dosage form is a relatively simple matter and formulation techniques are readily available to produce the desired release rate. The mechanism of absorption must always be evaluated when a sustained-release dosage form is considered. A drug that is passively absorbed throughout the GI tracts is an ideal candidate for sustained release. Drugs such as riboflavin, folic acid, aminopenicillins, amino-β-lactams and nucleoside analogs, which have windows of absorption due to site-specific and/or active transport processes, may have incomplete bioavailability when formulated in oral, sustained-release dosage forms.

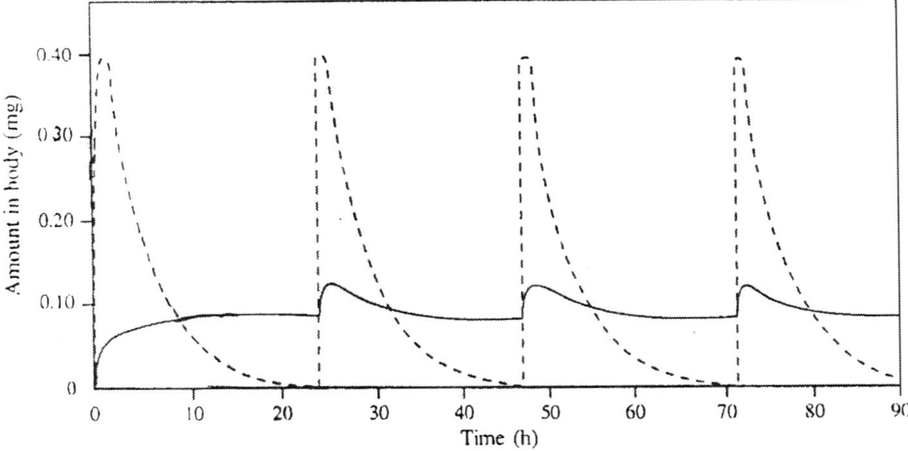

Fig. 5.3. Computer simulation of a plasma level-time profile of norethindrone from fast-releasing tablet (- - -) and sustained release tablet (—), from a dose of 0.5 mg/tablet and an elimination half-life of 3 h.

Prodrug Approach

An alternative to the formulation approach is the prodrug approach. A prodrug is defined as a drug that is prepared by chemically modifying a pharmacologically active species to form a new chemical entity that undergoes transformation to the active species within the body. The modification alters the physicochemical and biopharmaceutical properties of the drug in some beneficial manner. The ideal prodrug should have the following characteristics:

1. Possess no pharmacologic activity
2. Be eliminated more slowly than its rate of cleavage to the parent
3. Be non-toxic
4. Be inexpensive to prepare.

Prodrugs can be used to increase or decrease the aqueous solubility, mask bitterness, increase lipophilicity, improve absorption, decrease local side effects, and alter membrane permeability of the parent molecule. For example, chloramphenicol has an aqueous solubility of 2.5 mg/ml, but chloramphenicol sodium succinate, a prodrug, has an aqueous solubility of 100 mg/ml. Hydantoins also possess low aqueous solubilites that result in low and variable availability and precipitation following injection. In an effort to increase the aqueous solubility of phenytoin, Stella et al. prepared the ethyl and triethylamine esters of diphenylhydantoic acid. The esters improved aqueous solubility by adding an amine function to the molecule, and under physiologic conditions, the cyclization to phenytoin is irreversible, rapid, and complete.

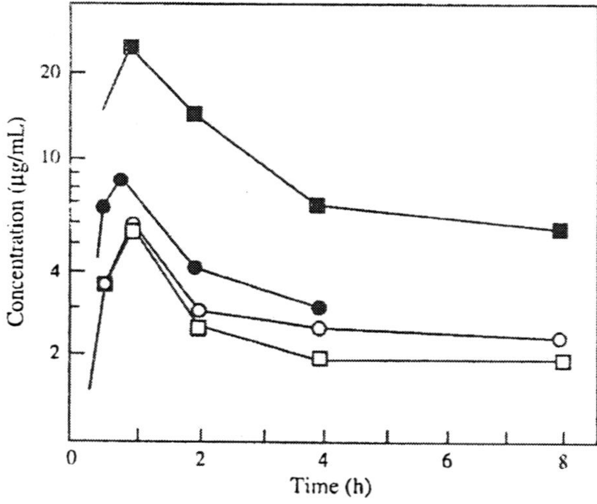

Fig. 5.4. Plasma acetaminophen concentration following the oral administration of acetaminophen and its ethyl vinyl ether prodrug.

The perception of taste requires that some minimum aqueous concentration be exceeded so that the taste can be detected (perceived). As a result, bitterness can be masked by reducing solubility. The technique has been applied to acetaminophen by blocking the phenolic substituent with ethyl vinyl ether. Chemical hydrolysis to acetaminophen is rapid in the acidic conditions of the stomach. Plasma acetaminophen concentrations in dogs following oral administration of acetaminophen and the prodrug were found to be similar.

Membrane permeability is governed in part by the lipophilicity of a compound. Highly polar compounds have low lipophilicities and, therefore, low membrane permeability. Epinephrine is a compound of this type. It is very effective in the treatment of glaucoma, but it produces a myriad of side effects. Ocular side effects include hyperemia, mydriasis, corneal edema, and allergic sensitivity. Systemic side effects, such as cardiac arrhythmias, elevated blood pressure, cerebral vascular accidents, dizziness, fear, and restlessness, are observed frequently. In an attempt to enhance the absorption and minimize the side effects of epinephrine, a prodrug, the dipivaloyl ester, was synthesized. It was found to be devoid of cardiac symptoms, with no effect on heart rate or blood pressure and was effective in *lowering intraocular pressure* (IOP).

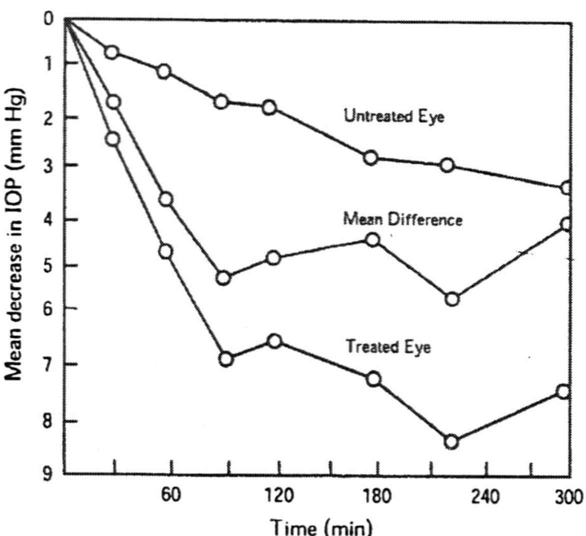

Fig. 5.5. The mean effect of one drop of 0.025% solution of the DPE of epinephrine on the intraocular pressure of nine glaucomatous individuals.

On the other hand, highly lipophilic compounds, such as hormones, can be solubilized via the prodrug approach. For example, the rate of transdermal absorption of the highly lipophilic drug, testosterone, was enhanced over 50-fold by forming water-soluble, yet lipophilic, prodrug ester. The prodrug testosteronyl-4-dimethylaminobutyrate was found to penetrate human skin tissue, in vitro, 54 times faster than testosterone itself. Furthermore, the prodrug was found to generate testosterone rapidly in biological fluids by enzymatic hydrolysis.

Oral administration of aspirin can result in gastrointestinal bleeding. The bleeding has been attributed to local irritation due to the acidic nature of the carboxylic acid substituent. In an attempt to reduce the gastric irritation of aspirin, acylal prodrugs were synthesized. In vitro, the prodrugs generated rapidly aspirin and in a pH-independent fashion. The conversion to aspirin was very sensitive to changes in dielectric constant: decreases caused a corresponding decrease in the reaction rate. This sensitivity is strongly indicative of an S_N1 mechanism. The authors postulated that GI irritation would be reduced due to blockage of both the charge and the acidic nature of the aspirin.

Device Approach

Controlling the release of medication at the site of action is often desirable, especially for compounds that are absorbed rapidly through mucous membranes or are removed rapidly from the site of action. The approach normally reduces the systemic side effects of the agent. The application of this approach can be illustrated with the Progestasert and Pilocarpine Ocusert dosage forms.

Diffusion-controlled devices may be designed for continuous release and usually use either a matrix or reservoir construction. In matrix systems, the drug is dispersed randomly throughout a polymer, whereas reservoir devices surround the drug with an intact rate-controlling membrane. Regardless of the method of construction, the system must be safe and biocompatible for biological application.

The Progestasert intrauterine device (IUD) is a contraceptive IUD marketed in the United States. It is a white, T-shaped unit constructed of ethylene-vinyl acetate copolymer containing titanium dioxide. It releases progesterone at a rate of 65 μg/day for 1 year, controlled by an outer coat of ethylene-vinyl acetate copolymer. Zaffaroni pointed out several advantages to the uterine progesterone system. It permits target-specific delivery of a fertility-control agent for up to 1 year by utilizing a single natural hormone at the lowest effective level of release of hormonal activity. The 1-year duration gives improved patient compliance while eliminating the pulsing seen with repetitive oral or injectable regimens. The efficacy of the Progestasert was investigated by Aznar and Giner. Their results indicated that the systems are highly efficacious in avoiding accidental pregnancy and result in decreased menstrual blood loss.

The Pilocarpine Ocusert is a contact lens-shaped device that is inserted into the lower cul-de-sac of the eye. It provides continuous release of pilocarpine at a rate of 10 or 20 μg/h, over a 1-week period, for the treatment of open-angle glaucoma. The system is capable of producing significant lowering of ocular pressure and constriction of the pupillary diameter. Its use greatly enhances patient compliance and the convenience of the therapeutic regimen while reducing local and systemic side effects.

Armaly and Rao examined the clinical effects of the Pilocarpine Ocusert systems with different release rates. The systems exhibited a dose-response relationship such that increases in the release rate above 50 μg/h resulted in increased ocular hypotensive effects with no appreciable change in ocular pressure. The reduction in pressure observed at the 50 μg/h rate was comparable with the changes seen after the administration of 4–8% of pilocarpine solutions.

Alternative Administration Routes

The administration of drugs by alternative routes avoids absorption and metabolic barriers that may be present in the GI tract. The routes can also provide systematic availability when oral administration is contraindicated due to a physiologic condition, or the route may provide for a concentration-time profile that approaches intravenous dosing profiles. The ophthalmic, nasal, pulmonary, buccal, transdermal, and rectal routes provide one or more of these advantages.

The ophthalmic route has been used traditionally for topical application for local effects. However, with the increasing number of peptide drugs being developed, the ophthalmic route has been considered for systemic drug delivery. After topical administration in the eye, peptides can be absorbed from the mucosa during tear turnover as well as via the blood vessels of the conjunctiva. The route suffers from the hesitancy of practitioners to place a drug into the eye for any reason other than to produce ophthalmic effects. Another drawback is the sensitivity of the eye to irritation by foreign substances.

Nasal administration produces rapid blood levels and rapid responses that approach those obtained from intravenous dosing. In addition, the absorbed drug does not pass through the liver before reaching the systemic circulation, and, thus, first-pass metabolism is avoided. In recent years, the nasal route has received a great deal of attention as a convenient and reliable route for the systemic administration of drugs, especially those that are ineffective orally and must be given by injection. Recently, butorphanol tartrate was introduced commercially in a nasal spray dosage form for the relief of pain, such as migraine headache. It would appear that the nasal route could be considered for drugs that meet the following criteria: are ineffective orally; are used chronically; are used in small doses; and are desirable to have rapid entry to the general circulation.

Published work carried out in many laboratories has shown that, with the notable exception of the peptides, drugs with a wide variety of chemical structures are well absorbed through the nasal membranes of animals and man. It is believed by many authors that in vivo nasal absorption of compounds with molecular weights less than 300 daltons is not significantly influenced by the physicochemical properties of the drug molecule. Factors, such as the size of the molecules and, in the case of peptides, their ability to hydrogen bond with the component(s) of the membrane, are more important than their lipopohilicity and their ionization state. For example, the in vivo rate of absorption of the very lipophilic drug progesterone is similar to that observed for sodium benzoate, and the in vivo rate of absorption of benzoic acid is independent of the pH of the medium.

Although many drugs are absorbed rapidly and quantitatively following nasal administration, peptides have generally shown low bioavailabilities. Hussain et al. examined the nasal bioavailability of leucine enkephalin. The low bioavailability of this pentapeptide was attributed to hydrolysis in the nasal cavity, with dipeptides causing significant inhibition of the hydrolysis. They concluded that polar compounds, such as peptides, can cross the nasal mucosa, and that administration of low concentrations results in extensive hydrolysis in the nasal mucosa and that hydrolysis of leucine enkephalin can be reduced by concomitant administration of peptidase labile peptides.

If the presence of a pharmacologic activity for a peptide is the only criterion for its use in therapy, then nasal administration may be employed, even though bioavailability is not 100%. However, when bioavailability, as determined by plasma level profiles, is considered, the nasal route for peptide administration is not optimal unless enhancers are employed. Enhancers may cause irritation and reduced membrane integrity. Other drawbacks of nasal delivery include the small volume permitted (i.e., 0.2 ml or less), the need for highly potent drugs with low doses, the potential for irritation, and the unknown consequences of long-term nasal administration of drugs, adjuvants, and other formulation components.

The buccal and sublingual routes of administration permit rapid delivery to the systematic circulation. Absorption from the buccal and sublingual vasculature and lymphatics bypasses hepatic circulation and, thereby, reduces first-pass metabolism. The driving force of absorption is the high thermodynamic activity of the compounds. Organic nitrates and testosterone have been administered by these routes to produce rapid plasma concentrations and to minimize hepatic metabolism.

The sublingual administration of methyltestosterone was examined by Alkalay et al. The sublingual tablet produced a 50% higher relative bioavailability when compared with the oral tablet or oral solution.

The increased bioavailability was attributed to the avoidance of first-pass hepatic metabolism due to absorption from the sublingual vasculature and lymphatics. The limitations of the buccal and sublingual routes include the requirement for successful candidates to possess high thermodynamic activities, the restrictive size of the buccal pouch and sublingual area, and the concern over the palatability and local irritation by the compound.

Transdermal administration can avoid first-pass metabolism as well as provide a large surface area for continuous–controlled administration of drugs with short biological half-lives and narrow therapeutical indices. The route has been used for nitroglycerin ointments, and transdermal therapeutical systems (patches) have been developed for scopolamine, nitroglycerin, clonidine, estradiol, and nicotine.

Scopolamine can cause side effects of dry mouth, drowsiness, tachycardia, central nervous system (CNS) disturbances, and amnesia if plasma concentrations exceed the levels required to alleviate motion sickness. The application of scopolamine to the posterior auricular areas (the most permeable anatomical site) via a microporous patch permits constant delivery of 0.5 mg over 3 days to prevent motion sickness and avoid side effects.

The transdermal route suffers from the inability of the skin to deliver large doses, the relatively slow plasma increase when compared with other routes, and the potential for irritation. However, several products utilizing this route of administration are currently on the market. Absorption can be enhanced with molecules that maintain an appropriate hydrophilic–lipophilic balance for efficient passage through the barrier of the stratum corneum.

Rectal administration of systemic effect has traditionally been limited to clinical situations where oral intake is restricted due to a physiologic condition (e.g., vomiting) or to compounds that are irritating to the gastric mucosa. The route has been utilized for aspirin, acetaminophen, aminophylline, promethazine, per- chlorpromazine, chlorpromazine, and indomethacin. The rectal administration of drugs is limited by increased interpatient variability and patient acceptability. This section has reviewed some of the dosage form design methods available to the pharmaceutical scientist that have been shown to improve the therapeutic efficacy of certain drugs. The key to optimal dosage form design lies in the prerequisite understanding of the physicochemical and biopharmaceutical properties of the drug and the available routes of administration. Once the compound has been characterized and the problem has been defined, the technology is available to optimize bioavailability.

Basic Preparations

The creation and manufacture of dosage forms has been at the center of pharmacy practice for the past thousand years. For American pharmacists of the nineteenth century, *secundem artem*, or the acronym "S.A." in physicians' prescriptions, instructed them to use their special skills "according to the art" of their profession to compound a medicine; it was out of this art, rather than science, that almost all of today's major dosage forms arose. Tablets, capsules, injectables, and oral solutions were all known to pharmacists and physicians a century ago. In addition, there were scores of specialized dosage forms that attempted to meet the medical needs of patients, even if the drugs administered in these doses were ineffective or designed to treat symptoms rather than the underlying disease. The origins of most of these dosage forms are lost in history. For this reason, the authors have elected to forego a contrived narrative tying together the few facts at hand with an equally large amount of speculation about the history of dosage forms. Rather, we have assembled a glossary of terms used in orthodox Western medicine to describe both common and unusual modes of drug administration.

For most of its history, the field of pharmacy was much more concerned with drug preparations than with the resulting dosage forms. Up to the sixteenth century, almost all drugs were derived from plants and were made into preparations that served as the ingredients for medicines; these preparations were called *galenicals*, after the great central figure of Western therapeutics, Claudius Galen of Pergamon. Strictly speaking, galenicals are pharmaceutical preparations obtained by macerating or percolating crude drugs with alcohol or some other menstruum to remove only the desired principles and leave the inert constituents undissolved. Examples of galenicals include decoctions, extracts, fluidextracts, fluidglycerates, infused oils, infusions, oleoresins, resins, tinctures, and vinegars. The term is used very loosely today to designate any type of simple pharmaceutical preparation, whether it is an extract of a crude drug or a solution of chemicals. Because galenicals were often administered without alteration, the pursuit of new extraction and other preparative techniques sometimes led to developments in dosage forms as well. The goal of medicine preparers since Galen's time has been to create dosage forms that are stable, free from inert material, therapeutically efficacious, and concentrated to facilitate handling and administration.

Preparations are divided into liquids and solids. The liquids are further subdivided as: (1) general aqueous solutions and preparations; (2) sweet or viscid aqueous solutions and preparations; (3) general nonaqueous solutions and preparations; (4) alcoholic or ethereal solutions and preparations; (5) oleaginous solutions and preparations; and (6) parenteral solutions and preparations. The solids are subdivided as: (i) medicated solids; (ii) medicated particulate solids; (iii) medicated solid applications; (iv) oral individual dosage forms; and (v) nonoral individual dosage forms. The dosage forms are arranged alphabetically and include Latin titles and synonyms. The historical development of individual dosage forms is traced to about 1950; it was about then that modern pharmaceutical science was applied in depth to the problems of dosage forms, and the term itself gained general currency in the literature of pharmacy.

Dosage Forms and Basic Preparations

Abstracts: Abstracts are powdered extracts of crude drugs prepared by percolating the drug with an appropriate menstruum, reserving a certain portion, evaporating the weak percolate to a thin extract, blending this extract with the reserve portion and lactose, and evaporating the mixture until dry. The mass is weighed and enough lactose added to make the finished product exactly half the weight of the drug from which it is derived. The resulting product represent twice the strength of the original drug. Although they were convenient for compounding prescriptions, abstracts gained little popularity.

Acids, diluted: Diluted acids are acid preparations, usually 5–10% strength, used for both internal and external medicines. Acids became official with the first United States Pharmacopoeia (1820). The term comes from the Latin acidus meaning "sharp" or "sour."

Aerosols: Aerosols are a system of finely divided liquid or solid particles dispersed in and surrounded by a gas. The roots of the modern aerosol go back to 1862 and J.D. Lynde, who received a patent for a valve, complete with dip tube, designed to dispense an aerated liquid from a bottle. In 1899, Helbing and Pertsch added liquefied gases. Patents in the early twentieth century usually were related to spraying perfumes. Aerosol fire extinguishers came into use in the 1930s, and insecticide sprays (bug bombs) appeared during World War II. Introduced in 1947, medical aerosol use increased greatly during the 1950s. In 1952, fewer than half a million such aerosols were produced; by 1963, this figure had risen to almost 40 million.

Ampuls: Ampuls are small, flask-shaped, hermetically sealed glass containers containing a sterile medicinal liquid intended for hypodermic injection, either subcutaneously, intramuscularly, or intravenously. Also, ampul is the class name adopted by the National Formulary V (N. F.) (1926) for the solutions in these containers. The ampul was invented in 1886 by the French pharmacist Stanislas Limousin (1831–1887) in response to a need by physicians to conserve their stocks of injectable solutions, which were difficult to transport and deteriorated rapidly due to the development of mold. In his classical essay, "Ampoules hypodermiques; nouveau mode de preparation des solutions hyperdermiques," published in Archives of Pharmacy (1886), Limousin outlined the essential directions for their manufacture: These ampoules have the form of a small ovoid balloon. They are terminated by a tapered glass tube, and their capacity is a little greater than one cc.

Although great advances have been made in the techniques and mechanics of ampul production, Limousin's simple rules capture the basic underlying principles. In the United States, ampuls, or "hermetically sealed containers which are filled with a medicinal liquid in a sterile condition, intended for parenteral use," became official in the National Formulary V (1926); that same year, the United States Pharmacopeia X included a chapter on sterilization but no monograph for individual ampuls. Iodine Ampuls, N.F., containing Iodine Tincture, United States Pharmacopeia, in sealed containers, intended to be broken and the liquid applied topically for the emergency disinfection of cuts or wounds, remained official through the National Formulary XIII (1970). The French term ampoule came from the Latin ampulla, which originally designated an earthen jar container for perfume.

Auristilla: Auristilla is a preparation used for medication of the ear canal. The National Formulary V (1926) Compound Oil of Hyoscyamus is an illustration of the type, closely resembling the Baume Tranquille of the French Codex (1908).

Bacillules: Bacillules are rod-shaped lozenges, prepared by massing the lozenge material, rolling it into cylinders or pill pipes, and cutting the cylinders into sections approximately twice the length of the diameter. Licorice lozenges are frequently prepared in this form, a popular example of which was formerly known as Wister's lozenge.

Balneum: Balneum is a bath for general application.

Balsams: Balsams are natural solutions of resin in an essential oil, which may also contain benzoic or cinnamic acids. The term has ancient roots in words referring both to spices and to embalming. In premodern times, balsams (baume in French) were any resinous vegetable juices or gums, acquiring their modern meaning in the 1800s. Several official preparations, such as Balsam of Copaiba, do not meet this definition but still carry the name because of their outward similarities with true balsams.

Bandages: Bandages are strips or ribbons of muslin gauze or other material employed in surgery for the retention of dressings and for the compression, protection, or support of diseased or injured parts. Bandages may be classified as inelastic, semielastic, elastic, or splint bandages. Inelastic bandages include muslin ribbon or roller bandages, gauze bandages, and water dressing bandages; semielastic bandages include flannel bandages; elastic bandages include rubber, rubberized, or crepe bandages; splint bandages include plaster-of-Paris bandages and crinoline bandages (gauze stiffened with dextrin) or starch bandages (gauze stiffened with starch paste), used to form the base upon which plaster-of-Paris is applied.

Baths: The word baths refers to the external application of water to the body, one of the oldest therapeutic techniques. Although some drugs were added, the simple water bath, or balneum, was most common. In the nineteenth century, when the therapeutic application of water was at its peak, baths were divided into hot or vapor (above 36.1°C), warm (29.4–36.1°C), tepid (18.3–29.4°C), and cold (0–18.3°C). The hot bath was a stimulant; the warm bath was soothing; the tepid bath was for treating skin problems; and the cold bath could be used as a stimulant, tonic, or sedative, depending on the administration technique.

Boluses: Boluses are large pills, over 325mg (5 grains) in weight. The term comes from the Greek bolos meaning "lump".

Bougies: Bougies are instruments or shaped, solid medications for insertion into the urethra or other body cavities. The term comes from the French bougie, signifying a thin wax candle named for the Algerian city, Bougie.

Cachets: Cachets are lenticular or spoon-shaped rimmed disks pressed from rice-flour wafer sheets, used to administer bitter or nauseating drug powders. The powder is deposited in dry concave cachets, and the rims are moistened with water; empty convex cachets are placed on top, sealing the cachets and enveloping the powder. The term "cachet" is from the French cacher, "to hide." The cachet de pain was invented by the French pharmacist Stanislas Limousin (1831–1887) in 1873 as an improvement over wafers and wafer envelopes. Limousin also developed a perforated board, accommodating three sizes of cachets, a powder measurer, powder funnels, and wooden "wetter and pressers" to speed extemporaneous cachet production by the pharmacist. A popular brand of cachets and cachet apparatus was manufactured around 1885 under the trade name Konseals by the J.M. Grosvenor Company of Boston around 188[illegible]. The Konseal apparatus consists of three perforated, nickel-plated metal plates, hinged together to form a cover plate, a base plate, and a shield plate. Saucer- shaped rice-flour Konseals are pressed into the perforations on the cover and base plates, while the shield plate is folded back over to protect the sealing edges of the Konseals in the base plate. The Konseals in the base plate are filled with powdered drug with the help of special funnels and are tamped down with thimble compressors. The shield plate is lifted, and a moistened roller is passed over the edges of the empty Konseals in the cover plate, which is closed over the base plate, sealing the Konseals. The Konseals are made of thinner material than ordinary cachets, and the finished product is less bulky and neater in appearance. Johann Schmidt later introduced rimless Dry Seal Cachets resembling flattened capsules, which were sealed by pressure without moistening.

Capsules: Capsules are telescoping, interconnecting shells of hard gelatin and sugar used for the administration of solids, masses, and liquids. The term comes from the Latin *capsula*, which is the diminutive of capsa, meaning "box." Successor to the soft capsules invented by the French pharmacist François Mothes in 1833, the telescoping hard gelatin capsule was invented and patented in 1847 by James Murdoch of London. In the United States, the New York firm of H. Planten manufactured two-part capsules sometime after 1836, but their usefulness was impaired by their poor fit. In 1863, the firm developed jujube paste capsules intended for dispensing powders alone, offering them to the trade before 1870. Another manufacturer, Dundas Dick, experimented in the same direction and secured a patent on cone-shaped capsules in 1865. Twelve years later, inspired by reports from Italy, the Detroit pharmacist F.A. Hubel made molds of iron wire mounted in blocks of wood, which could be dipped in a gelatin solution. Using pins of different diameters for the body and cap allowed Hubel to produce capsule sections which would telescope into each other, producing a small cylinder closed at both ends—the prototype of the modern hard gelatin capsule. Hubel sold his entire output to Parke, Davis & Co. in 1875, securing the first in a series of patents in 1877. Despite this protection, several small competing firms soon emerged that made capsules for other companies to sell or for their own sales organizations, most of which were consolidated by James Wilkie into the U.S. Capsule Company. Around 1901, this firm and its subsidiary, the M.L. Capsule Company, were purchased by Parke, Davis & Co., which expanded and improved its manufacturing processes under Wilkie's supervision. Wilkie is also credited with introducing phosphorbronze wire for capsule molds, a material superior to iron and one which remained in use until replaced by stainless steel in the 1 930s. Capsule manufacturing received its greatest impetus in the 1920s when automatic filling devices were perfected. Pharmacists extemporaneously fill capsules at the prescription counter by "punching" capsule bodies into a smooth layer of medicated powder and filler at a uniform level of compression, replacing the caps, and checking the weight of the filled capsule.

Capsules, soft: Soft capsules are elastic globular shells of gelatin, containing sufficient glycerin to retain permanent flexibility, and intended primarily for the administration of irritating or nauseating oily liquids. They were invented in 1833 by French pharmacist François Mothes; an improved capsule was patented by Mothes and Joseph Dublanc the following year and perfected in 1840 by the court apothecary Adolph Steeger of Bucharest. Soft capsules are easier to swallow than hard capsules and are desirable for administering large volumes of liquids. The original Mothes capsules were hollow globes of soft gelatin with an opening at the top for filling. Once filled, the capsules are sealed with a drop of hot gelatin. In 1846, Giraud introduced olive-shaped elastic capsules with an elongated neck, made by dipping molds into a warm glycerogelatin solution. After drying, the molds were stripped and the capsule necks sealed for future use. Pharmacists cut off the necks of the capsules as needed, filled them with a dropper or syringe, and sealed them with a drop of warm glycerogelatin or the blade of a hot spatula. The first official formula for the manufacture of soft gelatin capsules appeared in the French Codex Medicamentarius of 1866.

Cataplasms: Cataplasms are moist substances intended for external application and are of a consistency as to accommodate themselves accurately to the surface to which they are applied, without being so liquid as to spread over the neighboring parts, or so tenacious as to adhere firmly to the skin. Cornelius Celsus (50–25 B.C.) described early Roman softening ointments or malagma (from the Latin ma lasso, meaning "soften") made by boiling flour in water to make a stiff paste that was admixed with melted gums or wax. The word "cataplasm" derives from two Greek words, kata, meaning "down," and plasso, meaning "to mold." Modern cataplasms are made by rubbing together glycerin and a dry powder, such as kaolin, to make a very firm mixture. Since cataplasms (or poultices) were commonly used in the United States in domestic practice and made in the home, they were rarely prepared by pharmacists. A kaolin cataplasm became official in the United States Pharmacopeia VIII (1905) but was transferred to the National Formulary IV in 1916.

Caustics: Caustics are local remedies that destroy life on the part of the body to which they are applied. The term comes from the Greek kaustikos, meaning "to burn." The strongest common caustic (causticum commune acerrimum) was potassium hydroxide, or caustic potash, used to form issues on the body or to open abscesses. The United States Dispensatory (1836) advised that the most convenient mode of employing a caustic to form an issue was: To apply to the skin a piece of linen spread with adhesive plaster, having a circular opening in its centre corresponding to the intended size of the issue, and then to rub upon the skin within the opening a piece of the caustic previously moistened at one end. The application is to be continued until the life of the part is destroyed, when the caustic should be carefully washed off by a wet sponge or wet tow, or neutralized by vinegar.

Caustic potash was sometimes used to remove strictures in the urethra or, in solution, as an application to the spine in treating tetanus. A contemporary caustic, silver nitrate, was described in the seventh century A.D. by Geber; it remains official in the United States Pharmacopeia as Fused Silver Nitrate. Christopher Glaser, apothecary to Louis XIV, first prepared it in sticks for use as a caustic.

Cements: The 7th edition of the National Formulary (1942) listed a formula for a Cement of Zinc Compounds and Eugenol, which was widely used by dentists as a temporary filling. The cement was supposed to exert a sterilizing effect and protect the dentine from further destruction. The formula passed out of the National Formulary with its 9th edition (1950).

Cerates: Cerates are unctuous substances for external application as dressings for inflamed surfaces. Derived from the ancient Greek keroma (from keros, "wax"), cerates are generally made with oil, lard, or petrolatum as a basis, with sufficient wax, paraffin, spermaceti, or resin added to raise the melting point of the oils and fats employed. Cerates should be of such consistency that they may be easily spread at ordinary temperatures upon muslin or a similar material with a spatula and, yet, not so soft as to liquefy and run when applied to the skin. The most widely used cerate was Ceratum Cantharidis, a blistering plaster made of Spanish flies that was official in the United States Pharmacopeia and later in the National Formulary until 1950.

Cerecloths: Cerecloths are an early form of dipped plasters, described by William Salmon in his Pharmacopoeia Londonensis (1691), used chiefly to lay upon issues—small ulcers produced by caustics or cutting, the discharge from which was encouraged to fulfill certain therapeutic indications. Also known as spasma-draps or sparadraps.

Coatings, pill: Rhazes (850–923) used a mucilage of psyllium seed to coat offending pills: a century later, Avicenna (980-1037) introduced silver and gold coatings for pills not merely to mask bad taste but to enhance the supposed medicinal effect. Later, the influential seventeenth-century Parisian physician and pharmacist Jean de Renou recommended that pills with a bitter taste should be gilded and mixed among some powdered spices. Coating pills with gold and silver leaf was commonly practiced in France, other parts of Europe, and the United States until well into the nineteenth century but then fell into disuse. Mohr, Redwood, and Procter's classic Practical Pharmacy (1849) reported that foil-coated pills were "still occasionally administered, but much less frequently than formerly." Sugar-coated and gelatin-coated pills had their first acceptance as an indirect consequence of the invention of the gelatin capsule. In 1838, M. Garot, a Parisian pharmacist, coated offending pills with gelatin. A year earlier, the French pharmacist Labelonie had recommended that pills of cubeb and copaiba be covered with sugar, a process that was patented by Adolphe Fortin of Paris in 1837. Over the next several years, other French pharmacists (Deschamps, Bousquet, Mayer, and Roman) secured patents for coating pills with various combinations of sugar, honey, and acacia. By 1862, England's Bernard Proctor could list 45 distinct processes for coating pills with a variety of substances. In the United States, the first manufacture of sugar-coated pills was associated with the patent-medicine industry, probably as early as 1845. New Yorkers Cornelius V. Clickener and Zadoc Porter and a Philadelphia physician named Swayne all claimed to be the "inventor" of the sugar-coated pill but doubtlessly adapted French technology. By 1857, five different sugar-coated patent- medicine pills were available to American pharmacists, but no process was available for pharmacists who wished to sugar-coat pills extemporaneously. About that same time, Henry A. Tilden and William R. Warner independently developed processes for manufacturing sugar-coated pills and began selling them in bulk; in 1866, Warner began manufacture under his own firm name, William R. Warner & Company. That same year, Henry Wathew of Philadelphia developed and patented a prototype of the angled coating pans still employed today. By the mid-1870s, a variety of small mechanical coating pans were available to American pharmacists, although the quality of the extemporaneous coatings that could be achieved was generally inferior to that of the manufactured variety, which caused pharmacists to relinquish the practice.

Coatings, tablet: After the introduction and acceptance of the compressed tablet as a dosage form superior to pills, the same techniques that had been employed for sugar-coating pills were adapted to tablets. Moreover, compression coating techniques were also introduced by Charles Carter of Philadelphia as early as 1858. In 1896, P.J. Noyes invented an apparatus incorporating a movable die cavity into which the coating material was fed; the powder was compressed to form a coating around the pill or tablet by striking the upper punch with an automatic hammer. The following year, Noyes patented an improved machine that not only applied the coating but also performed the preliminary compression of the tablet. F.J. Stokes received a patent for a similar machine in 1917, although the compression coating of tablets did not become widely adopted until the 1950s.

Collodions: Collodions are liquid, external preparations with a base of pyroxylin dissolved in a mixture of alcohol and ethyl oxide or similar solvent. They were used medicinally soon after the discovery of gun cotton by Schoebein in 1846, first as a surgical dressing by Maynard in 1847.

Condita: Condita are comprised of candied or preserved roots or fruits. They are made by boiling the plant parts until tender, soaking them in hot syrup, and then pouring off the syrup; the procedure was repeated several times, reusing the syrup after boiling it down to a thick consistency. Condita can also be a compound of wine, honey, and spices (often pepper). Condita are also known as confitures or sweet-meats.

Cones, medicated: Cones are light, porous hemispherical masses of sucrose and egg albumin, used as a vehicle for homeopathic medications. The cones, also called disks, are designated (in millimeters) according to size by the diameter of the base. The common size should absorb about 2 drops of dispensing alcohol. Cones are medicated by adding a sufficient quantity of the dilution to saturate them and pouring off the excess liquid.

Confections: Confections are saccharine, soft solids, in which one or more medicinal substances are incorporated to provide an agreeable form of administration and a convenient method for preservation. In the thirteenth century, some apothecaries were called *confectionarii* from confectio meaning "a composition." Confections are made by adding medicinal ingredients in either the form of a smooth paste, a fine powder, or a liquid to a basis of finely powdered sugar. Confection of Rose and Confection of Senna were official in the National Formulary through the 5th edition (1926).

Conserves: Conserves are confections prepared from fresh medicinal agents and refined sugar, beaten into a uniform mass. The United States Dispensatory (1836) noted that "as active substances even thus treated undergo some change, and those which lose their virtues by desiccation cannot be long preserved, the few conserves now retained are intended rather as convenient vehicles of other substances, than for separate exhibition." Conserves are also known as preserves.

Cordials: Cordials are sweetened alcoholic preparations of high alcoholic content. They are also a tonic medicine formulated to stimulate the heart.

Creams: Creams are semisolid emulsions, usually medicated, intended for external application. The term "cream" has been used to refer to a wide variety of opaque, soft semisolids or thick liquids intended for external use. The British Pharmacopoeia classifies creams as medicated liquid emulsions consisting of a mixture of anhydrous lanolin, olive oil (or other fixed oil), and lime water; milk of magnesia is often referred to as a cream, and many cosmetic preparations are called creams. Claudius Galen prepared the first *unguentum refrigerans* or "cold cream," an ointment containing olive oil, rose oil, white wax, and a small quantity of water. This was a prototype for other cosmetic ointments introduced by Johann Mesue, Jr., in the thirteenth century. A modern version, consisting of almond oil, spermaceti, white wax, and rose water, passed into the United States Pharmacopeia as "Rose Water Ointment" or "Galen's Cerate." Pharmaceutical creams became official with the introduction of the formula for a "Sun Cream" in the National Formulary VIII (1946), a product designed to prevent sunburn but permit tanning. Cosmetic creams, which are usually not medicated, include preparations classified as all-purpose creams, baby creams, barrier creams, bleaching creams, cleansing (or rolling) creams, cold (or fatty) creams, foundation (or vanishing) creams, hair creams, and hand creams.

Cucufa: Cucufa is a cap, dusted on the inside with medicinal powder, which is applied to the head to strengthen the brain.

Decoctions: Decoctions are a solution of vegetable drugs, obtained by boiling the substances in water; they are also known as apozemes.

Dentifrices: Dentifrices are powders, pastes, washes, or medicated soaps used for cleaning the teeth. Dentifrices are usually flavored with aromatic oils, frequently contain soap, almost always some form of chalk, and are applied with a toothbrush. The National Formulary carried official formulas for a liquid dentifrice through its 5th edition (1926) and a powder dentifrice through its 11th edition (1960).

Douches: Douches are a column of fluid, of a certain nature and temperature, allowed to fall on a part of the body. Air can also be a used as a douche.

Dragees: Dragees are candied or preserved roots and fruits described by the Arab Najm ad-dyn Mahmoud in the eighth century and reintroduced in the eighteenth century by the famous French pharmacist Moyse Charas. By the middle of the nineteenth century, the term was extended to include a type of sugar-coated pill formed by repeatedly shaking slightly moistened, tiny 6-mg (1/10 grain) sugar granules (or nonpareils) in a basin of finely powdered drug mixed with sugar. After a sufficient number of layers had been built up, the dragées would receive a final coating of sugar or copal and tolu balsam, a painstaking process described by Ernest Agnew in the American Journal of Pharmacy (1870).

Draughts: Draughts are liquid medicines usually prepared to be taken in a single dose or "draught." Draughts are also known as potions.

Dressings, medicated: Medicated dressings are external applications resembling ointments in consistency but remaining semisolid at body temperature. Paraffin Dressing, formerly official in the National Formulary VI(1936), was employed as an air-excluding, soft, pliable, analgesic, splint-like covering for surfaces denuded by burns. A wide range of materials have been used as coverings or protectives to apply heat or medicaments to a diseased or injured part, to prevent wound infection, and to absorb and prevent decomposition of wound discharges. Antiseptic or Medicated Cottons include borated cotton, iodoform cotton, iodized cotton, and styptic cotton; Antiseptic or Medicated Gauzes include borated gauze, corrosive sublimate gauze, carbolated gauze, iodoform gauze, and picric acid gauze; Antiseptic or Medicated Lints include borated lint; Cellulose Waddings or wood wools include moss, peat, sawdust, jute, and oakum or marine lint.

Dressings, protective: Protective dressings are comprised of a wide range of materials employed as wound coverings, either to shield the parts from external infection or to prevent the escape of fluids contained in the dressing. Protective dressings are also used as a covering for poultices and for the retention of heat. Common protective dressings include oiled silk, oiled muslin or cambric, waxed paper, gutta percha tissue, rubber dams, mackintosh or jaconet, and rubber sheeting.

Drops: Drops are pharmaceutical mixtures meant to be given in small amounts. Before the twentieth century, the term applied to solutions used in small quantities expressed in "drops." These were commonly strong medicines "dropped" into water, such as Vinegar of Opium or "black drop." In modern pharmacy, the term became more associated with the need to get a medicine into an appropriately small amount of vehicle for application to the eye (ophthalmic), ear (otic), or passages of the nose (nasal). As a dosage unit, the drop is troublesome because it can vary greatly in size, depending on the size of the dropper orifice and the surface tension of the liquid. The United States Pharmacopeia IX (1910) set the official dropper at 20 drops per gram of water at 15°C ± 10%.

Drops, toothache: Drops for toothache are comprised of a solution of phenol in oil of cinnamon and methyl salicylate. The solution entered the National Formulary V (1926). A mixture of phenol, creosote, or volatile oils dissolved in paraffin, with a few filaments of cotton added, and molded into sticks constitutes Dental Wax.

Electuaries: Electuaries are confections prepared from dried medicinal agents, especially powders, combined with syrup or honey in order to render them pleasant to the taste and convenient for internal use. The United States Dispensatory (1836) noted that electuaries "should not be so soft... as to allow the ingredients to separate, nor so firm... as to prevent them from being swallowed without mastication." French writers recommend using brown sugar syrup to prepare electuaries, because it is less apt to crystallize than that made from refined sugar. The term comes from the Greek words ek, meaning "out," and leichein, "to lick".

Elixirs: Sweetened, hydroalcoholic, flavored liquid medicines, which became popular in mid-nineteenth-century America. The word is derived apparently from the Arabic al-iksir, which is an Arabic form of the Greek, xirion. Originally the term meant "dry powder." Elixirs came into medicine through their connection with alchemy. Elixir Rubrum, one of the most renowned alchemical compounds, could supposedly turn mercury to gold or prolong life. The term was picked up by followers of

Paracelsus and became applied to liquid preparations. European elixirs were generally bitter. One of the first American elixirs was Cordial Elixir of Quinine, made by John T. Heinitsh of Lancaster, Pennsylvania. After the Civil War an "elixir craze" began, which led to scores of companies competing for business. As much as any other development, the "craze" led to the publication of the first National Formulary in 1888.

Emulsions: Emulsions are a preparation consisting of two immiscible liquids, usually water and oil, one of which is dispersed as small globules in the other. Before the late seventeenth century, the term only applied to natural emulsions, such as ground almonds and water, which resembled milk. In 1674, a physician named Grew reported the preparation of oils and egg yolk to the Royal Society of Great Britain. In the 1700s, other emulsions were made with acacia, honey, tragacanth, and other natural emulsifying agents. In the 1800s, the wet-gum (ca. 1850) and dry-gum (ca. 1870) methods were established as standard preparation techniques. Interest in medicinal emulsions peaked in the early to mid-twentieth century with the development of several new emulsifying agents.

Enemas: Enemas are injections of liquid, either plain or containing drugs, into the rectum and colon to empty the lower intestine or to introduce food or medicine for therapeutic purposes. Enemas are one of the most ancient and widely used methods of introducing therapeutic substances into the body. The origins of use are lost in prehistory, but written records in Egypt before 1000 B.C. describe enemas being used to both cleanse the bowel and administer medicines. These early enemas consisted of three parts: a vehicle (usually water, beer, or milk), an emollient (usually oil or honey), and a medicinal substance. The Greek historian Herodotus (fifth century B.C.) attributed the general good health of the Egyptians to their use of enemas and claimed they had achieved their expertise through their experiences with injecting embalming fluids via the anus. Pliny (first century A.D.), however, argued that the Egyptians had learned to administer enemas by watching the ibis use its curved bill to inject itself with Nile River water as a purge. Hippocrates recommended enemas to treat fevers and constipation. Other authors of antiquity, such as Galen and Oribasius, wrote at length about what substances could be introduced via enemas. Enema apparatus was first described in detail by Arabian physicians of the eleventh and twelfth centuries. Albulcasis described a device made of an anal tube or funnel attached to a bag made from an animal bladder or sheep skin. The metal piston syringe came into use in the 1400s and supplanted these clumsy bags. The enema syringe soon became the object of much medical ingenuity, particularly in France. In 1480, Louis XI suffered a severe stroke and recovered, giving credit to the enemas he had received, beginning a 400-year period of fascination with the enema among the French, who refined the syringe apparatus. Molie're referred to enemas repeatedly in his works, and Ambrose Pare devised a syringe instrument about 1580 that allowed enema self-administration. During the seventeenth century, other special apparatus were designed to allow administrations of tobacco smoke via enemas. The Dutch anatomist Regner de Graaf completed the first book- length study of enemas in 1668. In the mid-eighteenth century, gum rubber began to be used in enema apparatus, replacing skin bags. In 1820, John Read developed a two-way syringe with ball valves (the first modern stomach pump), which was also used for enemas. Spring-loaded syringes and other advances followed, but by the late nineteenth century the dangers of improper enema use became apparent, especially the consequences of high-pressure administration. By the mid-twentieth century, enemas were again administered with simple funnels and gravity, a reflection of their prehistoric origin. Enemas are also known as clysters or glysters.

Enteric-coated doses: Enteric-coated doses are dosage forms that have been coated or chemically treated to prevent disintegration in the stomach but which disintegrate in the intestinal tract. Enteric coating is employed when the medicinal substances would be decomposed or rendered inactive by gastric enzymes or when they would irritate the gastric mucosa. The Pacific Medical and Surgical

Journal (1867) noted that collodion protects pills from dissolving in the stomach, but gastric insolubility as a basis for medication is generally credited to the German dermatologist Paul Unna, who introduced keratin-coated pills in 1884; Ceppi introduced salol as an enteric coating in 1891. Glutoid capsules are a special form of enteric coating prepared by subjecting soft or hard gelatin capsules to the action of formaldehyde until they become insoluble in the stomach but not in the intestine. The hardening process was developed in Switzerland by Weyland in 1895 and patented by Hausmann in Germany that same year. Pharmacists have extemporaneously coated capsules, pills, and tablets with salol, keratin, casein, and shellac, or with a mixture of n-butyl stearate, carnauba wax, and stearic acid to create enteric coatings. Early patented enteric coatings included keratin, fat-covered capsules enclosed in membranous sacs, and benzoin-coated capsules. Later patented coatings utilized cellulose nitrate and acetate, cellulose esters and ethers with saponifiable organic compounds, ammoniacal bleached shellac, stearic acid, carnauba wax, petrolatum, elm bark, and agar, and abietic, oleic, and benzoic acids with methyl abietate. Since 1940, research on enteric coatings has focused on the synthesis of resinous polymers, which are insoluble in acids, such as cellulose acetate phthalate and a glycerol-stearic acid-phthalic anhydride ester.

Epispastics: Epispastics are local remedies, the application of which produce a serous discharge beneath the cuticle, forming a blister. Epispastics are also known as vesicatories.

Epithema: Epithema consists or topical applications other than ointments or plasters. Liquid epithema include fomentations, soft epithema include cataplasms, and dry epithema include bags filled with dried drugs.

Essences: The term essences sometimes refers to a volatile oil or to a simple tincture; most often, the term is used interchangeably with spirits.

Extracts: Extracts are either pasty or semisolid masses or dry, solid, or powdered products prepared by exhausting drugs with appropriate solvents, carefully evaporating the products to fixed standards. An extract is intended to preserve the useful constituents of a drug in a concentrated, relatively uniform, permanent condition, and in a form suitable for medication. The Edinburgh Pharmacopoeia (1817) and Dublin Pharmacopoeia (1826) distinguish between extracts prepared from infusions, decoctions, or tinctures, and those prepared from the expressed juices of plants, calling the latter succi spissati or inspissated juices. Three forms of extracts are recognized: semiliquid or those of syrupy consistency; plastic masses known as pilular or solid extracts; and dry powders known as powdered extracts.

Fluidextracts: Fluidextracts are concentrated liquid preparations representing the therapeutically active principles of vegetable drugs. They are formulated in such a way that the activity of one gram of the drug is contained in one milliliter of the fluid- extract. They are generally prepared by some form of percolation, using alcohol in the menstruum. Fluid- extracts first became official in 1850 when five were entered in the United States Pharmacopeia by their heyday in the late nineteenth century, almost 100 were official. Joseph Remington called fluidextracts "American preparations," because they were developed by such native pharmaceutical scientists as William Procter, Jr., and Edward Squibb. Fluidextracts were perhaps the ultimate galenical class because of their permanence, concentrated form, and uniform relationship between the strength of the extract and the drug it contained. With the dominance of synthetic chemical drugs in the twentieth century, fluidextracts all but disappeared, except for those used for flavoring purposes.

Fluidglycerates: Fluidglycerates are a class of fluidextracts in which a mixture of glycerin and water is used as the primary menstruum during percolation instead of alcohol and water. The preparation of these extracts was suggested by Beringer in 1908. They were briefly official from the 5th–7th editions of the National Formulary (1926–1942).

Fomentations: Fomentations consists of an external application of cloths dampened with hot water or a medicinal decoction. Narcotic drugs were sometimes used. Dry fomentations were heated bricks wrapped in cloth and applied externally.

Frontalia: Medicines applied to the forehead.

Gargles: A gargle is a liquid medicine intended to be retained in the mouth and placed in contact with the back of the throat by throwing back the head and agitated by air released from the larynx.

Gels: Gels are semisolid organic or inorganic colloids rich in liquid, consisting of hydrated threads or granules of the dispersed phase intimately associated with the dispersion medium. Although Francesco Selmi studied inorganic colloids in the 1 840s, modern colloid science began in 1861 with the work of Thomas Graham, who investigated diffusion and dialysis and introduced such terms as colloid, glue, sol, gel, peptization, and syneresis. In the early 1900s, Freundlick introduced the terms *lyophilic* and *lyophobic* to describe colloids in which the dispersed phase has a high or a low affinity, respectively, for the dispersion medium. In 1950, Weiser divided gels into inorganic gels, which include gelatinous precipitates (such as Milk of Magnesia) and inorganic jellies (such as Bentonite Magma), organic gels or jellies (such as Pectin Paste), and crystalline or amorphous jellylike networks in which both solid and liquid phases are continuous.

Glycerites: Glycerites are solutions of medicinal substances in glycerin introduced in the 5th revision of the United States Pharmacopoeia (1873). Glycerites afford a rapid and simple method of making aqueous solutions of phenol, tannic acid, tar, and other substances that are not otherwise easily soluble. This class of preparations is called glycerins in Great Britain.

Glycerogelatins: Glycerogelatins are soft, medicated masses, usually molded into the form of blocks, which melt at body temperature and have as a base a mixture of gelatin, glycerin, and water; Glycerated Gelatin United States Pharmacopoeia is generally used as a base. At the time of application, the blocks are melted, and the liquid applied to the skin with a soft brush. Four glycerogelatins were introduced into the 3rd edition of the National Formulary (1906), and a general formula remained official through the 8th edition (1946). Under the title Gelatinum, the British Pharmaceutical Codex (1922) included preparations that were either similar to glycerogelatins, that more closely resembled dermatologic pastes, or that were intended for internal administration and called *jellies*.

Granules: Granules are small spheres of sugar pellets that are saturated with liquid medication before being swallowed. They can also be very small pills of 0.06 g or less, sometimes called parvules, made by slightly moistening sugar granules (or nonpareils) with a syrup in which an active ingredient has been dissolved. Granules containing 1 mg of powerful medications, such as arsenious acid or aconite, found favor among physicians in Europe, particularly in Italy, because they provided powerful drugs in small, precise doses.

Gums: Gums are mucilaginous, amorphous, transparent, or translucent glucosidal principles of plants used internally (as demulcents or expectorants), externally (as emollients or protectives), or for their emulsifying action. Three distinctive types of gums are recognized: arabin, which is completely soluble in water; bassorin and cerasin, which are partially soluble or swell in contact with water; and mucilages and pectins, which swell to form jellies. Many gums are complex mixtures of several of these types.

Infusions: Infusions are aqueous solutions obtained bysoaking vegetable drugs in cold or hot (not boiling) water.

Inhalants: Inhalants are products consisting of finely powdered or liquid drugs that are carried into the respiratory passages by the use of powder blowers or low-pressure aerosol containers holding a suspension of the drug in a liquefied propellent. A dry inhalation is a product consisting of finely powdered drugs that are carried into the respiratory passages with the help of special devices. Inhalants can also refer to drugs or a combination of drugs which, by virtue of their high vapor pressure, can be carried by an air current into the nasal passages where they exert their effect. In the latter form of inhalant, the drug is absorbed on fibrous material and enclosed in an inhaler—a plastic or metal tube fitted with a cap to prevent loss of medicament when not in use. The patient removes the cap, inserts the nasal tip into a nostril, and breathes the air drawn through the inhaler to obtain the drug.

Inhalations: Inhalations are medicinal agents administered by breathing in gases and vapors. A wide variety of techniques and purposes fall under this category. The isolation of pure gases by Priestley, Scheele, and others in the late eighteenth century motivated Thomas Beddoes to found the Pneumatic Institute (1798) in England to treat lung diseases. The gases used for inhalation therapy included oxygen, nitrous oxide, and ether. Gases were applied as surgical anesthesia in the 1 840s largely through the efforts of the Americans Crawford Long, Horace Wells, and W.T.G. Morton; their innovations were the first great contributions to medical science by citizens of the United States. The therapeutic use of gases continued throughout the nineteenth century, especially for the treatment of tuberculosis. During this period, devices were designed to vaporize liquid drugs with steam for the treatment of lung disorders. The first apparatus developed to atomize medicinals, made by Berson in 1860, was a combination inhaler and atomizer operated by steam that was generated by heating water in a closed vessel. These devices were quite popular for home use, and their modern counterparts remain a part of home health care. The term inhalation has also been applied to preparations more properly called inhalants, such as Compound Eucalyptus Inhalation, or sprays, such as Epinephrine Inhalation.

Injections: Injections are sterile solutions or suspensions used for administering pharmaceutical preparations by intravenous, subcutaneous, intramuscular, and intraspinal injection. The term injections is also the class name adopted by the 5th edition of the National Formulary (1926) for solutions in ampuls intended for hypodermic injection. Although ancient humans may have invented the concept of introducing drugs through punctures in the skin by attempting to recreate the effects of venomous snake and insect bites through the use of poisoned arrows, perhaps the first introduction of medication through the skin for medicinal purposes was inoculation for smallpox. Human inoculation with the smallpox virus by pricking the body with needles dipped in pus from an active case of the disease was practiced for centuries among people of the Orient but was only introduced into Western medicine about 1717. In 1796, Edward Jenner (1749–1823) performed his first vaccination with material from a cowpox sore. In 1657, Sir Christopher Wren was the first to inject a drug intravenously, a practice successfully adopted by the English practitioner Johan D. Major in 1662 under the title "chirurgica infusoria." Physicians experimented with the injection of water, opium, arsenic, cinnamon, oil of sulfur, and other substances with limited and often fatal results. Injections of purging medicines, such as jalap resins, were particularly popular in the treatment of syphilis. Nevertheless, the successful utilization of intravenous injection awaited the proof of the germ theory of disease and the discovery of sterile methods by Pasteur, Koch, Lister, and others in the latter half of the nineteenth century; the introduction of the hypodermic syringe, which was suggested by Charles G. Pravez of Lyons in 1853, popularized by Alexander Wood of Edinburgh and Charles Hunter of London in 1855–1858, and improved by Luer in 1894; and the invention of the ampul by Stanislas Limousin in 1886. A committee of the Royal Medical and Chirurgical Society of London gave approval to hypodermic injections in 1867, the same year the British Pharmacopoeia published a monograph for the first official injection, Injectio Morphinae Hypodermica. No attempt was made to sterilize these solutions, but E.R. Squibb (1873) and others recommended that parenteral solutions could be preserved by the addition of small amounts of carbolic acid, salicylic acid, chloroform, or camphor. At about the same time (1875), John Tindall developed the process of sterilization by discontinuous heating, which bears his name. Nevertheless, hypodermic routes of administration were slow to gain widespread recognition, for physicians became increasingly aware of fevers and other toxic symptoms following the use of crudely prepared injections. Ehrlich' s introduction of hypodermic injections of salvarsan for syphilis (1910) provided the strongest impetus for the development of parenteral administration, stimulating a series of rapid advancements in technique. In 1911, Martindale and Wynn discussed the pharmaceutical manipulation of salvarsan, emphasizing sterilization and aseptic techniques. That same year, Hort and Penfold applied the term pyrogens to describe substances that cause a febrile reaction upon injection. They found that distilled water sealed in sterile containers gave rise to toxic symptoms, whereas freshly distilled water caused no reaction; later that same year, Wechselmann showed that febrile reactions could be eliminated if solutions were made from sterile distilled water. Seibert confirmed these findings in 1923, noting that poorly constructed stills could produce pyrogenic distilled water. In 1930, Rademaker formulated a rigid set of aseptic precautions and rules, governing the preparation of parenteral fluids, which are still valid today, and setting the stage for modern intravenous medicines. Injections are also known as *parenterals*.

Insessia: Insessia refers to a vapor bath, usually administered by having the patient sit on a perforated chair, beneath which is placed a large container filled with hot water or a hot decoction of a plant drug.

Insufflations: Insufflations are powders used for blowing into the nose, preferably by means of one of the various kinds of powder blowers or insufflators made for the purpose. They may also be applied directly in the way in which snuff is usually taken. Also, a snuff. The term comes from the Latin insufflare meaning "to breath into" or "to blow into."

Inunctions: Inunctions are ointments applied with friction, intended for local application and quick absorption. The term was formerly applied to preparations consisting of wool fat in which mercury or other medicinal agents were incorporated. A Compound Menthol Inunction remained official in the National Formulary until 1960.

Juices: Juices are liquids obtained by expression from the fresh parts of plants. The British Pharmaceutical Codex (1949) contained monographs for the juices of garlic, lemon, and taraxacum. In the United States, Cherry Juice remained official through the 16th edition of the National Formulary (1985) as a flavoring agent.

Juleps: A julep is a sweet drink, usually a demulcent, acidulous, or mucilaginous mixture. Much more popular in Europe than in the United States, a typical julep of the late nineteenth century (*mistura gummosa*) contained 10 parts acacia triturated with 30 parts syrup of acacia, 100 parts water, and 10 parts orange flower water.

Konseals: Konseals is a trade name for the brand of cachets and cachet apparatus manufactured by the J.M. Grosvenor Company of Boston about 1885, originally introduced as "Morstadt's cachets" by Karl Morstadt of Prague.

Lamels: Lamels are small disks, about 3 mm in diameter, cut or stamped from thin films of glycerinated gelatin, containing definite quantities of various medicaments used in ophthalmology. Lamels, or eye disks, are applied with a camel's-hair brush to the inner surface of the lower eyelid, where they are immediately dissolved in the lachrymal fluid. Four lamels were official in the British Pharmacopoeia until 1953.

Linctus: A linctus is a thick viscid liquid that must be licked from a spoon or licorice stick, from the Latin lingere, "to lick".

Liniments: Liniments are external preparations of a consistency thicker than water, but thinner than ointments, usually applied to the skin with a gentle rubbing of the hands. Liniments are among the oldest of dosage forms, along with related forms, such as plasters and ointments. The term came to its present use about 1600. Drying liniments are preparations which dry when smeared on the skin, forming a medicated film removable by water.

Liniments, dental: Dental liniments were introduced in the National Formulary V (1926) through cooperation between dental and pharmaceutical authorities: these concentrated, often poisonous liniments, were designed to be rubbed into the gums.

Lohochs: Lohochs are thick syrupy medicines, usually used to fight a cough, to be sipped slowly or licked, sometimes called a looch. If in the latter dosage form, it is usually called a *linctus*.

Lotions: Lotions are fluid preparations, usually containing suspended insoluble material and applied externally. They are different from liniments by being aqueous, rather than oleaginous or alcoholic in nature. Lotions were official in the first National Formulary (1888). In the mid-nineteenth century, lotions were often applied by wetting linen and placing on the affected area.

Magisteries: Certain precipitates from saline solutions bore this title, but it was usually applied to secret remedies.

Magmas: In modern pharmacy, the term magma means an aqueous preparation containing precipitated inorganic material in a fine state of subdivision. Magma Bismuthi and Magma Magnesiae (milk of magnesia) were the first official magmas in the United States Pharmacopeia IX (1916). In the nineteenth century and previous eras, this term referred to the residue obtained after expressing organic substances to extract their fluid parts, usually referred to as a marc.

Masses: Masses are plastic, semisolid pharmaceutical preparations composed of active medicinal substances combined with a diluent or filler and an excipient, capable of being shaped into pills with little or no further treatment. The three essential requirements of a pill mass are: adhesiveness (the mass must be sufficiently adhesive to retain its shape and yet be soft enough to be worked by the fingers or suitable apparatus into the desired form); firmness (the mass must possess sufficient firmness to permit the pills to retain their shape); and plasticity (a natural result of the proper degree of adhesiveness and firmness). Two masses appear to have survived the changes in modern medicine: Mass of Mercury (or Blue Mass), a cholagogic preparation last official in the National Formulary IX (1950), and Ferrous Carbonate Mass (or Vallet's Mass), a hematinic last official in the National Formulary X (1955).

Milks: Historically, the term milk has been applied generally to any liquid that possesses the outward appearance of milk, such as milk of magnesia. Legend holds that the class of beauty preparations called toilet milks may have arisen from Cleopatra and her milk baths. The modern milks are oil-in-water emulsions, named for their appearance and use as additives to baths. Moreover, actual milk was used and modified, especially with the addition of malt, as a medicinal beverage. Fermented Milk, or kumyss, is fresh cow's milk, to which sugar and yeast are added for fermentation. Fermented milk was official in the 3rd through the 5th edition of the National Formulary (1906–1926). Humanized Milk was a combination of cow's milk and fresh cream, plus Humanizing Milk Powder, which contained a small amount of Compound Pancreatic Powder and lactose, made official in National Formulary III (1906).

Mixtures: Mixtures are aqueous preparations for internal use containing insoluble, nonfatty substances. They differ from emulsions in containing no fat and from liniments in being used internally. Both mixtures and emulsions were originally grouped under Mistura in the United States Pharmacopoeia: in the 7th revision (1890), emulsions were given separate recognition. Examples include Compound Mixture of Opium and Glycyrrhiza (Brown Mixture), Carminative Mixture (Dalby's Carminitive), Mixture of Copaiba (Lafayette Mixture), Mixture of Copaiba and Opium (Chapman's Mixture), Mixture of Magnesia, Asafetida, and Opium (Dewees' Carminative), Oleobalsamic Mixture (Hoffman's Balsam), Compound Mixture of Opium and Chloroform (Squibb's Diarrhoea Mixture), and Expectorant Mixture.

Moxa: Moxa are cones of combustible matter used for cauterization by burning. Moxibustion, the burning of moxa, was an ancient method of counterirritation or cautery arising out of China. Small cones of combustible organic material (originally Artimesia moxa or common mugwort) were placed on certain areas of the skin, ignited, and allowed to burn down, leaving a blister. Moxa entered Western medicine in the seventeenth century as a treatment for gout but fell into disuse a century later along with other forms of cautery.

Mucilages: Mucilages are viscid preparations made by dissolving or suspending gummy substances in water. The term comes from the Latin *mucus*. The gummy substances, if natural, are carbohydrates obtained from the exudates of trees or shrubs. Gums have been used since ancient Egypt. Hippocratic works (ca. 400 B.C.) mention acacia. Mucilage of Acacia was official in the first United States Pharmacopoeia (1820), with Mucilage of Tragacanth becoming official in the 1st revision (1830). Both have been used as thickening agents or to prevent the creaming of emulsions.

Mulls: Mulls are ointments of high fusion points, containing the desired medicinal agent, and spread on soft muslin or mull in a manner similar to that of ordinary spread plasters. The most suitable base for preparing mulls is a mixture of suet and lard, with the occasional addition of wax or lead oleate plaster. Mulls are prepared extemporaneously by tacking unsized mull over a sheet of moistened parchment paper and spreading a melted, partially cooled ointment over the mull with a broad, flat bristle brush and smoothing the surface with two warmed elastic spatulas. When cooled, the mull is covered with waxed paper and rolled into a cylinder for dispensing. Salicylic Acid Mull, Salicylated Creosote Mull, Corrosive Mercuric Chloride Mull, and Zinc Mull were last official in the National Formulary V (1926).

Oil sugars: Mixtures of sugar with fixed and volatile oils, rendering the oils miscible to water to an certain extent, offered as a convenient mode of administering medicines to children. The National Formulary offered a general formula for 2% oil sugars through its 7th edition (1946).

Oils: Any liquid that greases; i.e., leaves, when dropped on a cloth, a stain which water does not wash out; this stain makes paper translucent. If a solid substance exhibits similar properties, it is called a fat. Oils are called volatile or fixed, according to whether this stain disappears on warming or is permanent because of the nonvolatility of the oil. A few medicated oils, such as Phenolated Oil N.F. and Phosphorated Oil N.F., were briefly official.

Oils, infused: Oleaginous preparations for external use made by macerating a drug with alcohol and ammonia water, and digesting the mixture with sesame oil at 60–70°C until the alcohol and ammonia water have evaporated. The most common, Infused Oil of Hyoscyamus, was used to make Compound Oil of Hyoscyamus. This preparation was popular in France for the treatment of earache under the name baumetranquille.

Ointments: Semisolid preparations intended for application to the skin with or without inunction. In addition to serving as vehicles for the topical application of medicinal substances, ointments may also serve as emollients for the skin and as protectives to prevent contact of the skin surface with aqueous solutions and skin irritants. Ointments are made by fusion, incorporation, or chemical reaction. Ancient humans attributed special powers to the fats of animals and humans, and their mixtures with resins, waxes, powdered herbs, and minerals represent one of the earliest dosage forms employed. A greaseless ointment, consisting of hartshorn beaten up with incense and flour and mixed with sweet ale appears in the Ebers papyrus (1500 B.C.)

The Greeks did not distinguish between liquid or semisolid preparations used for an ointment, but rather according to use or ingredients. For example, malagma were softening ointments, whereas keroma were wax ointments, the predecessor of the later cerates. Plant mucilages, balsams, and oils mixed with wax were also classified as ointments. Galen's rose water ointment (or cold cream) was an early departure (second century A.D.) from the entirely fatty type of preparation. By the thirteenth century, pharmacists distinguished between olea or oils (liquid oily ointments), emplastra or plasters (masses sticking firmly to the skin), and unguenta or ointments (semisolid smears), a concept that remained unchanged for nearly 500 years. The first United States Pharmacopoeia (1820) recognized lard as the chief ingredient of the first official ointments, which were rendered to the consistency of butter by the addition of suet, wax, or spermaceti. By the middle of the nineteenth century, however, natural ointment bases began to be replaced by artificial bases, introduced with special regard to the purposes they were to serve.

Schacht introduced Glycerite of Starch in 1858, a translucent jelly prepared by heating glycerin and starch in certain proportions to a certain temperature, and W.A. Miller introduced Petrolatum in 1873 as "Cosmolin and Paraffin Ointment," both of which preparations were adopted by the United States Pharmacopeia in 1880. In 1885, the pharmacologist Oscar Liebreich rediscovered the therapeutic value of wool fat, the oesypus of the ancient Greeks, which he called lanolin; it was recognized by the Pharmacopeia in 1893. Later, the Russian chemist Lifschuetz discovered that the emulsification power of lanolin depended upon the free alcohols he had isolated as a group (1895–1898). In 1907, the dermatologist Paul G. Unna introduced eucerin, a new ointment base consisting of 1 part of Lifschuetz's alcohols, 20 parts of paraffin ointment, and 20 parts of water, the forerunner of the American "Aquaphor." Between 1920 and 1944, hydrogenated oils, sulfated and sulfonated hydrogenated oils, as well as stearic acid, sodium stearate, self-emulsifying glyceryl stearate mixtures, polymers of glycols (such as polyethylene glycol 4000), and esters of these glycols (such as polyethylene glycol monostearate) became important, followed by such modern bases as Plastibase, attapulgite, Veegum, guar gum, Carbopol, and the silicones, which were introduced between 1945 and 1959.

Ointments, ophthalmic: Sterile ointments designed for application to the eyelids. Petrolatum, petrolatum- mineral oil, and petrolatum-anhydrous lanolin bases are often used in ophthalmic ointments because of their low irritating potential. Finely powdered, sterile active ingredients are aseptically incorporated into a sterile base, using sterile utensils, and dispensed in sterile ophthalmic-tipped tubes to reduce the possibility of contamination.

Oleates: Usually liquid preparations made by dissolving alkaloids in oleic acid. Oleate of Mercury, however, is an ointment-like product of mercuric oxide in oleic acid. Oleic acid was named by the pharmacist Chevreul after olives.

Oleoresins: Extracts of plant drugs prepared by percolation using a selective solvent (usually ether or acetone), followed by complete removal of the solvent by evaporation. The term first arose in the 1820s (Buchner and Peschier), and the oleoresins first appeared in the United States Pharmacopeia of 1860 through the efforts of William Procter, Jr.

Oleovitamins: Preparations using fish liver oil, fish liver oil diluted with an edible vegetable oil, or a solution of vitamin concentrate in fish liver oil or in an edible vegetable oil. Oleovitamins were created during World War II to fill a therapeutic gap created by the interruption in cod liver oil supplies. The class became official in the second supplement to the United States Pharmacopeia XI (1942) as a source of vitamins A and D.

Paints, medicinal: Liquid medicinal preparations possessing antiseptic, caustic, soothing, or stimulating properties, usually applied by means of a brush. Paints intended to remain in contact with a specified surface are usually prepared with collodion, glycerin, glycerin and water, egg albumin in alcohol, or gutta percha. Paints intended to be absorbed are prepared with oleic acid or fatty oils. Caustic substances are usually applied dissolved in distilled water, alcohol, or ethereal vehicles, whereas resinous substances, such as benzoin, storax, tolu balsam, or sandarac dissolved in ether, are employed as bases for medicated varnishes, and used for application to the skin and raw mucous surfaces.

Papers, medicated: Preparations intended primarily for external application, either by saturating paper with medicinal substances or by applying the latter to the surface of the paper by the addition of some adhesive liquid. Potassium Nitrate Paper remained official in the National Formulary through its 5th edition (1926), but the most widely used paper is Mustard Paper, commonly called mustard plaster, a mixture of powdered black mustard and a solution of rubber spread on paper, cotton cloth, or other fabric, which remained official in the National Formulary through its eleventh edition (1960). Mustard poultices or cataplasms were formerly called *sinapisms*, after the botanical name for black mustard, Sinapis nigra, and were described in the United States Dispensatory (1836) as Powerfully rubefacient ... usually becoming insupportably painful in less than an hour.... As a general rule, the poultice should be removed when the patient complains much of the pain; and in cases of insensibility should not, unless greatly diluted, be allowed to remain longer than one, or at most two hours, as violent inflammation, followed by obstinate ulceration, is apt to occur.

Home-made mustard plasters (equal parts of mustard and flour, moistened with tepid water to form a paste and applied to the skin in a muslin bag) still play a role in folk medicine.

Papers, waxed: Parchment-like paper treated with melted wax or paraffin used largely as an economical substitute for more expensive protective dressings.

Parvules: Small sugar-coated pills, of 0.06 g or less, sometimes incorrectly called *granules*.

Pastes: Ointment-like mixtures of starch, dextrin, zinc oxide, sulfur, calcium carbonate, or other medicinal substances made into a smooth paste with glycerin, soft soap, petrolatum, lard, or other fats, and medicated with antiseptic or astringent agents, designed for external use. Early pastes, such as Pasta Glycyrrhizae and Pasta Althaeae, were internal preparations, most of which were of gum-like consistency. The modern pastes were introduced by the noted dermatologists Paul G. Unna and Oskar Lassar around 1900. Dermatologic Pastes normally contain a higher proportion of powdered material than that included in ointments and are less greasy but more absorptive than other preparations for external application. The British Pharmaceutical Codex groups Witch Hazel Cream, Vanishing Cream, Tannic Acid Jelly, Catheter Lubricant, and a wide assortment of "medicated preparations for external application, employed principally as antiseptic, caustic, cooling, protective or soothing dressings'' under the title "Pastes.'' Pastes entered the National Formulary III in 1906.

Pastilles: A form of lozenge, particularly those which are chocolate flavored; also, combustible cones of aromatic drugs used for fumigation. The term came into English usage around 1650 from the French pastille, which was derived from the Latin pastillus, meaning "little loaf.''

Pearls: Round or oval capsules made by enclosing liquids, solids, or tablets in a shell of glycerogelatin material. Pearls are less elastic than soft capsules and contain no air space, the glycerogelatin shell being completely filled with the medicinal substance. Pharmacists made pearls extemporaneously by laying a softened sheet of glycerogelatin over a warmed molding plate containing a specified number of semicircular (or other shaped) depressions. The sheet was covered with a measured quantity of medicinal liquid, and the liquid with a second sheet of glycerogelatin to exclude air. The whole assembly was covered with a matching molding plate, and compressed with a mechanical press to form the pearls, an exacting and time-consuming process requiring special apparatus. This process has been superseded in industry by a continuous automated process in which a liquid is injected between two ribbons of gelatin while passing between revolving dies.

Pellets: Small spheres of sucrose saturated with an alcoholic tincture, primarily used in homeopathic medicine. Pellets are made in different sizes, designated according to the diameter of ten pellets measured in millimeters. Remington's Practice of Pharmacy (1926) states that pellets "should be made of the purest materials, should be perfectly white and odorless and able to withstand all the tests prescribed for sucrose or cane sugar".

Pencils, medicated: Cylinders used in dermatologic practice to apply medicinal agents directly to the skin. The medicinal agent is incorporated into a paste consisting of starch, dextrin, tragacanth, and sucrose with sufficient water to form a plastic mass, which is rolled into cylinders about 5 mm in diameter, cut into sections about 5 cm long, dried on parchment paper at room temperature, and wrapped in tinfoil. Medicated pencils intended as a caustic application, such as sticks of silver nitrate, are sometimes referred to as escharotica. Salicylic Acid Pencils, the last official medicated pencils, appeared in the National Formulary V (1926); also known as Antiseptic, Astringent, Caustic, Salve, or Styptic Pencils.

Pessaries: Medicated vaginal suppositories, globular or oviform in shape, weighing between 4 g (if made from oil of theobroma or cocoa butter) and 10 g (if made from glycerated gelatin). The term derives from a Greek word describing the small stones used for playing the game of draughts.

Petroxolins: Fluid preparations for external use with a base of liquid petrolatum and ammonium oleate. The preparations became official in the 6th edition of the National Formulary (1936).

Pills: Small, solid masses of a globular, ovoid, or lenticular shape intended for oral administration. Pills are prepared by incorporating medicinal agents with other materials to form a cohesive, plastic mass, which is divided into the requisite number of portions, each of which is formed into the desired shape. Pills usually range in weight from 0.10 to 0.30 g. Exceptionally large pills of 0.60 g or more are referred to as boluses; very small sugar-coated pills of 0.06 g or less are known as parvules or granules; pellets, globules, or orbicules are small spheres of sugar saturated with an alcoholic tincture, largely used in homeopathic medicine. When the pill came into use in ancient Mesopotamia and Egypt, it offered for the first time a definite dose corresponding with a desired therapeutic action. The Greeks named the little balls of medicine *katapotia* ("something to be swallowed"), later Latinized to *catapotium*; by the first century A.D., the term *pilula* came into use In Rome. Pills persisted as a major dosage form for a remarkably long period of time. For example, over half of the prescriptions dispensed at a Charlestown, Massachusetts, pharmacy during the years 1872–1875 were for pills. Moreover, certain combinations of drugs persisted for thousands of years in pill form. The Pills of Rufus, for example, were originally a hiera (bitter powder) made into pill form by the Arabs and popularized by Avicenna (980–1033); a modern version, Pills of Aloe and Mastic, were last official in the 8th revision of the United States Pharmacopeia (1905).

Plasters: Substances intended for external application, made of such materials and of such consistency as to adhere to the skin. Adhesive plasters afford protection and mechanical support, whereas medicated plasters furnish an occlusive and macerating action, bringing the medication into close contact with the skin; when spread on perforated cloth, the product is called a porous plaster. Plasters are among the most ancient of all pharmaceuticals. Primitive humans may have used plasters of mud and leaves to help heal wounds or relieve pain. The Ebers papyrus (1500 B.C.) describes several plasters and poultices for treating burns, and the Greeks assigned a special place within their temples where plasters were prepared. Indeed, the word plaster is derived from the Greek emplastron meaning "to smear on" or "to mold on." The famous diachylon plaster, made from oil, litharge, and certain plant juices was compiled by Menecrates, physician of the Emperor Tiberius about 39 A.D. and passed on in verse form to Claudius Galen (131–201), who developed a number of practical formulas for plasters and procedures for their preparation which endured for centuries. A modern version of diachylon plaster survived as Lead Oleate Plaster (or Lead Plaster) in the United States Pharmacopeia and later in the National Formulary through its 8th edition (1946). Originally, plasters were spread directly on the affected part of the body; by the sixteenth century, plaster material was being spread on linen or leather or dipped. In 1514, Giovanni da Vigo popularized spread plasters called sparadraps or spasmadraps; in 1691, William Salmon described dipped cerecloths in his Pharmacopoeia Londonensis.

Plasters were spread with the aid of an offset spatula or plaster iron heated by means of a spirit lamp, an arduous and time- consuming process which exhausted the patience of pharmacists who struggled trying to keep the refractory plaster masses warm and malleable. Although Elisha Perkins of Baltimore is credited with obtaining the first American patent for a manufactured plaster (1830), John C. De La Cour of Camden, New Jersey, is generally credited as among the earliest producers of machine-spread adhesive plasters (1836), one of the first commercially prepared dosage forms manufactured in the United States. In 1852, an English apothecary named Mather patented a method of spreading plasters on leather by the use of heated rollers, producing a thinner and more uniform product, leading Edward Parrish to observe in his classic text, American Pharmacy (1856), that "the spreading of plasters which was formerly an important part of the business of the apothecary has now... been monopolized by manufacturers who bring machinery to their aid." The only plaster which still finds significant use today is Salicylic Acid Plaster, United States Pharmacopeia—the common corn plaster (also see Plasters, adhesive, and Plasters, porous).

Plasters, adhesive: A mixture of rubber, resins, and waxes, with a filler of absorbent powder, such as zinc oxide, orris root, or starch, mechanically mixed and spread on cotton cloth. Early adhesive plasters were composed of resin and litharge or diachylon spread on calico, muslin, or linen. In 1843, B.C. Rowland of Liverpool, England, reported on an "India Rubber Court Plaster" made by dissolving India rubber in naphtha or turpentine and spreading the liquefied rubber on silk or satin. Two years later, Horace Day and William Shecut of New York City patented a combination of India rubber and gums as a plaster mass. In 1852, Benjamin Nickels of Surrey, England, patented an "elastic plaster" combining adhesive material on an elastic fiber. In 1863, Joshua Melvin of Lowell, Massachusetts, patented the manufacture of adhesive plaster in roll or cylindrical form. By the early twentieth century, two types of rubber-based adhesive plasters emerged: surgeons' adhesive plaster, a plain yellow-colored mass, and zinc oxide adhesive plaster, a white mass containing zinc oxide. Modern adhesive plasters, consisting of vinyl resin, plasticizers, and other chemical additives have an excellent ability to remain adhered under severe conditions of moisture and heat, and rarely cause skin irritation. Adhesive plaster remained official through the 19th revision of the United States Pharmacopeia (1975).

Plasters, Blister: Plasters designed to produce inflammation, blisters, or issues (running sores). Many blistering agents were used to prepare blister plasters, but the potent and powerful cantharides (or Spanish flies), was the most widely applied. It was used internally by the ancients, who were well aware that it produced hematuria even when applied externally. Aretaeus introduced an external preparation of cantharides as a blistering agent in the second century to the shaved head to relieve headache. This treatment was also used for epilepsy and vertigo, and persisted through the centuries, but only after the patient had been given milk to drink for 3 days to protect the bladder from injury. "In many constitutions the strangury will ensue, especially where the discharge of serous juice is too great," an English textbook on materia medica advised in 1730. "But, however it be, such applications are necessary when a patient proves delirious, as frequently happens in high fevers." A century later, the United States Dispensatory (1836), in discussing the use of Cerate of Cantharides, "the common blistering plaster of the shops," remarked that "When the full operation of the flies is desirable, and the object is to produce a permanent effect, the application should be continued for twelve hours.... It should then be removed, and followed by a bread and milk poultice, or some other emollient dressing, under which the cuticle rises, and a full blister is usually produced. By this management the patient will escape strangury, and the blister will very quickly heal after the discharge of the serum."

Elisha Perkins of Baltimore obtained a patent in 1830 for an apparatus to prepare blister plasters. George W. Carpenter of Philadelphia sold and recommended Perkin' s blister cloth in 1831 as "a very convenient article for the country physician, being ready spread for immediate use." Ceratum Cant ha rides was official in the United States Pharmacopeia and, later, in the National Formulary until 1950.

Plasters, porous: Adhesive plasters spread on perforated cloth. Sir William Butts, royal physician to Henry VIII, devised a "spasmadrap or dypped plaster" which was to be poked "full of smalle hoolys."In 1845, Horace Day and William Shecut of New York City patented a rubber-based "porous plaster" rendered full of minute holes to "allow the free escape of the perspiration." In 1854, Somerville Scott Alison of London patented a porous or "perforated Lambskin... prepared according to the process called chamois curing." The porosity is considered a mechanical advantage in that it prevents the plaster from slipping from the point of application, each opening serving as a stop. Porous plasters are also far more comfortable than the nonporous variety, which they have superseded (also see Plasters and Plasters, adhesive).

Politzer plugs: Greased pellets of cotton about the size of a coriander seed with a thread attached, for insertion into the ear as a protective. The pellets were named after Adam Politzer (1835-1920), an Austrian otologist.

Poultices: Originally spelled "pultes" in sixteenth- century England, the term came from the Latin puls or pultes meaning "a pottage of meal".

Powders: Intimate mixtures of dry, powdered medicinal substances reduced to a fine powder by the processes of comminution and trituration. Bulk powders are divided into two categories: simple, consisting of one substance, and compound, consisting of two or more powders mixed together. One of the most ancient compound powders was *hiera picra* ("sacred bitters"), a mixture of aloe and canella introduced about 500 B.C. as a laxative, the prototype of a large number of bitter powders containing aloe as the principal ingredient and bearing the general title Hiera. This powder was listed in various pharmacopoeias and was last recognized in the 4th edition of the National Formulary (official until 1926). Powders were designed originally as a convenient mode of administrating hard vegetable drugs such as roots, barks, and woods; powders were also found to be convenient for the dispensing of insoluble chemical compounds such as calomel, bismuth salts, mercury, and chalk. Famous compound powders of the past include: Compound Powder of Glycyrrhiza, a variant of Compound Senna Powder recognized by the first London Pharmacopoeia (1618); Powder of Ipecac and Opium, or Dover's Powders, introduced by the English physician Thomas Dover as Pulvis Diaphoreticus in the early eighteenth century; Aromatic Powder of Chalk, a simplified version of a complex confection devised by Sir Walter Raleigh during his imprisonment and introduced into the London Pharmacopoeia of 1721 as Confectio Raleighana; and Antimonial Powder, patented in 1747 as Dr. James's Fever Powder. The United States Dispensatory (1836) noted that "the form of powder is convenient for the exhibition of substances which are not given in very large doses, are not very disagreeable to the taste, have no corrosive property, and do not deliquesce rapidly on exposure." Today, drugs not available in capsule or tablet form can still be conveniently administered in powdered form by placing them on the back of the tongue and swallowing them with water. Flavored powders are particularly useful for children who might have difficulty swallowing a tablet or capsule.

Powders, divided: Intimate mixtures of dry, powdered medicinal substances intended for oral administration, divided into single doses, each of which is folded into a small sheet of glassine paper. One of the oldest of dosage forms, divided powders have largely been replaced by capsules or tablets. Nevertheless, the preparation of powders permits the drugs to be reduced to a very fine state of subdivision, a physical condition which frequently intensifies their therapeutic activity, a factor in increasing the efficacy of homeopathic triturations, calomel and sodium bicarbonate mixtures, and Dover's Powder (Powder of Ipecac and Opium). Divided powders also furnish a convenient means for administering drugs that are not excessively bitter, nauseous, or otherwise offensive to the taste. One of the most durable divided powders is Seidlitz Powders, a saline cathartic originated and patented by Thomas Savory in 1815. Savory claimed that the powders owed their value to the mineral properties of the Seidlitz spring in Germany, which contains magnesium sulfate. The powders consist of sodium bicarbonate (wrapped in blue paper) and tartaric acid and potassium and sodium tartrate (wrapped in white paper), each of which are dissolved separately in water and then mixed. The formula was exposed in a book of recipes for patent medicines published by the Philadelphia College of Pharmacy in 1824, and remained official as Compound Effervescent Powders in the United States Pharmacopeia, and later in the National Formulary through its 12th edition (1965); also known as *Powder papers*.

Precipitates: Drugs prepared by separating particles from a previously clear liquid by physical or chemical means. Precipitation usually occurs when a hot saturated solution of an amorphous substance is allowed to cool or when a liquid in which the dissolved substance is insoluble is added to its solution. Pharmacists formerly used the process of precipitation as a convenient method of obtaining solid substances in fine particles (precipitated calcium carbonate), to purify solids (precipitated calcium phosphate), or to prepare mercury salts. White precipitate (ammoniated mercury) was first described by Beguin in 1632, a soluble double chloride of mercury and ammonium known to the alchemists as sal alembroth and sal sapientiae, respectively. Red precipitate (red mercuric oxide) was known to alchemists as hydra gyrum precipita tum per se or "*precipitate per se*;" yellow precipitate is a synonym for yellow mercuric oxide.

Resins: Solid preparations consisting chiefly of the resinous principles from vegetable bodies. The officially prepared resins differ from alcoholic extracts in that the latter contain all of the alcohol-soluble principles in the drugs, whereas the resins contain only the alcohol-soluble principles that are insoluble in water. The term probably arose from the Greek rheos, "to flow," referring perhaps to the flow of pine resin commonly observed.

Rubificients: Local remedies which produce redness and inflammation of the skin. The word comes from two Latin words: ruber, meaning "red," and facio, meaning "to make."

Saccharures: Preparations made by saturating sucrose with a tincture, drying it, and grinding the mixture to a powder.

Salts: Compounds formed by the union of acids and bases, by the action of alkalies upon metals, or by the direct union of elements. The term is often incorporated in the common name of salts used as pharmaceuticals: bitter salts, epsom salt, or Seidlitz salt (magnesium sulfate), preparing salt (sodium stannate), Preston's salts (ammonium chloride), Rochelle salt or Seignette's salt (potassium and ammonium tartrate), salt of Mars (ferrous sulfate), salt of Saturn (lead acetate), salt of tartar (potassium carbonate), salt of tin (stannous chloride), salt of wisdom (mercury bichloride and ammonium chloride), sore-throat salt (fused potassium nitrate), vinegar salts (calcium acetate), and vomiting salt (zinc sulfate). The term is also applied to some acids, such as salt of lemon or sour salt (citric acid), salt of sorrel (oxalic acid), and spirit of salt (muriatic acid).

Salts, artificial: A mixture of the more important chemical salts naturally present in several of the well- known mineral springs of Europe. "These are properly labeled artificial," notes Remington's Practice of Pharmacy (1926), "and if used to prepare effervescent salts or mineral waters they should be sold only as an imitation of the genuine."

Salts, effervescent: Granular effervescent salts were formerly made by mixing dry powders with dry tartaric acid and sodium bicarbonate and moistening the mixture with strong alcohol. The pasty mass was passed through a sieve, and the granules dried quickly in a hot room, sifted, and filled into bottles, which were hermetically sealed to prevent the access of moisture. This method was greatly improved upon by mixing the powders in a flat enameled dish and heating in an oven to about 100°C or by heating the mixture in a deep jacketed kettle or in a pill- coating pan, heated, as it revolves, by a gas flame. When the mixture becomes moist, it is manipulated with a wooden spatula to make it uniform in consistency, and rubbed through a coarse tinned iron sieve; the granules obtained are dried slowly at a low heat in an oven.

Salts, smelling: Ammonia-based preparations used as a restorative in "*hysterical syncope*" (fainting). Dry smelling salts (or vinaigrettes) are composed of ammonium chloride and potassium carbonate, perfumed with lavender; liquid smelling salts are composed of ammonium carbonate dissolved in stronger ammonia water and alcohol, and perfumed with oils; solidified smelling salts are similar preparations solidified with stearic acid.

Salves: This term probably arose from the Anglo- Saxon sealf or the German salbe, both meaning "ointment".

Scutum: Abbreviation for scutum stomachicum, a large plaster, applied to the breast or stomach.

Serums: Serum therapy came into prominence in the 1890s when Emil von Behring (1854–1917) extended Pasteur's theory of attenuated viruses. Behring demonstrated that the serum of animals immunized against attenuated diphtheria toxins can be used as a preventive or therapeutic inoculation against diphtheria in other animals through a specific neutralization of the toxin of the disease. In 1894, Behring began to produce his new antitoxic serum on a grand scale; it soon became recognized as the specific treatment for diphtheria. Antisera act by combining with the toxin in the blood of the patient, rendering it inert. Scarlet fever, tetanus, erysipelas, botulism, and gas gangrene have been successfully treated by antitoxic serums prepared in this manner. Antibacterial serum is produced by injection of an animal with successive doses of bacteria. The immune substances thus formed act by enhancing phagocytosis, destroying the bacteria. Pneumonia, streptococcic infection, and spinal meningitis have been aided by the use of this type of serum. Mixed serum contains both antitoxic and antibacterial immune bodies; the serum used to treat scarlet fever is of this type.

Shampoos: A wash for the hair or soap for hair washing. The term comes from the Hindustani word tshampa, meaning "to squeeze" or "to press," probably associated with hot oriental baths.

Silk, oiled: A thin, very soft, and pliable protective dressing made of fine silk, coated with a flexible linseed-oil varnish. Oiled Silk is available in semitransparent or opaque form, made by the addition of talc or starch in the final coating. Oiled Muslin or Oiled Cambric is similar to oiled silk, except that the basic fabric is of glazed cotton; it is thicker and heavier and consequently less pliable than oiled silk.

Soaps: A class of chemical substances which are metal salts of fatty acids. Pliny (first century A.D) records that the ancient Romans learned the preparation of soap from Nordic tribes, who used a pomade prepared from goat fat and the calcined ashes of beech- wood. Sapo, the Latin word for soap, is derived from the Nordic sepe. The chemistry of soaps was elucidated in the early nineteenth century by French chemist M.E. Chevreul (1786–1889). Soaps may be divided into two classes: soluble soaps (or detergent or cleansing soaps), which are compounds of fatty acids with alkali metals, particularly sodium and potassium; and insoluble soaps, which are compounds of fatty acids and metals of any other group, such as Lead Oleate Plaster or Lime Liniment, a calcium soap of lin-seed oil. Soluble soaps include Hard Soap (or Castile Soap), prepared from olive oil and sodium hydroxide, official through the 11th edition of the National Formulary (1960), and Soft Soap (or Green Soap), prepared from linseed oil, glycerin, and dekanormal solutions of sodium and potassium hydroxide; the latter continues to hold official status.

Solutio: Dental preparations official only in the 5th edition of the National Formulary (1926) consisting of a solution of a resinous material dissolved in chloroform.

Solutions: Liquid preparations that contain one or more substances dissolved in a solvent and, by reason of their ingredients or method of preparation, do not fall into some other category of preparation

From the seventeenth century on, the term liquor denoted liquid solutions. By the early twentieth century, *liquor* usually referred to aqueous solutions of nonvolatile substances. For example, Solution of Magnesium Citrate, United States Pharmacopeia, had the Latin title Liquor Magnesii Citratis. Beginning with the United States Pharmacopeia XVI and the National Formulary XI (1960), the term liquor was dropped and solutions were listed by their active ingredient or ingredients.

Solutions, irrigating: A preparation to be applied continuously by means of a special device for the purpose, as in the treatment of wounds with Dakin's solution.

Solutions, nasal: Solutions of drugs for instilling in the nose rather than spraying are generally a modern development. The first nasal solutions were formulated with menthol and thymol dissolved in light mineral oil. Later isotonic aqueous solutions were designed as drops.

Solutions, ophthalmic: Originally called collyria, ophthalmic solutions arose from the eye washes of the ancient world. Early preparations were not the sterile, buffered solutions of today. The term collyrium comes from the Greek kollurion, which Hippocrates used to designate fatty suppositories for gynecological purposes. They were formed into sticks, from which a paste was made with a liquid. Eventually, more liquid was added and the paste thinned to a lotion. This lotion was used as an eye wash, and term came to be used exclusively for this type of preparation. Remington's formula for a collyrium of 260mg (4 grains) of sodium borate in 30mL (1 oz) of camphor water was a standard from 1886 into the mid-twentieth century.

Spasmadraps: Pieces of linen or other cloth dipped in or spread with a medicinal plaster, popularized in 1514 by Giovanni da Vigo (1460–1525), physician to Pope Julius II. From the Latin spasma meaning "healing powder" and the French drap meaning "cloth." Also known as sparadraps or cerecloths.

Spirits: Solutions of volatile substances (usually volatile oils) in alcohol. Some editions of the National Formulary stated that "spirits of volatile oils" contained 6.5% of the volatile oil, but that figure was later rejected as too low. Although used internally, several spirits were used medicinally by inhalation or as flavorings.

Sprays: Medicated liquids prepared for dispersal by atomizers or nebulizers, usually on external surface or mucous membranes of the respiratory tract. In the United States Pharmacopoeia, sprays were called inhalatio; the National Formulary referred to them as nebulae. Sprays of the early twentieth century were formulated with aromatics dissolved in light mineral oil. As injuries from inhaled oils became apparent, especially among children, these sprays were displaced by buffered aqueous solutions.

Stilus dissolubilis: Dissolving pencils. Pencils containing a caustic or an astringent.

Suppositories: Conical or ovoid medicated solids intended for insertion into one of the several orifices of the body, excluding the mouth. Suppository use has been known as early as 2600 B.C., and was recom-mended in the works of Hippocrates (ca. 400 B.C.). The term derives from the Latin suppositus, meaning "to place under." Premodern suppositories were made by hand using soap or other semisolid fatty substances as the main vehicles. They were not commonly used until the seventeenth and eighteenth centuries and did not become popular until the mid-nineteenth century and the advent of cocoa butter as vehicle. In 1766, Antoine Baumé described a suppository mold which used liquefied cocoa butter. This technique was popularized in America by Alfred B. Taylor about 1852 using paper cones as molds. Metal molds were introduced about 1860, although many pharmacists continued to form suppositories by hand without heat. Cold compression of cocoa butter was made possible through the introduction of metal suppository presses about 1868, although the first popular compression mold was not introduced until 1879. After 1870, mixtures of glycerin and gelatin came to be used as vehicles for suppositories, beginning a quest for the perfect vehicle that continues to the present.

Suspensions: Heterogeneous systems containing coarsely dispersed material that settles. A wide variety of pharmaceutical preparations have been used as suspensions, for example, White Lotion,

Magma of Bismuth, and Compound Mixture of Opium and Glycyrrhiza (Brown Mixture). In addition, several official ointments are suspensions of solids in a semisolid base. A large number of suspensions are categorized as mixtures in the United States Pharmacopeia and the National Formulary.

Swabs: Ampuls containing Iodine Tincture, United States Pharmacopeia, covered with gauze or other absorbent material, and used for first-aid treatment. Iodine Swabs, later called Iodine Ampuls, were official in the National Formulary through its 13th edition (1970). When iodine tincture is required for first aid, the tip of the ampul is broken and the gauze absorbs the iodine and provides a means of applying it directly to the wound. Some Iodine Ampuls are in the form of fine capillary tubes, which are broken when needed and the tincture applied directly.

Syrups: A nearly saturated aqueous solution of sugar (usually sucrose) with or without medicinal or flavoring ingredients. Syrups are usually divided into flavored, containing a fruit or aromatic substance for a pleasant taste, and medicated, containing a drug. Simple Syrup, United States Pharmacopeia was commonly used in the preparation of pill masses and other mixtures.

Tablets: Dosage forms prepared by molding or compressing medicinal substances in dies. Tablets vary widely in shape, the most common form being discoid, and range from 0.06 to 0.60 g in weight. Jean de Renou applied the Latin word tabella to a special type of troche in 1608; Burroughs Wellcome & Company coined the term "tablet" in 1878 to refer to its brand of compressed pills; the term is derived from the French tablette, meaning "shelf" and the Latin tabula, meaning "board." In 1843, the English apothecary William Brockedon patented a device for compressing medicinal agents commonly employed in pills and lozenges without the use of liquid adhesive agents; the resulting product was known as compressed pills.

The Philadelphia druggist Jacob Dunton invented a similar device in 1864, marketing his own compressed pills in 1869; Joseph Remington devised a similar machine in 1875 to allow the retail druggist to "manufacture his own medication called for on prescription."Each of these devices consisted of a compression cylinder and lower die (to hold the medicinal substance) as well as an upper die which was struck with a mallet to compress the material. More reliable compression was achieved by using the screw devices invented by Germany's Professor Rosenthal (1874) and perfected by Austria's Carl Engler (1907). Another advancement was the lever device introduced by Philadelphia's Bennett L. Smedley (1879). The first rotary tablet machine was developed in 1872 by Henry Bower, an employee of the Philadelphia drug manufacturer John Wyeth; two years later, Joseph A. McFerran received a patent for the first fully automatic tablet machine.

Tablets, hypodermic: Molded tablet triturates intended to be dissolved in water to make a solution to be injected parenterally. The usual weight of hypodermic tablets is about 0.03 g, which distinguishes them from ordinary tablet triturates that weigh about 0.06g. Formerly prepared extemporaneously by pharmacists, modern compressed hypodermic tablets are not intended to be sterile, although they are manufactured under strict conditions as a precaution against contamination.

Tablets, poison: Tablets of mercury bichloride in an angular, not discoid shape, blue in color, each having the word "POISON" and the skull-and-crossbones design distinctly stamped upon it. A unique one-product classification, poison tablets (or Toxitabellae) first became official in the United States Pharmacopoeia IX (1916), and two strengths remained official in the National Formulary through its 10th edition (1950); the larger tablets remained official through the 12th edition (1965). Diluted in a solution of 1:1000 concentration, mercury bichloride is an antiseptic used chiefly for the disinfection of inanimate objects and the unabraded skin.

Tablets, solution: Molded or compressed tablets containing large amounts of potent substances not intended for administration, but rather as a convenience in dispensing; also known as Dispensing Tablets.

To lessen the risk of their being dispensed by mistake for other tablets, dispensing tablets are always of angular rather than discoid shape. They are usually scored to facilitate division into more or less accurate fractions. Also tablets to be dissolved in water for external use.

Teas: Coarsely powdered mixtures of dried herbs intended for medicinal teas or poultices; also known as Species. The National Formulary recognized an Emollient Species, used as a cataplasm; a Laxative Species (St. Germain Tea); and a Pectoral Species (Breast Tea) for a "catarrhal condition of the respiratory tract" through its 5th edition (1926). Similar teas from home-grown herbs persist as common household remedies. True tea from China was introduced to England by Christopher Borough in 1379. The English word probably comes from the Dutch thee.

Tinctures: Alcoholic or hydroalcoholic solutions of drugs, usually of plant origins. The term comes from the Latin tingere, "to dye or soak in color." Tinctures, as alcoholic solutions, entered medical practice in the thirteenth century through the efforts of Raymond Lull and Arnald of Villanova. Paracelsus (1493–1541) was a strong advocate for tinctures; inasmuch as he was controversial, his advocacy probably discouraged their incorporation into compendia until the 1700s. In the 1800s, wine remained the prime hydroalcoholic vehicle in the United States. After the turn of the century, however, tinctures (and elixirs) displaced those wines because of their wide variation in strength. Moreover, prohibition impeded their widespread use. As galenicals declined throughout the twentieth century, tinctures lingered on as an official class, mainly as flavorings, for example, Tincture of Orange Peel. Homeopathic Tinctures are generally prepared by long maceration of freshly dried succulent plants or their parts in alcohol, the completed tincture being made to represent one part of the dry crude material in each ten parts of the completed preparation.

Triturates, tablet: Small, disk-like masses of medicinal powders prepared by forcing a moistened tablet mass into a die by manual pressure and allowing them to dry and harden. The basis of tablet triturates is usually a mixture of lactose and sucrose in a 5: 1 ratio, moistened with a volatile liquid such as alcohol. Tablet triturates were introduced in New York in 1878 by Dr. Robert W. Fuller as a palatable and convenient means of administering potent drugs by mouth. Fuller's original triturates consisted of triturations of metallic, mineral, and vegetable matter, mixed into a paste with alcohol or water, and molded into the desired shape. In 1882, Fuller described a perforated, hard rubber tablet triturate mold with a corresponding pegged plate, which was practically identical to those available today. Tablet triturates served the purposes of homeopathic physicians well and undoubtedly helped to further the use of homeopathic doses. Twentieth-century pharmacists also prepared hypodermic tablets (used for preparing hypodermic injections) utilizing the technique. Today, tablet triturates and hypodermic tablets are formed by compression and are termed molded tablets.

Triturations: Dilutions of potent powdered drugs prepared by intimately mixing them with a suitable diluent, usually lactose, in a definite proportion by weight, usually 10%, used as a dispensing aid. Such poisonous substances as strychnine sulfate, arsenic, mercury bichloride, and atropine are much more accurately dispensed using this technique, the pharmacist weighing a multiple of the prescribed drug in a triturated form. Homeopathic triturations were formerly prepared by triturating one part of a drug into 99 parts of lactose over a period of at least one hour; homeopathic tincture triturations were prepared by mixing 10 mL of a homeopathic "strong tincture" with 10g of lactose and triturating the mixture gently until dry. Although such powdered triturations were being replaced by commercially prepared tablet triturates by the mid-1920s, a general formula for triturations, specifying geometric dilution, remained official in the United States Pharmacopeia through its 14th revision (1950).

Troches: Solid dosage forms in the form of small disks, cylinders, or tablets, intended to be placed in the mouth and allowed to dissolve or disintegrate slowly. The term is derived from the Greek trochos, meaning "round" or "circular." They were subsequently called pastils in French and lozenges in English. One of the earliest troches (500 B.C.) was terra sigillata, or sealed earth, a product composed of clay from the island of Lemnos and goat's blood, rolled and cut into disks and impressed with a seal; by the Middle Ages, a variety of troche presses were employed. In 1856, Edward Parrish described an apparatus for rolling and cutting troches consisting of a rolling-board, wooden roller, and cutting punch. During the next two decades, F.L. Slocum (1879), F.E. Harrison (1880), Wallace Procter (1894), and nearly a dozen others patented similar machines. The 4th edition of the National Formulary (1916) featured nine formulas for troches; by the mid-1930s, troches were being replaced by tablets: the 6th edition (1936) featured only Troches of Elm. Modern troches consist of powdered drugs bound with sugar and tragacanth or incorporated into a hard candy or glycerogelatin base.

Vapors: Steam, plain or medicated, generated by the use of steam or boiling water or by the use of a specially constructed apparatus.

Vesicatories: Local remedies, the application of which produces a serous discharge beneath the skin, forming a blister. Also known as *epispastics*.

Vinegars: Infusions or solutions of drugs in vinegar or acetic acid; one of the oldest methods of drug preparation. Ancients knew that vinegar was often a better solvent than water and a preservative as well. The first preparation listed in the first United States Pharmacopeia (1820) was Acetum Opii, or Vinegar of Opium. The English word derives from the French vin, "wine," and aigre, "sour."

Wafer envelopes: Preformed envelopes of rice flour used to administer bitter or nauseating drugs. Developed by Johann Schmidt as *saccelli amylacei*, wafer envelopes marked an improvement of convenience over wafer sheets. Pharmacists often furnished empty wafer envelopes to their patients, who transferred doses to them from prepared powder papers.

Wafers: Flat sheets of rice flour used to administer nauseating drugs. When dry, wafer sheets are nonadhesive, stiff, somewhat brittle, and slightly thicker than ordinary cardboard. Powders are administered by floating a piece of wafer sheet upon water until it becomes thoroughly softened, passing a tablespoon underneath and lifting it out, and depositing the powder in the center and folding over the corners to thoroughly enclose the powder. If water is poured into the spoon, the concealed powder can be swallowed without any disagreeable taste being perceived. Wafer sheets are made by pouring a mixture of rice flour and water upon hot greased plates or rolling it between two hot, polished, revolving cylinders.

Washes: Aqueous preparations designed to cleanse specific parts of the body. Examples include enemas, eye drops, mouth washes, and nasal washes. General washes made official include Alkaline Aromatic Solution N.F. and Antiseptic Solution N.F.

Washes, mouth: Hydroalcoholic solutions of soap flavored with essential oils for cleansing the oral cavity; they became first official in the National Formulary V (1926).

Waters, aromatic: Saturated solutions usually of volatile oils or similar substances in distilled water. Aromatic waters such as rose water were used in antiquity. Distilled waters containing volatile oils reached their therapeutic peak in the early sixteenth century. Although their therapeutic use declined in modern times, they continued to be used as flavorings. Hamamelis water (witch hazel) has lingered on as an aftershave and astringent.

Wines: Alcoholic liquids prepared from drugs by the process of solution, maceration, or percolation. differing from tinctures only in that wine is used as a solvent or menstruum instead of various strengths of alcohol; one of the oldest liquid preparations, since the alcoholic content of the wine improved its solvent characteristics in many cases. The National Formulary IV (1916) recognized 15 wines, but the passage of Prohibition convinced the revisors to drop red and white wine, as well as all medicated wines, from that compendium.

Lipid Excipients

Biologically, lipids function as structural elements in plants and animals, transport vehicles, mediators of chemical reactions, energy sources, and as messenger molecules. It is from an understanding of these functions that lipids have been applied to pharmaceutical applications. Lipids can be appropriately manipulated to conform to various physical states such as solutions, suspensions, emulsions, creams, gels, or solids. Because a combined lipid-drug formulation will present a very different conformation and/or molecular size than the drug alone when introduced into a biological environment, changes in both the distribution and the recognition of the drug by the host defense system will occur. These changes may be either intended or undesired.

Overall, the uses of lipids in pharmaceutical dosage forms can be grouped into four categories: (1) improvement in the processing or stability of the formulation in the preferred physical state; (2) enhancement or reduction in cellular or systemic absorption of the drug from the formulation; (3) more effective drug targeting; and (4) sustained or more controlled delivery of the drug. In this article, the problems and opportunities in utilizing lipids for these applications will be explored from various aspects of pharmaceutical formulation, analysis methods, and other commercial issues.

Categories of Lipids in Pharmaceutical Preparations

Categories shown are: fatty chain acids, salts, alcohols or amines, oils and waxes, phospholipids, glycolipids, neutral lipids, and non-linear chain compounds, such as sterols.

Fatty acids and derivatives

Fatty acids, salts, alcohols, and amines have been utilized in pharmaceutical formulations. Fatty acids are present in cosmetics, ointments, and suppositories and are used in tablet coating applications and as carriers in inhalant products. Fully saturated fatty acids are solid materials at chain lengths above eight, whereas longer chain polyunsaturated forms may exist as liquids, unless the double bonds are conjugated. Fatty acid salts are used widely in tableting applications and often include magnesium, calcium, and aluminum stearates. The handling properties and physical interaction with other solids make them ideal as conditioning agents to effect even distribution of particles, improve compressibility, and control the eventual release of active agent. The fatty alcohols, including cetyl and palmityl alcohol, are well known and are used extensively in ointments or creams as an emollient or emulsion modifier. Fatty amines are generally utilized as precursor compounds in coupling reactions to produce lipophilic drug derivatives. Fatty amines, like the acids, are solid at higher

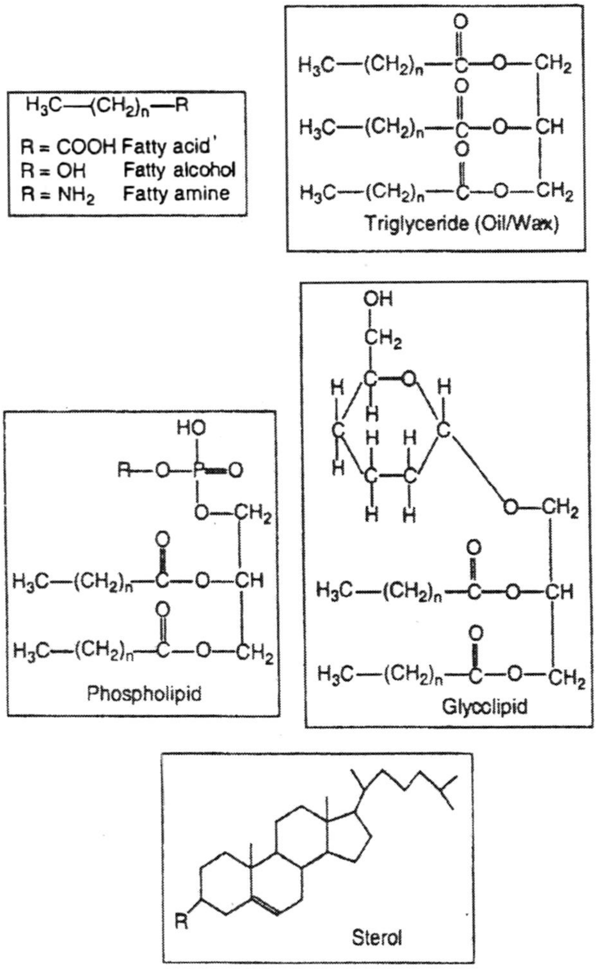

$H_3C-(CH_2)_n-R$

R = COOH Fatty acid
R = OH Fatty alcohol
R = NH_2 Fatty amine

Triglyceride (Oil/Wax)

Phospholipid

Glycolipid

Sterol

Fig. 5.6. Lipid structures.

chain lengths and insoluble in aqueous solution. Finally, aldehydes of fatty chain compounds have application in fragrances and flavorings. The unsaturated liquid forms of fatty aldehydes are most often employed.

Oils, waxes, and neutral lipids

Fatty acids, when esterified to glycerol, form mono-di-and triglycerides. Depending on the number of substituted fatty acids, the carbon chain lengths and the unsaturation level, the resultant product may exist in either liquid state (oil) or solid state (wax). Products in this category may either be naturally derived or synthetically produced and, thus, a wide diversity of products is commercially available. Oils have drug- carrying and solubilization functions in oral, topical, or injectable products. Waxes are presently used in topical and oral preparations to improve desired physical properties and control dissolution of the final product. Common materials in this group that are present in commercialized pharmaceutical preparations include castor oil, hydrogenated vegetable oil wax, paraffin, carnauba wax, white wax, olive oil and olive oil ethyl ester, mineral oil, petrolatum, cetyl ester wax, and beeswax. Neutral lipids, such as steroids, are also of value in pharmaceutical practices. For example, cholesterol and cholesterol esters can be exploited to broaden liposome phase transitions and to allow easier manipulation and or emulsification.

Phospholipid compounds

The complexity of glycerides advances by modification of the terminal hydroxyl with phosphate linked head groups to form phospholipids. Common phospholipid head groups include choline, ethanolamine, serine, inositol and inositol phosphates, glycerol, and glycerol esters. As with the triglycerides, numerous species are possible by various combinations of different head- groups and fatty acyl substitution at the 1st and 2nd positions of the glycerol backbone. Fluidity differences are evident as a function of the gel to liquid crystalline transition temperatures. Solubility of phospholipids is intimately linked to the conformation of the aggregate material rather than strictly a chemical function of the molecule. Monoacyl phospholipids, which tend to form micelles, are usually more readily soluble in aqueous solution. Diacyl phospholipids generally form liquid crystalline suspensions as long as the temperature is held at or above the phase transition. Overall, because phospholipids are amphipathic, they function well as emulsifying or dispersing agents. Although most often found in topical products, phospholipids have been employed in oral capsule formulations as well as in liposomal parenteral formulations.

Glycolipid compounds

Glycolipids include compounds formed by the linkage of a sugar moiety to a glyceride backbone. Classical glycolipids such as glycosyl glycerides or ceramides are not common in pharmaceutical preparations primarily due to low abundance and high cost; however, glycosyl modifications can be used to impart targeting mechanisms to aggregate lipid formulations.

Lipid Conformation

The colligative and solubilizing properties of lipids have been known since the early part of the 20th century. What had been perceived as clusters of amphipathic molecules (soaps) in aqueous solution are now better understood as micelles. Micellar solubilization of pharmaceuticals is now a familiar classical technique. Additional understanding of drug dissolution and impact of lipid conformations can be gained from studies that utilized macro and microemulsions to solubilize drugs.

Beyond the concept of micelles and emulsions, the combination of lipid and aqueous components can result in formulations that exhibit a variety of physical states. These result from lipid orientations, which may be either random, in thermotropic crystalline lattices, or in aggregate structures with long-range order (lyotropic liquid crystals). Lipid molecules are also capable of packing tightly together to give more ordered states, such as a bilayer. In fact, depending on the components in the formulation, lipids may contribute to distinct phase diagrams containing up to at least six different regions. The "neat" or lamellar (liposomal) phase physically can appear as a suspension to a highly viscous cream, depending on the final volume. Lamellar organizations further include liquid crystalline, gel state, and interdigitated phases. The middle phase (hexagonal) is a cylindrical arrangement with a hydrocarbon core, surrounded by an interfacial layer of hydrated polar groups. This orientation can be reversed to yield the hexagonal II structure, which appears stiff, and suspends as hard particles in water and will not dilute in additional aqueous solution. Lipids can also organize into cubic structures that appear clear, brittle, and viscous in character. Mixed conformations of lipids have also been observed, as is the case for lipidic particles, with inverse micelles distributed between a lamellar matrix.

These different aggregated states are sometimes reached by transitions through other phases simply by changes in temperature or by nature of the external environment (such as solvent concentration). Phase transitions of lipids can be regulated by changes in pH, temperature, cation concentrations, and presence of amphipathic additives. A comprehensive database on lipid phase transitions has been recently compiled by Caffrey. Polymorphic transitions are common in the preparation of lipid-containing formulations and can account for the differences in physical handling properties of the material during manufacture in which varying amounts of solvents, or energy input, are encountered at the different process steps. Geometric preferences of lipids can be better understood by considering the relative volume occupied by each portion of the molecule.

The various macromolecular aggregates of lipids also make it possible to associate with drugs through physical entrapment. In these cases, the concentration of lipid associated drug is dictated by the size or conformation of the drug and the spaces created in the lipid aggregate. Entrapment levels of drug can vary from less than 1% to as high as complete encapsulation. Excluding chemical interactions or solubilization phenomena, drug encapsulation efficiency is linked to both the lipid conformation and the manufacturing method. which juxtaposes the two components. This is particularly true of liposome formulations in which factors of temperature, pressure, solute concentration, solvent volumes, or energy application all contribute to the final amount of drug incorporated within the lipid matrix.

Manufacturing of Lipid-containing Products

Manufacturing issues should be evaluated as part of overall lipid formulation development. Although lipid addition may be desirable for pharmacological purposes there are often commercial issues which present hurdles to eventual marketing. Among those factors are the availability and cost of raw materials, handling of intermediate mixed-phase systems, particulate control, stability of the lipid ingredients, sterilization, packaging interactions, qualification of non-compendial ingredients, and development of validated methods for analysis of either raw material or product.

Availability and cost of lipid raw materials

For commercial formulations, raw material sources should be of high purity and quality consistently meeting defined specifications, preferably compendial when available. Fortunately, high-purity lipids have become increasingly available in large supply, and in particular, phospholipid supply has advanced in recent years due to the approval and marketing of parenteral liposome formulations.

Large supply of naturally derived lipids can be obtained from plants in which many oils and fatty acids can be readily extracted and purified. Animal sources (e.g., eggs or milkfats) are used to derive complex lipids such as phospholipids and cholesterol. Yield from natural sources is dependent on the weight- percent composition and the efficiency of the extraction procedure. The constitution of fatty acids in vegetable oils varies widely from different sources. For example, oleic acid is present at 64.6% by weight in olive oil but is present at only 0.7% in palm kernel oil. Similarly, castor oil triglyceride is comprised of almost entirely ricinoleic chains. There are numerous raw material suppliers of oils and oil fractions worldwide. As such, the relative cost of bulk purified fractions and their derivatives such as salt forms and alcohols is quite low (~$50–150/kg). Costs for high purity synthetic phospholipids (>97%) continue to drop when compared to prices 8 to 10 years earlier. This is primarily due to the advent of marketed liposome products. Phospholipids are available worldwide from companies such as Genzyme, Avanti Polar Lipids, Matreya Inc., American Lecithin Co., Lipoid GmbH/Vernon Walden, Lucas Meyer, Nichiyu Liposome/Nippon Oil and Fat and Northern Lipids. Also now available in larger supply are PEGylated phospholipids, lysopholipids, and various cationic lipids used in gene therapeutic applications.

Compounding of lipids into formulations

Lipids may be supplied either as lyophilized or dried powders, as liquids, or dissolved or suspended in an appropriate solvent. Dried powders are typically waxy or sticky in character, making aliquoting of the product troublesome. Lipid lyophilates can also be hygroscopic, thus presenting some difficulty for fluidized bed operations. Fluid bed applications however, may be successful if the concentration of lipid is held fairly low. Handling of lipid products in a liquid state allows for more accurate compounding. Solubilization vehicles may involve dissolution into either polar or non-polar solvents or surfactant solutions. Aside from safe handling, a primary concern when introducing lipids from solvent environments is the compatibility of the solvent with processing equipment, in particular the gaskets and seals found in the pumps, transfer lines, mixers, and extractors. Elevated temperatures, which are used to dissolve or maintain the phase transition of the lipid or to initiate solvent evaporation, can further induce problems for gaskets and seals. In systems with nonvolatile solvents and detergents, removal of the dissolution vehicle can be achieved with flow centrifugal separation, chromatography or diafiltration. Introducing a lipid-containing solvent to an aqueous solution of drug will require some means for energy input to mix the components, whether by simple rotating blade stirring, more vigorous homogenization, or milling, by sonication and filtration, or by high-pressure extrusion. Unless cosolvation is achieved a suspension of non-miscible aqueous and non-polar phases will offer more resistance to flow and may present problems for extrusion through filters, which tender a surface that is of opposite character to one of the phases. Binding of active agent, such as proteins, must also be considered. The conformational state of the lipid and the concentration also will govern the workability of the formulation. Lamellar orientations will flow fairly readily at concentrations below about 400 mg/ml whereas cubic or hexagonal phases will present difficulty even at very low concentrations.

Particulate and particle size control

For lipids dissolved in solution, particulate control may be necessary, depending on administration route. For parenterals the large- or small-volume parenteral particulate tests of the USP are applicable, as would be the Ph. Eur. clarity test and JP foreign matter insoluble test. For suspended or opaque lipid formulations, compendial particle size tests and specifications for suspensions will apply (i.e., light obscuration or microscopy). Size reduction of lipid formulations can be achieved with a variety of processing equipment including paddle stirrers, homogenization and high shear mixers, Microfluidizer, colloid mills, ultrasonic and piezoelectric emulsifiers, and pressurized filtration or membrane extrusion.

Lipid stability

A characteristic of lipid products, particularly those with unsaturated lipids is peroxide formation with oxidation. Free radicals such as ROO•, RO•, and OH• can damage the drug and induce toxicity. Lipid peroxides may also form due to autoxidation, which increases with unsaturation level. Hydrolysis of the lipid may be accelerated due to the pH of the solution. or from processing energy such as ultrasonic radiation. Antioxidants (i.e., α-tocopherol, propyl gallate, ascorbate, or BHT) may be required.

Sterilization methods

Because of possible oxidation, steam or heat sterilization of lipids may not be an attractive option. Validations at non-standard autoclave cycles or F_0 values may prove valuable. In some instances, as in ophthalmic ointments made with white petrolatum or oleagenous components, the base can be sterilized by dry heat (160–180°C for 1–3 h) and combined aseptically with the sterile drug and additives. Ointments with lipids such as lanolin, petrolatum, and mineral oil have been terminally sterilized by cobalt-60 gamma irradiation with success. In less viscous solutions, end terminal filtration with aseptic fill is often necessary, requiring justification to regulatory authorities for lower sterility assurance levels. High pressures may be required to force lipid through membranes, thus adequate filter integrity checks are critical. High-pressure extrusion through straight channel membranes (polycarbonates/ceramics) may reduce the pressures and improve flow rates.

Packaging and processing surface considerations

Lipids will be attracted to hydrophobic surfaces where losses might be expected. Overall binding will be affected if the molecule also contains ionic regions. Generally, lipids are chemically compatible with most plastics or glass used in packaging. Residual solvents that partition into the lipid phase may interact with plastic resins such as polystyrene or polycarbonate or with rubberized seals. Extractables from plastic packaging may be accelerated by the presence of lipid. Extraction of silicone polymer into lipid phases also occurs from silanized surfaces or coated gaskets. Compendial tests and regulations on extractables and impurities will apply here. Presence of metals coming from process or package surfaces are a potential source of catalysis leading to degradation of lipid components. In addition, reducing oxygen headspace should be considered to minimize potential degradation. Inert gas purging can improve lipid stabilities.

Analysis of Lipid Pharmaceutical Products

Because lipids exhibit primary through quaternary conformations, the analysis of lipid-containing pharmaceutical products must therefore involve both chemical and physical determinations to define the product on the molecular level as well as the aggregate state of the product. Stability-indicating assays can be developed from both approaches.

Chemical determinations

Lipids can be measured by standard analytical methods such as wet chemistry, HPLC, thin-layer chromatography, and gas chromatography. Because lipid formulations may have several components and because the formulation may have an overall aggregate structure, it is usually necessary to develop further strategies for isolation and detection of the lipid ingredients. Dissociation of the individual components using temperature, solvents, detergents, reducing or oxidizing agents, or mechanical disruption prior to analysis may be necessary. Further separation or extraction of the components before analysis is required if interference is encountered. With lipid solvent extraction, there is a greater likelihood for losses of material. More often than not, a combination of techniques will be required for validation of the product. There are worldwide compendial procedures for analysis of various lipids by wet chemistry procedures to determine concentration, end group analysis, acid value, hydroxyl value, iodine value, and saponification value.

HPLC methods

Analysis of non-polar lipids by HPLC is best carried out using normal phase columns. However, for mixed phases with polar drug or drug within an aqueous phase some compromise may be necessary. Good separation of polar and neutral lipids with a C8 column and a four-solvent mobile phase has been reported. Elution of neutral lipids like triglycerides from C18 columns is slow, however, good resolution can been achieved. Mobile-phase development is usually necessary to effect a high degree of separation and resolution of similarly eluting components. Heated columns are beneficial for increasing temperature above the phase-transition temperature of the lipid and thus minimize clogging. Lipids with predominantly saturated chain lengths will have poor ultraviolet (UV) absorption even at the lower wavelengths (190 nm). Alternative detectors should then be considered.

Thin layer chromatography

One- and two-dimensional thin-layer silica gel chromatography remains a cornerstone of lipid analysis. Sensitivity by this method is typically as low as 2 μg/ spot. Lipid visualization can be achieved by many methods, including iodine vapor or charring of plates following exposure to sulfur-dichromic acid, cupric reagents, Phospray, or α-naphthol. Other useful reagents include stains and dyes such as fluorescamine, rhodamine 6G, bromothymol blue, molybdenum blue, phosphomolybdic acid, and silver nitrate, which may be impregnated into the silica. Validation of lipid purity and quantitation is performed using gel or plate scanners.

Gas chromatography (GC)

Capillary and packed (GC) columns are of value in the analysis of complex mixtures of lipids. The best capillary column length will depend on the complexity of the material injected, however, 30-m columns are often employed. In packed columns, many types of stationary phases are available for lipid separation, and these include silicone and alkylated or cyanogenated derivatives, polyesters, polyglycol, and carboranes. It is also common to derivatize the fatty-acid side chains to the corresponding methyl esters by reaction in BF_3/methanol prior to chromatographic analysis to achieve more distinct and uniform separations.

Physical determinations

The aggregate states of lipids are discernable from measurements provided by a host of analytical devices, which yield information on physical properties. These techniques may also be used to give clues as to the interaction of the lipid carrier and the drug.

Particle sizing

Lipid particulate analysis can be achieved with most commercial laser particle counters. Compendial requirements for suspensions also allow for sizing via electron microscopy determinations, which can provide for qualitative assessments in addition to quantitation. Lipid suspension particles can be detected by negative-stain, freeze-fracture, critical-point drying and scanning techniques.

Nuclear magnetic resonance (NMR)

NMR is a valuable technique in the analysis of lipid phases. More specifically, proton, deuterium, carbon-13, fluorine-19, and phosphorus-31 NMR have been utilized for analysis of the dynamic and motional properties of lipids, lipid diffusion, ordering properties, head-group hydration, lipid asymmetry, quantitation of lipid composition, and head-group conformation and dynamics. Cullis et al. and Gruner et al. have shown the importance of P-31 NMR as a tool in the determination of phase properties and lipid asymmetry and the identification of bilayer, hexagonal, and isotropic phases.

Electron spin resonance (ESR)

ESR is used to give information on the local environment of a lipid molecule. In normal state these molecules inherently do not exhibit ESR spectrums. However the necessary signal can be generated from reporter labels such as nitroxide or doxyl probes, which can either be linked directly to the lipid molecule or prelinked to a lipid chain and then partitioned into the lipid aggregate formulation. Data from ESR spectrums are valuable for determining molecular properties of the formulation, such as phase transitions and separations, order parameters (anisotropy), polarity, lateral diffusion, segregation and clustering, surface and transbilayer potentials, permeability and internal volumes, surface determinants (antigens), pH gradients, lipid asymmetry, flip flopping, and fusion.

Differential scanning calorimetry

Differential scanning calorimetry is a well known technique in the study of the thermal behavior of lipids and can be used to assess purity and stability of lipids, perturbation of aggregate structures, phase transition temperatures, lipid mixing behavior, and influence of other molecules and ions on structure.

X-ray and neutron diffraction

Diffraction patterns of lipid solutions can yield strong evidence for the presence of specific repeating conformational structures as well as the spacing between lipid molecules in organized films or layers.

Spectroscopic analysis

Appraisals of the optical properties of lipid solutions and dispersions will provide information on concentrations, aggregation and stability, phase transitions, densities, and repeating structures. Measurements of refractive index, scattered light intensity (polarized and depolarized), and birefringence are relatively easy laboratory methods on which certain product specifications may be based. Also, fluorescent techniques can readily provide information on lipid movements and transfer of lipid between particles.

Commercial and Experimental Lipid Dosage Forms

The key purposes of lipid materials in dose forms include: (1) improving the solubility or physical workability of the drug for ease of administration or to enhance stability; (2) augmentation or reduction in absorption of the drug from the formulation; (3) specific drug targeting to maximize response and minimize side effects; and (4) controlled or slow delivery of the drug from the formulation. Currently, the largest use of lipids in pharmaceuticals is in products for oral or topical dosage administration, although there is growing use in parenteral, pulmonary and nasal products.

The mechanics of drug delivery from lipid systems is governed by five structural features: primary structure, that is, chemical or molecular interactions, secondary organization into aggregate structures such as inverse micelles, tertiary organization of the aggregate projected into three dimensions such as three dimensional inverse micelles or hexagonal phase tubules; quaternary associations, agglomeration or interaction of the three dimensional structures such as lateral stacking of hexagonal tubules, and final packing of the molecules in solution (concentration effects) to produce liquids, creams, solids, etc. Mammalian systems have natural degradative pathways for the rapid metabolism of most lipid raw materials. However, the release of drug to a biological system will be controlled at least as much by these structural features as by simple-natural degradative mechanisms.

Lipophilic derivatives and prodrugs

Lipophilic derivatives and prodrugs are a prudent tactic to alter the normal interaction of drug compounds with cells and cellular barriers. The type of modification desired may be a permanent one if the drug compound maintains its activity following conjugation, or a reversible type subject to biological cleavage. A variety of strategies for chemical coupling of lipids to drugs can be developed to produce the desired modified product. Briefly, non-reversible reaction approaches include conjugation to drugs with amine residues either via glutaraldehyde, lipid anhydrides or halides, or succinimidyl derivatives of the fatty acyl chain via carbodiimide activation. Non-reversible conjugations have also been accomplished via carbodiimide-activated carboxyl moieties of drugs reacted with amine containing lipids. Permanent conjugation to phenolic residues of drugs can be accomplished with diazo derivative of lipids bearing available amines. This approach has been successfully employed to prepare lipophilic derivatives of peptides containing tyrosine residues. Lipid conjugation reactions have also taken advantage of available sulfhydryl groups on drugs, particularly for modification of antibodies. On the other hand, bioreversible conjugates have been made via use of the Schiff base reaction to couple an aldehyde-bearing lipid to amines present on the drug. It is possible to convert the hydroxyl groups of mo abundant glycolipids to the corresponding aldehydes using periodate. An extension beyond the Schiff base reaction is the Mannich base condensation, which introduces a nucleophilic reactant such as an enolate anion or amide to the reaction between the aldehyde and amine. In these reactions the amine component is generally a lipophilic primary or secondary amine. Extensive literature is available on the production and biological activities of lipophilic N-Mannich base derivatives and stabilized *a*-acycloalkyl forms.

Permeation enhancers

There are a number of excellent reviews on the requirements for enhancing drug permeability across lipophilic biological barriers, with particular reference to the importance of the lipophilic properties of formulations. Administration sites include buccal, oral, nasal, ocular, transdermal, rectal, and pulmonary.

Vehicles for dispersion

There is fairly extensive use of lipid materials in oral liquid dose forms strictly as vehicles. Primary applications have been as surfactants to promote drug suspension or dissolution (fatty glycols and fatty acids), as flavoring agents (natural or synthetic oils), and as thickening agents (hydrogenated oils). Aspects of pharmaceutical oral suspensions have been discussed in greater depth. Solution based-lipid vehicles have been applied in softgel applications, the primary category being oils that are compatible with gelatins and that that have had applications as both lubricants for processing of the gelatin sheets and as drug vehicles for liquid fill operations into the softgel. High lipid concentrations may allow for higher ethanol content in softgel fills.

Lipids may also be used to create solutions for injectable products, particularly intravenous preparations. Fatty acids, fatty glycols, and fatty alcohols may be used to enhance the dissolution of certain insoluble drugs, act as preservatives, or function as active agents as demonstrated by Scleromate injection, a mixture of fatty acid salts derived from cod liver oil. As another example, benzyl alcohol preservative has been useful in formulations for water insoluble drugs such as etoposide and is a primary active agent in Zilactin gel. Polyoxyethylated fatty-acid derivative has been used in the dissolution of phytonadione, a lipid-soluble vitamin for subcutaneous or intramuscular injection. Injectable amphotericin B is solubilized with sodium desoxycholate in Fungizone. Polyoxyethylated or PEGylated castor oils are also used in dissolution of injectable drugs such as cyclosporine, paclitaxel, and teniposide and miconazole. Clear colloidal dispersions are also possible using a wide varity of phospholipids, cholesterol esters, and tocopherol esters.

Solid- and liquid-crystalline suspensions, creams, and gels

Suspensions and creams are most often developed for aqueous insoluble drugs, as typified by ophthalmic and otic preparations of corticosteroids. In suspensions such as Cortisporin or Pediotic, components such as cetyl alchol, glyceryl monostearate, mineral oil, and propylene glycol are commonly used to effect a homogeneous suspension of drug particles.

The creation of fine suspensions may also be necessary to administer a highly insoluble product by parenteral injection. In these instances lipids may be used as either wetting agents or suspension vehicles. Lecithin (phosphatidylcholine) is a suitable agent for wetting or suspending of drug particles in either aqueous or non-aqueous solutions. This common formulation additive is used for injectable long-acting IM suspensions of penicillin for the bronchodilator inhalation aerosol, Atrovent, and for the otic suspension Cipro HC. Naturally derived and synthetic lecithins, in mixtures with neutral lipids, also serve as the active ingredient in lung surfactants products such as Exosurf, Survanta, and Infasurf.

Lipid materials are used extensively as vehicles in topical creams, ointments, gels, and lotions, and usually serve as the base material for many such preparations. These formulations are principally presented as emulsions and may contain fatty acids, fatty-acid salts, fatty alcohols, petroleum based and natural oils, waxes, fatty glycols, lanolin, and other hydrophobic surfactants. Such emulsions are common in dermal topicals, for which the list of products is too numerous to elaborate. Some of these ingredients also are present as vehicles in suppositories such as semi- synthetic glycerides existing in Nembutal, hydrogenated vegetable oil as found in Dulcolax (Novartis Consumer Health), and glycerides of fatty acids or oils that can be found in vaginal suppositories such as Prostin E2 and Crinone Gel. Mineral oil is frequently present in transdermal products such as Catapres-TTS and Estraderm. In addition, numerous ocular or topical ointments, such as TobraDex and Nitro-Bid, use white petrolatum and mineral oil as a base. Short-chain triglycerides such as triacetin can be found in products such as Prepidil Gel, a cervically administered prostaglandin.

Oil-in-water emulsions have also been applied for intravenous use. Commercial parenteral emulsions include Dizac and Diprivan. Many commercial or experimental parenteral products have been based on vegetable oil (most often soybean, safflower, or cottonseed) stabilized with phosphatides and monoglycerides, which nicely match the hydrophile–lipophile balance (HLB) requirements of those oils (~6–7). Further prospects for expanded non-toxic parenteral emulsions may come with use of other phosphatide-based surfactants with high HLB values. Drug delivery from oil/phosphatide emulsions stems from earlier development and marketing of intravenous nutrient emulsion products such as Intralipid and Aminosyn II, which are sterile and non-toxic. The development of these emulsions as well as distribution profiles of these and similar emulsion compositions have been studied. A cursory scan of the literature on parenteral oil emulsion formulations will obtain studies on amphotericin B, prostaglandin E1, halothane, pregnanolone, paclitaxel, perilla ketone, penclomedine, F-octylbromide, flurbiprofen axetil (Lipfen), lasalocid, lignin, podophyllotoxin, tacrolimus, doxorubicin, epirubicin, menatetrenone, chlorpheniramine maleate, naproxin, cyclosporin A, propranolol, testotsterone, benzocaine, phenylazoaniline, palmitoylrhizoxin, pilocarpine, diazepam, and various peptide and proteins for vaccine delivery.

Liposomal dosage forms

Extensive studies on liposomes date back to the 1960s. Many good comprehensive review references exist on compositions and manufacturing of liposomes including the article "Liposomes as Pharmaceutical Dosage Forms" in this volume. The earliest commercial liposomal formulations were developed for veterinary application or over-the-counter cosmetic creams promoted for improved hydration. More recently, parenteral liposome formulations of amphotericin B, doxorubicin, and daunorubicin have been approved and marketed, with others on the horizon for applications in photodynamic therapy. Although the vast majority of liposome preparations are constructed from phospholipids, other nonphospholipid materials can be used either alone or in mixtures to form bilayer arrays. One such example is Amphotec, which utilizes sodium cholesteryl sulfate as the primary lipid. Other liposome forming materials may include but are not limited to fatty-acid compositions, ionized fatty acids, or fatty acyl amino acids, longchain fatty alcohols plus surfactants, ionized lysophospholipids or combinations, non-ionic or ionic surfactants and amphiphiles, alkyl maltosides, α-tocopherol esters, cholesterol esters, polyoxyethylene alkyl ethers, sorbitan alkyl esters, and polymerized phospholipid compositions.

Low density lipoprotein carriers

Lipoproteins are naturally occurring particulate emulsion carriers for the transport of cholesterol and other lipids such as triglycerides in the blood. Because low- density lipoprotein (LDL) particle clearance is receptor mediated, they have been proposed as drug carriers for targeting applications, specifically for targeting of cytotoxic agents to tumor cells, delivery of antiviral agents to parenchymal liver cells, targeting of immunomodulators, antiviral and antiparasitic drugs to Kupffer and endothelial cells, and as gene vectors.

Solid dosage forms

The main use of lipids in solid form has been for oral tableting applications. Fatty-acid salts such as magnesium and calcium stearates, and various waxes and glycerides are most often used as conditioners and binders during compaction and provide more even, controlled, or slower disintegration of the tablet once administered. Extensive literature is available in which these materials are discussed in context of the preparation of oral tablets or capsules. The use of lipids for solid-implant formulations has also been investigated. Materials such as cholesterol, and high-melting-point fatty-acids, fatty anhydrides, and glycerides have been utilized in compressed implants to prolong systemic delivery of drugs. Lipids are also well suited for suppository and vaginal insert formulations.

Safety of lipid products

The safety of a lipid product will in part be a reflection of: (1) the purity of the compounds administered; (2) biological toxicity of the basic chemical ingredients; and (3) reactions to structural presentations of the lipid. Noncompendial lipid materials will necessitate significant toxicology testing.

Contaminants and impurities

Sensitive analytical procedures will be required to distinguish contaminants from lipid peaks within the preparation. By-products may be present from the synthetic processes used to produce the lipids or if copurified from the natural source. For example, common impurities in synthetic diacyl chain lipids are the monoacyl forms, which are generally more toxic to biological systems. Endotoxins and pyrogens either may be detectable in a lipid preparation or difficult to detect due to the lipids shielding against the analytical reagents.

Immune reactivity

Consideration should be given to immune reactivities when administering lipids to mammalian systems. Oils are well known for their adjuvancy; different oils will produce varying levels of reactivity. Biological responses such as leukocyte attraction, encysisting of the oil, and edema reactions vary in severity simply as a function of the chemical nature or purity of the oil itself. Importantly, most lipids, including normal endogenous compounds possess antigenic potential to varying degrees. These possible reactivities should be monitored as part of the overall clinical design.

Conformational considerations

There may be biological sensitivities to the conformational presentation and sizing of the lipid formulation. For example the ability of antibodies to distinguish between lamellar organizing lipids and hexagonal-phase lipids are known and may form the basis for certain types of autoimmune dysfunction. Biological factors such as reticuloendothelial cell recognition of particles provide further impetus for control of the particle size and stability.

NON-PARENTERALS

Dosage form is a drug delivery system designed to deliver the active ingredient to the body and, upon administration should deliver the drug at a rate and amount that assures the desired pharmacological effect. Such dosage forms are manufactured under current good manufacturing procedures (cGMP), using equipment and packaging to ensure product stability. The dosage form must produce the same therapeutic response each time it is administered. To maintain this reproducibility between and within batches, manufacturing procedures are validated under a specific quality assurance program. Non-parenteral dosage forms can be categorized based on the route of administration or physical form. Based on physical form they can be classified as solids, liquids (homogenous and heterogeneous systems), semisolids, and aerosols. Dosage forms can also be categorized based on the route of administration. Solid dosage forms include different types of compressed tablets, granules, troches, lozenges, coated dosage forms, and hard and soft gelatin capsules. Liquid dosage forms include solutions, suspensions, emulsions, and buccal and sublingual sprays. Topical dosage forms are applied to the skin and include ointments, pastes, creams, lotions, liniments, and transdermal patches. Some dosage forms are formulated for application to body cavities, viz. rectal and urethral suppositories and vaginal pessaries. Inhalation aerosols, using metered dose inhalers (MDIs), dry powder inhalers (DPIs) and nebulizers, are used to deliver drugs to the respiratory tract. Nasal route uses solution and suspension dosage forms. Occular route is used to administer solutions and suspensions to the eye for local and systemic effects.

Solid Dosage Forms

Powders and granules

Powders are intimate mixtures of dry, finely divided drugs and/or chemicals that are intended for oral administration or external use. Powders may also be formulated as larger particle sized, free-flowing granules to aid in handling and administration. Bulk powders usually are packed into a suitable wide-mouth container and contain relatively non-toxic medicaments in large doses, e.g., compounded magnesium trisilicate oral powder. Insufflations are medicated powders blown into ear, nose, or throat.

Tablets

Flowability and compressibility are two important parameters essential for successful manufacture of tablets. Flowability determines ease of material flow from tablet hopper to the press. Inadequate flow gives rise to arching, bridging, or rat-holing in hoppers. Powder flow can be improved mechanically by use of force feeders. Flowability can also be increased by incorporation of glidants like fumed silica and talc. Another method involves the conversion of powder to spherical particles by spray drying or spheronization. Tablets are manufactured by dry and wet methods. Dry methods consist of direct compression, slugging, and roller compaction of drug-excipient blends. Directly compressible excipients may be disintegrants with poor flow, e.g., microcrystalline cellulose (Avicel PH102); free-flowing materials which do not disintegrate, e.g., dibasic calcium phosphate (DiPac); or free-flowing powders which disintegrate by dissolution (e.g., spray-dried lactose, anhydrous lactose, dextrose, sucrose, amylose, etc.). The drug is mixed with excipients in a blender and then compressed directly on a tablet press. Dry granulation by compression or slugging is used for moisture or heat sensitive actives. The powder blends are compressed into compacts or slugs. An alternative method is to squeeze the powder blends into solid cake between rollers called roller compacts. These slugs or compacts are milled and screened in order to produce granules with improved flow. Granulation is the process of particle size enlargement of homogeneously mixed powder ingredients and simultaneously increasing bulk density, flowability, and compressibility of the system.

Wet granulation process involves the massing of the powder mix, using a binder and solvent. The solvent should be volatile non-toxic, and removed by drying. This process is not suitable for hydrolysable and thermolabile drugs. The binder is added in the form of a solution, or added dry or its mucilage incorporated with the powder blend. The choice of liquid depends on the properties of the material being granulated. Water is widely used alone or along with a binding agent. Commonly used non-aqueous liquids are isopropanol and ethanol. Massing process is usually performed in a low or high shear granulator where the liquid is poured or sprayed onto a moving powder bed until a moist mass of finely divided material is formed. This is passed through an oscillating granulator with the appropriate screen size to obtain the required granule particle size. Sometimes both intra and extra-granular portions are divided to prevent incompatibility between excipient material hiding or better distribution, tableting or dissolution. Tablets require different functional excipients for their manufacture. Diluents are inert bulking agents added to actives to make a reasonably sized tablet. Generally, a tablet should weigh about 50–60 mg and therefore very low dose drugs will require these diluents to make at least a 50 mg tablet. Adsorbents such as fumed silica and kaolin are sometimes used for holding large amounts of fluids in an apparently dry state. Binders are used as adhesives to bind powder in wet granulation and give strength to compacts during compression. Binders may be incorporated into the dry blend or added as a solution to the mixed powder during wet granulation. Disintegrants are usually added to promote rapid breakup of tablets to increase surface area and aid drug dissolution. Disintegrants can act by different mechanisms such as like swelling and capillary action. Glidants are materials that are added to tablet formulations to improve flow properties of the granulation. They act by reducing inter-particulate friction (e.g., fumed silica). Lubricants are added to prevent the adherence of granules to the punch and die faces of the tablet press. Many lubricants also facilitate flow of granules. Talc and magnesium stearate are more effective as punch lubricants. Stearic acid works better as a die lubricant.

Specific types of tablets

Lozenges: These are compressed tablets formulated, without a disintegrant and must be allowed to dissolve in the mouth. They are used for local activity (throat lozenges) or for systemic effect (vitamins).

Effervescent tablets: These tablets undergo quick dissolution of actives in water due to internal liberation of carbon dioxide. By combining alkali metal carbonates or bicarbonates with tartaric or citric acid, carbon dioxide is liberated when placed in water.

They are prepared by the heat fusion technique. Usually a water-soluble lubricant is used to prevent scum formation at the water surface. Sweetness is achieved by the addition of saccharin, since sucrose is hygroscopic and increases the bulk of the tablet, e.g., Rochelle Salt.

Chewable tablets: These tablets are preferred for pediatric and geriatric patients who have difficulty swallowing whole tablets. Another advantage is that they do not need water for administration. Mannitol is normally used as the base diluent because of its pleasant taste and texture, and because it can effectively mask the taste of objectionable actives. They are usually prepared by wet granulation and are not compressed very hard. High amounts of flavor are added to increase palatability. Antacids are typically formulated as chewable tablets.

Sublingual and buccal tablets: These tablets are placed under the tongue (sublingual) or the cheek (buccal) and can produce immediate systemic effects by enabling the drug to be directly absorbed through the mucosa by preventing the first pass effect (e.g., isoprenaline sulphate and glyceryl trinitrate). Tablets are small, flat, without a disintegrant, and are compressed lightly to produce soft tablets.

Molded tablets: These are prepared from mixtures of medicinal substances and a diluent usually consisting of lactose and powdered sucrose in varying quantities. The powders are dampened with solutions containing high proportions of alcohol depending on the solubility of the active and filler. The dampened powders are pressed under low pressure in die cavities. Solidification depends upon crystal bridging during the subsequent drying process, and not upon the compaction forces.

Multi-layered tablets: A multilayered tablet consists of several different granulations compressed on top of each other to form a single tablet. They may also be bi-layer when incompatible drug substances are used, e.g., phenylephedrine HCl in one layer and ascorbic acid and paracetamol in another.

Modified release dosage forms

Modified release (MR) has been used to describe dosage forms having drug release characteristics based on time, course, and/or location and are designed to accomplish therapeutic or convenience objectives not offered by conventional or immediate release dosage forms. Drugs for chronic conditions with short half- lives, possessing a good therapeutic index and uniform absorption pattern are ideal candidates for such dosage forms. These are either delayed release or extended release (ER) preparations. ER dosage forms allow at least a twofold reduction in dosing frequency as compared to the conventional dosage form. Delayed release dosage forms are designed to release all or a portion of drug at times much later than the time of administration. The delay may be time based or environment specific, as in enteric-coated dosage forms. Some other MR dosage forms include repeat action and targeted release dosage forms. Most controlled release products are good examples of ER dosage forms. These dosage forms can be classified by their mechanism of release and/or type of formulation. Coated beads, granules microspheres, and other particulate systems are pellet type controlled release dosage forms, where the drug is usually coated onto non-pareil beads (low dose) or made from granules composed of the drug (high dose). These pellets are further coated with functional coating agents (Eudragits, HPMCs, Surelease, etc.) to provide various release characteristics.

These pellets can be used to fill capsules (e.g., Ornade Spansules) or compressed at low pressure into tablets (e.g., Theo-Dur). In some cases small mini-tablets of about 3–4 mm diameter can be compressed. These tablets function like pellets and can be used to fill capsules. Microencapsulation is a process of encapsulating microscopic drug particles with a thin wall of coating material. Several coating materials have been used including gelatin, ethylcellulose, and polyvinyl alcohol, e.g., Micro-K-Extencaps. Matrix systems are dosage forms where drug substance is combined with hydrophilic cellulose polymers (excipient material), which slowly erode in the presence of body fluids. On hydration, the polymers behave like a gel and prevent the fast disintegration of the tablet. Diffusion from the gel controls the drug release (e.g., Oramorph SR tablets).

A multi-layered tablet consists of several different granulations compressed on top of each other to form a single tablet composed of two or more layers. Each layer is fed from a separate feed frame with individual weight control. Precompression tamping helps in good binding of layers. Also, reduced pressures prevent intermixing of granules during compression. They may be bilayer where IR/ER combination are used or mainly when incompatible drug substances is used. Sometimes the release from individual layers is controlled to give a drug delivery system, such as, Geomatrix system. In some cases if the bulk density of the tablet is less than one, it floats in the gastric fluids thus extending the residence time in the gastrointestinal tract (GIT). Such dosage forms are called Hydrodynamically Balanced Systems (HBS), an example being Valrelease (Roche). In some cases the drug is embedded inside inert polymeric matrices with materials such as polyethylene, polyvinyl acetate, and polymethacrylates. The granulations are then compressed into tablets. These inert matrices are excreted in the feces unchanged (e.g., Ferro Gradumet (Abbott).

Some drugs form complexes resulting in slower dissolution and behave as extended release dosage forms, e.g., Rynatan. A slowly eroding tablet may be granulated with hydrophobic excipients (waxy lipophilic material) so that the drug leaches out over an extended period with an outer shell containing the IR dose (buffered aspirin). In some cases a cationic or anionic drug solution can react with an insoluble resin to form a complex. This complex can be tableted, encapsulated or suspended in a vehicle, e.g., Tussionex Pennkinetic Extended Release Suspension (Medeva). Osmotic pump drug delivery systems consist of a core tablet coated with a semipermeable membrane with a fine orifice made by laser beams. The core usually forms two layers containing the active and osmotic agents. In the gastric fluids water is imbibed by the osmotic agent (pull) and then exerts pressure on the drug (push) in solution, out through the orifice. Such dosage forms are independent of pH of the gastric fluids and are termed as gastrointestinal therapeutic systems (GITS), e.g., Procardia XL (Pfizer). Repeat action tablets consist of slow release inner core and a immediate release (IR) as in Repetabs (Schering) or as bilayer IR/ER tablets. Delayed release dosage forms are used for drugs that are destroyed in the gastric fluids, or cause gastric irritation, or are absorbed preferentially in the intestine. Such dosage forms are enterically coated using materials such as cellulose acetate pthalate, shellac, and waxes. The coating allows the drug to release at higher pH (pH dependent) or by enzyme catalyzed reactions, e.g., Erythromycin or Aspirin delayed release dosage forms. Several forms of oral controlled release systems are available in the market; however, most of them are dependent on the rate at which the system passes along the gastro-intestinal tract. This can be overcome by regulating the release of the drug by physical chemical means, or by a process related to the environment in which the delivery system is present at the specific time.

Capsules

The word "*capsule*" is derived from the Latin word *capsula* meaning a small box. Gelatin, a substance of natural origin with unique properties, is the major component of capsules. Gelatin is used because it is non-toxic and readily soluble in biological fluids at body temperature. It has good film forming properties and, as a in water and water–gylcerol systems, undergoes reversible phase change from a solution to gel at only a few degrees above ambient temperature. There are two forms of gelatin (A and B) based on the method of manufacture from animal bone and skin. The properties important for capsule shell manufacture are viscosity and bloom strength. Hard gelatin capsules are firm and rigid while soft gelatin capsules are soft and flexible. This is because soft capsules contain a larger proportion of plasticizers like glycerol, sorbitol, propylene glycol, acacia, and sucrose. Varying proportions of plasticizers are added depending on the intended use of soft gelatin capsules. The colorants used consist of soluble and insoluble dyes. Titanium dioxide and iron oxide pigments are common, although recently aluminum lakes are being used. Preservatives are added to capsules to prevent microbial contamination. Moisture levels are also maintained at low levels to prevent bacterial growth on storage.

Hard gelatin capsules (HGCs)

Hard gelatin capsules are available in sizes ranging from size 000, (the largest) to size 5 (the smallest). The fill weight of capsule and tapped bulk density of the powder blend determines the selection of capsule size. Recently, better techniques for capsule sealing, like, self-locking and have made it possible for a range of materials. The filler material should not react with gelatin. Aldehydes lead to gelatin cross-linking affecting the integrity of the shell and water in the formula can act as a plasticizer. On the other hand, hygroscopic agents can make the capsule shell brittle. Powders filled into hard gelatin capsules should have good flow properties to maintain uniform fill weights during filling operations. Granules and pellets of spherical shape making them free-flowing and non-friable are good candidates for capsule filling using gravitational systems or specialized dosing chambers to maintain uniform fill weight. In some instances, minitablets (filmcoated, non-friable) can be filled into capsules to produce specialized dosage forms or to separate incompatible ingredients. A recent innovation in hard gelatin capsule filling is a revival of the old practice of filling liquids or semisolids. The main problem encounted is product leakage. This difficulty was overcome by using self-locking capsules and formulation techniques. The use of mixtures of material which are either thermosoftening or thixotropic in nature has become prevalent. These materials are liquefied by heat or shearing force, and revert to solid state within the capsule shell after filling. Filling machines have been developed to handle such formulations with existing powder filling equipment. This system works with solid, liquid, semisolids, and potent drugs. The application of semisolids filling is also getting prevalent. A more recent innovation in HGCs to fill liquid dosage forms with the use of new machines which heat-seal the caps permanently to prevent leakage as observed with liquid filled HGCs in the past. A good example is the introduction of Licaps (Capsugel) for liquid fills. Capsules made of non-gelatin ingredients for materials not compatible with gelatin are also available, e.g., cellulose (Vegecaps).

Soft gelatin capsules (SGCs)

SGCs or softgels are continuous gelatin shells surrounding a liquid or semi-solid fill. These capsules are formed, filled, and sealed, all in one operation. These capsules are available in different shapes and sizes. SGCs are preferred for drugs with poor compressibility, poor powder flow, mixing problem, unstable or poor solubility in gastric pH, and bioavailability problems. Such drugs can be solubilized or dispersed in a liquid, where dosage uniformity is more accurate. Some drugs that are liquid or that melt during compression are good candidates, if other means of tabletting are expensive. Gelatin used in SGCs has lower bloom strength than HGCs. The plasticizer type and concentration controls the mechanical strength of the shell. In general, plasticizer amounts are larger, making them more flexible than HGC shells. Preservatives, colorants, and opacifiers are used in the same manner as in HGCs. Sometimes softgel capsules are enteric coated for drugs which are absorbed in the small intestine. Once the capsule shells dissolve in vivo, the drug is available in a liquid or semi-solid form that dissolves or disperses into fine particles with enhanced bioavailability. SGCs can be filled with several materials such as aqueous solutions, non-aqueous solutions, suspensions, pastes, oily solutions of drug, self-emulsifying system, and water-miscible liquids. Materials that cause migration of water or plasticizer from the shell cannot be filled. Surfactants and systems with extreme pH should be avoided.

Liquid Dosage Forms

Solution

A solution is a homogenous single-phase system consisting of two or more components. Solutions are easier to swallow and are acceptable dosage forms for pediatric and geriatric use. The drug in solution is readily available for absorption and therapeutic response is faster. Solutions, however, are bulky and inconvenient to transport. The stability of actives is poorer than in solids and they provide suitable media for microbial growth. Aqueous solutions are preparations made with water as solvent. Purified Water USP is widely used for most preparations. Some drugs are unstable in water or sensitive to the presence of carbon dioxide or oxygen. Not all substances are completely soluble in water and may lead to precipitation. Several other techniques are used to increase solubility of drugs in solution. Cosolvency is a process of increasing solubility of a drug by using a combination of solvents. Some suitable cosolvents are ethanol, isopropyl alcohol, sorbitol, glycerol, and propylene glycol. If a drug is a weak acid or base, then its solubility in water is influenced by pH. The pH for optimum solubility may not give a stable product. Thus, a compromise must be reached to ensure proper formulation and bioavailability. Suitable buffer systems may be used if necessary. Solubility of insoluble or poorly soluble drugs can also be increased by addition of surface-active agents. Most surfactants are miscible with solvent system and compatible with other ingredients. Hydrophilic surfactants with HLB values > 15 are generally preferred. In some cases complexation of a drug with a material may result in formation of soluble molecular complex. However, such complexation needs to be reversible for the active to cross the biological barrier. Chemical modifications of the drug can also result in more water-soluble derivatives. However, these modified drugs are regarded as new chemical entities. Non-aqueous solutions are used when complete solution is not possible in water or if the drug is unstable. Ethyl alcohol is the most widely used water-miscible solvent for external preparations. Ethyl ether is occasionally used as a co-solvent, in combination with alcohol in the preparation of some colloidons. Other solvents such as isopropyl myristate and isopropyl palmitate are solvents with low viscosity and are ideally used in cosmetics preparations. Xylene is present in ear drops for human use to dissolve ear wax.

Liquid formulation additives used include buffers, colorants, flavoring agents, and preservatives. Buffers are dissolved in solvents to resist pH changes. The choice of buffers depends on the pH and the buffering capacity. Most pharmaceutically acceptable buffer systems include carbonates, phosphates, citrates, gluconates, and lactates. Colors are added for attractiveness and product identification. Flavors are added to solutions to increase their palatability, particularly for drugs with unpleasant taste. This is especially useful in pediatric formulations. Flavors also help in product identification and are of natural or synthetic sources. Fruit juices, peppermint oil, and menthol are some examples of flavors. Some flavors are preferred for specific products, e.g., mint is associated with antacid formulas. Similarly, flavors are preferred by specific patient groups, e.g., children prefer fruity tastes and smell, while adults prefer flowery and acid flavors. Preservatives help prevent microbial growth. The choice of preservatives should be based on their performance from a microbial challenge test. Care should be taken to ensure there is no adsorption of preservatives onto product containers or packaging material. Antioxidants are added to prevent degradation of the drug in solution; the amount and type can be determined after careful determination of the degradation pathway and stability testing with different agents. Sucrose is widely used as sweetening agent, because it is water soluble, and stable at a wide range of pH. It has a pleasant texture and soothing effect on the throat. There are several other sweeteners that are less widely used. Artificial sweeteners like sugar alcohols and aspartame are used by diabetic patients.

Types of liquid preparations

Draught and elixirs: Draught is a mixture by which one or two large doses of about 50 ml are given. Traditionally, elixirs are solutions of potent or nauseating drugs containing alcohol as a cosolvent (60–70%).

Linctuses: A linctus is a viscous preparation usually prescribed for relief of cough. They usually consist of a simple solution of active in a high concentration of sucrose, often with other sweetening agents.

Mouthwashes and gargles: These are aqueous solutions for prevention and treatment of mouth and throat infections. They usually contain antiseptics, analgesics, and/or astringents. These solutions are used directly or diluted with warm water.

Nasal drops: These are small volume aqueous solutions. They are usually buffered to pH of 6.8 and are isotonic solutions. These drops are used locally as antibiotics, anti-inflammators, and decongestants.

Ear drops: These are simple solutions of drugs in water, glycerol, and propylene glycol for local use in the ear and include antibiotics, antiseptics, cleaning solutions, and wax softeners (xylene).

Enemas: These are available as solutions (aqueous or oily) as well as suspensions for rectal administration of drugs for cleaning, diagnostic, or therapeutic effect.

Lotions: These are available as solutions and suspensions to be applied topically without friction. They may either contain humectant, so that moisture is retained on the skin after application, or alcohol, which evaporates quickly imparting a cooling sensation to the skin.

Liniments: These are intended for massaging the skin. They may contain ingredients such as methyl salicylate or camphor as counter-irritants.

Colloidons: These are prepared from volatile solvents that evaporate quickly leaving a tough, flexible film on the skin that seals small cuts and or holds the active in intimate contact with the skin.

Intermediate solutions: Pharmaceutical solutions are used as intermediates for manufacturing other preparations. Aromatic water is used as a flavoring agent and peppermint and anise waters have some carminative properties. These are manufactured as concentrated waters and are diluted before use. Infusions are prepared by extracting the drug using 25% alcohol without heat. Extracts are similar to infusions, but are concentrated by evaporation. Tinctures are alcoholic or hydro-alcoholic solutions prepared from vegetable materials or from chemical substances. They are relatively weak compared to extracts. Spirits are alcoholic or hydro-alcoholic solutions of volatile substances prepared by simple solution or by admixture of ingredients. These are used as flavoring agents and may have medicinal value. Syrups are concentrated solutions of sucrose or other sugars to which medicaments or flavoring agents are added. These are bacteriostatic by virtue of their osmotic effect, e.g., simple syrup, USP.

Suspensions

These are liquids consisting of insoluble solid particles dispersed throughout a liquid phase. Most suspensions are ready to use while some are prepared as solids to be reconstituted just before use. Ideally, suspension should be homogenous between the time of shaking and dispensing the required dose. The suspended particles should be small, uniformly sized to give a smooth elegant product free from grittiness. Some insoluble solids are not easily wetted by water and thus need wetting agents to be able to disperse readily throughout the medium. Some wetting agents include surfactants, hydrophilic colloids, and solvents. Surface active agents or surfactants possessing HLB value between 7 and 9 are suitable as wetting agents. Most surfactants are used at concentrations of 0.1%. For oral use Tweens and Spans are commonly used, while sodium lauryl sulphate (SLS) is used for external applications. Some wetting agents may cause foaming and formation of deflocculated systems. Hydrophilic colloids like acacia, bentonite, tragacanth, alginates, and cellulose derivatives function as a protective colloid by coating the surface of the particles and thus imparting hydrophilic character to the solid particles. Solvents such as alcohol, glycerol, and glycols are water-miscible and reduce the liquid/air interfacial tension, increasing wetting.

Flocculation and deflocculation

Flocculation comes from the Latin word *flocculate* meaning loose and woolly. Flocculated systems result in rapid rate of settling because each individual unit is composed of many particles and is therefore larger. However, due to the loose packing of flocs they are easily dispersible on shaking. Deflocculated systems on the other hand are made up of smaller particles whose settling rate is slower, but the settled particles tend to form an irreversible compact and are difficult to redisperse. This phenomenon is called *caking*. For coarse suspensions, a deflocculated suspension will have better uniformity of dose but poorer stability due to formation of cake. Thus, a stable suspension is obtained by preparing a partially flocculated suspension with controlled viscosity so that settling is minimal. Controlled flocculation is achieved by a combination of particle size control, electrolytes to control zeta-potential and by the addition of polymers.

Inorganic electrolytes, added to an aqueous suspension alter the zeta-potential of the dispersed particle. Lowering the zeta-potential sufficiently will result in flocculation. Some of the commonly used electrolytes include sodium salts of acetates, phosphates, and citrates. Use of ionic surfactants may also result in flocculation by neutralization of particle charges. Starch, alginates, tragacanth, and cellulose derivatives are sometimes added to control the degree of flocculation so that the suspension is in a flocculated state and the sedimentation volume is large. Suspensions should exhibit high viscosity at low shear rate and vice versa. Also, the viscosity should be low enough to be poured from the container but should spread evenly, if it is intended for external application. Suspensions for injection should be able to pass through hypodermic needles. Acacia gum is used as a thickening agent for extemporaneously prepared suspensions.

Tragacanth forms viscous aqueous solutions, and its thixotropic and pseudoplastic properties make it a better thickening agent than acacia. Sodium alginate is used as a suspending agent but is incompatible with cationic materials. Several cellulose derivatives, such as methyl-cellulose (Celacol), hydroxy-ethylcellulose (Natrasol 250), sodium carboxymethylcellulose, and microcrystalline cellulose, disperse in water to produce viscous colloidal solutions and are suitable, as suspending agents. Montmorillonite clays or hydratyed silicates like bentonite, veegum, and hectorite readily hydrate and absorb upto 12 times their weight of water. The gels formed are thixotropic and therefore have wonderful suspending properties. Carbopols are synthetic polyacrylic acid copolymers that function as thickening agents at higher pH values.

Buffers are included in suspensions to maintain chemical stability and control tonicity. Density modifiers like sucrose and propylene glycol can be added to prevent large differences in densities that could result in sedimentation. Flavors, colors, and perfumes may be added to improve palatability and appearance of the product. Humectants like glycerol and propylene glycol are added in concentrations of 5% for external applications to prevent the product from drying out after application to the skin. Addition of preservatives is important, particularly when using naturally occuring adjuvants. In some situations sweeteners may be added but their affect on final product viscosity and degree of flocculation should be well understood. Suspensions are normally manufactured using colloidal mills with rotor-stator mechanism to ensure free flowing and evenly dispersed particles. Oral suspensions usually have flavoring agents intended for oral administration. Good examples are milk of magnesia, bentonite, magma, and jellies. All these systems swell and form a gel like consistency with non-Newtonian characteristics. Topical suspensions like Calamine lotion are for external use only.

Emulsions

These are dispersions of one liquid (dispersed phase) in the form of uniformly divided droplets in another liquid (dispersion medium). Depending on which liquid is the dispersed phase oil-in-water (o/w) or water-in-oil (w/o) systems are obtained. To test the identity, emulsion miscibility, staining and conductivity tests are performed. The choice of emulsion depends on the route of administration and the end use. For oral administration, o/w emulsions are used while for external use, both o/w and w/o systems can be employed. Semisolid o/w emulsions are termed as "creams," and are easily washable after application. Water-in-oil emulsions have an occlusive effect and are therefore preferred as moisturizing lotions and cleansing agents. The choice of oil depends on the application with some oils like castor and cod liver oil having a therapeutic value. Thus, w/o preparations are greasy, with high apparent viscosity while o/w emulsions are less greasy and readily absorbed and washable. Ideally emulsions should exhibit pseudoplasticity and thixotropy, that is, high viscosity at low shear rates and vice versa. They should be dispensable from containers, bottles, and tubes but at the same time should spread on the skin with light pressure. The rheological properties of emulsions are controlled by the concentration, particle size, and viscosity of dispersed phase, concentration of dispersion phase, and the nature and concentration of the emulsifier.

The choice of emulsifying system depends on the route of administration, its HLB value and its toxicity. There is no approved list of emulsifiers but pharmaceutical companies employ emulsifiers approved for use in the food industry. Emulsifiers with surface activity reduce the interfacial tension between the phases, thereby decreasing the need for energy to disperse the internal phase. The surfactants used can be anionic like sodium, potassium, and ammonium salts of long chain fatty acids (e.g., sodium stearate), soaps of di- and trivalents metal ions (e.g., calcium oleate and amine soaps, sulphated and sulphonated compounds (e.g., SLS). Cationic surfactant, amphoteric surfactants like lecithin, and non-ionic surfactants, like glycol and glycerol esters (e.g., glycerol monostearate), sorbitan esters, polysorbates, fatty alcohol polyglycol ethers (e.g., cetyl or cetostearyl alcohol), fatty acid polyglycol esters are also used. Sometimes naturally occurring materials and their derivatives, such as acacia, semi-synthetic polysaccharides (e.g., methylcellulose), sterol containing substances (e.g., beeswax), and wool fat (anhydrous lanolin), can also be employed as emulsifiers. Other ingredients used in emulsions are finely divided solids, antioxidants, such as butylated hydroxy toulene (BHT) and butylated hydroxyanisole (BHA), humectants and preservatives like benzoic acid, parahydroxybenzoic acid esters, chlorocresol, and phenoxyethanol. Emulsions can be used orally (o/w) with the therapeutic agent included in the internal phase (as for taste masking bad tasting medicaments). Externally, they can be used as lotions either with therapeutic agents or without (as in cosmetics). Emulsions are made using a variety of equipment depending on the stability requirement and the kind of process used. Both batch and continuous processes can be used. Colloid mills have been used traditionally. However, high-pressure homogenizers, microfluidizers, and ultrasonic homogenizers are being used for manufacturing emulsions.

Semisolid Dosage Forms

Ointments, creams, and pastes are semisolid dosage forms intended for topical application. They may be applied to the skin, used nasally, rectally, and vaginally. Most of them contain some form of medicament. Medicated ointments are semi-solid preparations intended for application to skin or mucous membranes. Non-medicated ointments are used as protectants, lubricants, and emollients. Ointment bases used for- ointment preparation are of fourtypes, hydrocarbon bases, absorption bases, water-removable bases, and water-soluble bases. Hydrocarbon bases have emollient properties and are effective as occlusive dressings (e.g., Petrolatum, USP). Absorption bases permit the incorporation of aqueous solutions to form w/o emulsions (e.g., hydrophilic petrolatum and lanolin). Water-removable bases are also o/w emulsions and are water washable (e.g., hydrophilic ointment). Water-soluble bases have no oleaginous component and are referred to as greaseless water-washable bases (e.g., polyethylene glycol ointment). The potential for absorption depends on the choice of the bases, and intended use of the medicament. Appropriate selection of ointment bases is important fordermal therapy. Ointments for rectal preparation (e.g., Tronolane ointment for hemorrhoidal analgesia) and vaginal preparations (e.g., Mycelex-7 ointment as antifungal) are available in the market. Creams are semisolid emulsions with one or more medicinal agents intended for external use.

The so called *vanishing creams* are o/w emulsions with stearic acid and cold creams are w/o emulsions with an oily base. Creams spread more easily than ointments and are preferred by some patients. Gels are semisolid systems with dispersions of small or large molecules in an aqueous vehicle with a gelling agent e.g., high molecular weight Carbopols that are cross-linked polyacrylic acid. Some gels like milk of magnesia or magma has two phases. These behave as thixotropic systems with the viscosity changing due to a gel–sol transition on shaking. Pastes are ointments with large amount of powder levigated into the base and are intended for application to the skin. Pastes are more hygroscopic than ointments and are used to absorb serous secretions. (e.g., zinc oxide paste). Plasters are solid or semisolid masses spread on backing paper, plastic, or fabric.

Non-medicated forms are termed as adhesive plasters while medicated plasters provide a therapeutic effect at the site of application. Some medicated plasters are termed as cataplasm, e.g., ibuprofen and salicylic acid plasters. Transdermal drug delivery systems (TDDS) are used for delivery of actives through the skin into the systemic circulation. Several methods have been used to facilitate the transport of active through the barriers of the skin. Certain absorption enhancers are used to temporarily increase permeability of the skin for increased delivery. More recently, iontophoretic techniques have allowed the delivery of charged chemicals across the skin using an applied electric field (e.g., amino acids and proteins).Sonophoresis or high-frequency ultrasound is also being studied as a means of effectively enhancing trans-dermal delivery of drugs.

Transdermal delivery systems are of two main types the monolithic matrix system that contains the excess drug dispersed in the polymeric matrix and cast into a matrix with a backing layer and frontal membrane, e.g., Estraderm (Novartis). Membrane-controlled transdermal patches contain drug reservoir in the form of a gel or saturated solution of drug with a backing adhesive and a rate controlling membrane e.g., Transderm-Scop (Novartis). Currently, the market is flooded with a variety of transdermal systems for smoke cessation and hormonal delivery patches. More recently efforts are on to develop transmucosal delivery patches.

Other Dosage Forms

Suppositories are solid dosage forms intended for insertion in body cavities like rectum, vagina, and occasionally in the urethra for local or systemic effects. The length, shape, and weight of these depend on the body cavity it is used for. These melt, soften, or dissolve after application depending on the type of suppository base applied. Cocoa butter base suppositories usually melt in contact with the body temperature. Other bases, such as polyethylene glycol, glycerin, and soap based suppositories solubilize. Cocoa butter suppositories are hydrophobic, and dissolve oil soluble drugs but absorption is poor in the aqueous rectal fluids. Thus, better absorption is obtained with water-soluble bases. Rectal suppositories can be used for local (hemorrhoids) or systemic effects. Systemic bioavailability is poor and the amount of drug required is more than oral administration. Vaginal and urethral suppositories are usually used for their local effects (e.g., anti-infectives). Rectal suppositories weigh about 2 g and have varying shapes like bullets and torpedoes. Urethral suppositories are thin pencil- shaped with tapered ends. Vaginal suppositories are globularized and weigh about 4–5 g. Generally absorption from suppository bases rectally is better when the rectum is empty. Particle size of solids plays an important role in absorption. Most importantly rectal absorption allows to bypass the first pass effect. Most suppositories are manufactured by molding from melts or by compression.

Aerosol Dosage Forms

Aerosols are pressurized dosage forms containing one or more active drug dissolved, suspended, or emulsified in a propellant or a mixture of solvent and propellant, which is released on actuation of the valve as a fine dispersion of liquid or solid in a gaseous medium. Aerosols are intended for topical administration; for administration into body cavities; for administration orally or nasally as fine solid particles or liquid mists through the pulmonary airways, nasal passages, or oral cavity (buccal or sublinual). Those that provide an airborne mist are called space sprays; those intended for carrying actives to surface are termed as surface sprays and other are termed foam aerosols. Aerosol consists of product concentrate and the liquefied propellant. The pressure depends on the types and amounts of propellants and the nature and amount of active present. Propellant is a liquefied gas or mixture of liquefied gas, which serves as the solvent, or vehicle. In some cases non-liquefied gases like nitrogen, and carbon dioxide are used. Space aerosols (85% propellant) operate at 30–40 psig at 70°F. Surface aerosols (30–70% propellant) operate between 22–5 5 psig at 70°F. Foam aerosols operate at a slightly higher pressure. Foam aerosols are emulsions of the propellant and product concentrate. Aerosols can be two-phase systems comprising of a solution of drug in liquefied propellant and a vapor phase of propellant/gas.

Some of them are present as three-phase systems, comprising of water-immiscible propellant, an aqueous product concentrate or drug in suspension/emulsion and a vapor phase. Aerosol containers are made from glass (coated and uncoated), tin, aluminum, and stainless steel containers. There are various forms of spray valves and metered valves (for more accurate dosing of potent drug). Oral aerosols are mostly used via the buccal route, e.g., Nitrolingual spray that emits nitroglycerin at a dose of 0.4 mg per metered dose. The respiratory tract offers several advantages for administration of drugs. Inhalation systems should be capable of producing fine particles, usually < 10 μm for effective drug delivery. Inhalation drug delivery has been traditionally used to treat respiratory disease, but in recent times the lung has been used as a portal for administering drugs to the systemic circulation. With their large effective surface area, the lungs offer an attractive route for systemic drugs.

Three main dosage forms, viz. metered dose inhalers (MDIs), dry powder inhalers (DPIs), and nebulizers have gained prominence. Metered dose inhalers are pressurized systems consisting of drug suspension in a propellant and may contain other additives such as surfactants, antioxidants, and solvents, although some solution systems are available. Traditionally MDIs have been formulated using chloroflurocarbons (CFCs). These propellants are now being phased out under the terms of the "Montreal Protocol" due to their ozone depleting potential. This has resulted in an increasing urgency to reformulate existing MDI formulations with alternative hydroflurocarbon (HFC) propellants such as HFC-143a and HFC-227. Formulations using the new propellants have recently won FDA approval. To offer better coordination between actuation and patient inhalation of the emitted dose, several spacer devices are available with marketed MDI formulation. Recent trends in devices include the breath actuated MDI, where the patient inhalation triggers the dose.

Due to the phase out of CFCs and extensive difficulties in reformulating using HFCs, dry powder inhalers, and nebulizers are becoming popular. Dry powder inhalers consist of mixtures of micronized drug and a large particle size carrier (usually lactose). These drug-carrier ordered mixtures are packaged in unit doses (capsules or blisters), as in Spinhaler and Rotahaler or as pure drug bulk powder, which can be metered into single doses. In many instances the patients inhalation maneuver causes the active particles to separate from the carrier in the air stream. More recently, to overcome intra-patient variability in dosing, active DPIs have been designed. In these devices, the patient's breath triggers a deaggregation mechanism, which separates the drug particles from the carrier, which are then inhaled. Newer fine particle generation technologies, such as spray drying and supercritical fluid extraction, are being used to produce fine particles of drug including proteins and peptides for delivery to the deep lung. This can facilitate the use of inhalation delivery systems for systemic drug delivery. Nebulizers generate fine mists from aqueous and non-aqueous drug solutions, using either compressed air or ultra-sonication. Their main disadvantage is that they are bulky and are not portable. Recent developments in this field have focused on the development of battery operated portable devices, which can nebulize aqueous solution containing minimal, or no preservatives.

Pediatric and Geriatric Dosage Forms

Physiology plays an important role in the development and performance of different functions in the body. It is important to determine their consequence on dosage form development. Pediatric dosing is usually determined by weight and age. FDA classifies the pediatric groups into neonates, infant, child, and adolescent. There are several excipients that have been reported to cause adverse reactions, e.g., azo dyes cause bronchoconstriction, lactose may cause prolonged diarrhea and intolerance, and sweeteners such as saccharin are weak carcinogens. Alcohol is a common solvent for most pediatric OTC liquid products. However, limits on the alcohol content of OTC products have been set to minimize toxicity in children. Oral administration is the preferred route for children. However, children younger than 5 years have difficulty swallowing solid tablets. Thus, oral liquid is the most preferred dosage form in pediatric patients. Liquids are often unstable and have short expiration and accurate dosing is difficult. Recently, there has been increased interest in chewable tablets and "*sprinkle*" powders in capsule formulations as they are well received by children with dentition. Rectal administration is not popular because of wide variability in absorption. Pulmonary administration is emerging to be a popular delivery mode for children, but needs to be studied further for systemic effects. Transdermal route may be another area to explore for children, since the stratum corneum is well developed in children as in adults. This may be beneficial as an alternate route for children. Pediatric drug therapy has very few drug delivery systems. There has been some in-roads made with OTC cough and cold products. However, most industries do not have resources to perform separate studies for safety and efficacy in children (smaller consumer than adults) for new chemical entities. Perhaps FDA should take initiatives to provide pharmaceutical companies with returns like tax break or patent extension and specific market for such developmental work especially for life threatening diseases.

Apart from alterations in the pharmacodynamics (PD) and pharmacokinetics (PK), the geriatric population suffers from a number of chronic conditions and physical limitations. Clinical monitoring becomes very important to titer dosing accurately. Most of their PK and PD processes take a down turn. Absorption is slower from the oral cavity. In general, the aged skin is more permeable to water and other chemicals. However, the clearance to the blood stream is lowered thus distribution may not be complete.

Physically, impairment or decline in vision may hinder one's ability for self-medication. Also, swallowing and chewing may be a problem in elderly patients. For example, patients suffering from dry mouth may have difficulty swallowing a tablet or capsule. Similarly, elderly patients who are edentulous (i.e., toothless) are incapable of chewing any tablet dosage form. Although sublingual and buccal tablets are used by the elderly population there is very less emphasis on its effect on bioavailability with aging. Patients with dry mouth condition may feel local irritation with such dosage forms. Capsules like tablets may hinder swallowing and are not advisable for elderly patients. Liquids are easier to swallow, but are usually not packaged as unit dosages. Patients with impaired vision and dexterity may not be able to accurately self-administer the required dose.

The trans-dermal route seems to offer better compliance with elderly patients but bioavailability needs to be determined before using this route. Several alternative dosage forms and packaging techniques are emerging to improve compliance of dosage form in elderly patients. Several types of packaging aids like dosett tray, calender-packs and med packs are used to remind the dosing schedule for elderly patients. Granules of drug may be easy to swallow. They can be mixed with water or food and swallowed easily. Unit dose packs may still be difficult to use for some elderly patients. Effervescent tablets provide an alternative dosage form. These tablets dissolve in water to form a ready-to-use product. The use of an irregular shaped tablet that prevents it from lying flat may be another form that can help patients with impaired dexterity.

Similar to granules the drug may also be presented in the form of a small amount of concentrated solution for the entire dose, e.g., 5 ml Rapamune concentrated oral solution. Such products can be mixed with food or drink. This is similar to the use of a dispersible tablet that forms a uniform stable suspension when dispersed in water. Emerging technology has focussed on newer dosage forms like the use of quick or rapid dissolving technology (RDTs), wherein, the dosage form quickly dissolves in the mouth and rapid absorption of the drug can occur systemically or even from the mouth. Furthermore, compliance in elderly patients has also resulted in the availability of sugar and sodium-free products that are beneficial for such age groups.

New Drug-delivery Technologies

Newer technologies are emerging as we move into the new millenium. These technologies promise to have lots of benefits such as simplifying administration regimens, enhancing compliance, improving clinical benefits, and reducing overall healthcare costs. Rapid-dissolving tablets (RDTs) are designed for patients who have difficulty in swallowing standard tablets/capsules, such as pediatric and geriatric patients. These include the lyophilized foam from Zydis, Flashtab, Orasolv, Wowtabs, and Flashdose. Hydrogel based technology offered by Professor Neil Graham of British Technology group for development of several systems including morphine suppositories. Nanocrystal technology offered by Elan Corporation where the crystalline drug (<400 nm) is thinly coated with a surface modifier to impart physical stability. Liquitard is a liquid taste masking sustained release granules as a suspension and is offered by Eurand America. Inhale Therapeutics offers proprietary technology for pulmonary delivery of proteins and peptides, using innovations in powder processing to develop formulations for deep lung delivery for systemic and local indications. Jago Pharma developed the Geomatrix systems which involves the use of multilayered hydrophilic matrix systems. Several newer excipients are now available as matrices for controlled delivery. These include polysaccharides from Galactomannan such as guargum and locust bean gum. Considerable research efforts have been towards the development of safe and efficient chitosan-based dosage forms. The development of solid-lipid nanoparticles (SLN) have made it possible for delivering drugs with less side-effects, better targeting, and protection from enzymes. Zambon group in Europe has developed Timeclock technology that involves coating solid drug with hrdrophobic surfactant.

Chronotropic drug delivery, which targets delivery to a specific absorption window for local as well as systemic effect. Emisphere technology uses a carrier that binds to drug molecules non-covalently to form a complex. These complexes easily cross the membranes and then dissociate to release the active. Theratech uses the Theriform microprinting technology to develop oral and implantable dosage form for making Microdose tablets. Delsys Corporation has revolutionized their Accudep technology of electrostatic deposition of dry powder to any surface with great accuracy. Labopharm Inc. has developed Contramid technology obtained by cross-linking of high-amylose starch in three dimensional network which is combined with the active. Once in the stomach, the tablet surface turns into a gel and the active diffuses at an even rate. PORT (Programmable Oral Release Technology) is a technology platform to resolve drugs with biopharmaceutical problems. PORT is a capsule based system with opportunity to provide multiple prolonged release of one or more drugs. This technology is applicable to a wide variety of drug classes and can be used to achieve difficult PK profiles, e.g., zero order with burst system. Quadrant Healthcare has engineered micron-sized particles with enhanced stability and PK profiles. Solidose technology is based on chemically modifying oiligosaccharides to make them more hydrophobic. In contact with body fluids they undergo phase change and release the drug. Several self-emulsifying and lipid- based systems have been developed that form micro-emulsions of water-insoluble drugs for oral delivery. DanBiosystems has developed a proprietary Targit technology, which involves enteric coating with azo polymers, which degrade only at specific sites by bacterial enzymes. Ethypharm is another company involved with coating of nano- and micro-particles, using supercritical fluid (CO_2) technology, suited for fragile water-soluble molecules (peptides and proteins). Protarga is another company which is involved in the development of dosage form by covalently attaching fatty acids (docosahexaenoic acid or DHA) to actives to create new compounds that can be taken up by cells targeted for treatment. A lot of focus has been directed to tissue engineering that is used to design biological substitutes or regenerate natural tissues for defective or lost tissues and organs through the use of cells and their scaffolds. Fentanyl Oralet (Abbott labs) is a lollipop that has painkillers used as preoperative sedative. Several forms of intra-vaginal drug delivery systems like Progestasert system and Dinoprostone vaginal insert have been developed. Implants like the levonorgestrel Norplant device that is incorporated as contraceptive on the upper arm. Similarly, Gliadel wafers are implanted in the brain tumor cells.

Non-parenteral dosage forms can be administered by different mechanisms. In recent years there has been a plethora of emerging drug delivery technology companies. Most of these technologies are addressing issues related to unique delivery systems and selectivity of these systems for affected organs or diseases. However, rarely it recognized that improvements in drug therapy are a consequence of not only the new chemical entity but also the combination of active and the delivery system (dosage form). Currently the trend is to develop a delivery system and then look for suitable drug candidates to apply. This needs to be changed to gain understanding of what unmet medical need is the active aimed for, the rate, time and site for the active to be delivered and then provide a suitable delivery system. More emphasis should be made on the improvement of drug effect profile. Thus, the future of drug delivery will depend on how they can contribute to drug therapy for unmet medical needs.

Parenterals

Parenteral is derived from the two words "para" and "enteron" meaning to avoid the intestine. Parenteral articles are defined according to the USP 24/NF19 "as those preparations intended for injection through the skin or other external boundary tissue, rather than through the alimentary canal, so that the active substances they contain are administered using gravity or force directly into a blood vessel, organ, tissue, or lesion. Parenteral products are prepared scrupulously by methods designed to ensure that they meet pharmacopeial requirements for sterility, pyrogens, particulate matter, and other contaminants, and, where appropriate, contain inhibitors of growth of microorganisms. An injection is a preparation intended for parenteral administration and/or for constituting or diluting a parenteral article prior to administration." Parenteral drug administration is an attractive route of administration when oral administration is contraindicated, and it has been traditionally used in institutional settings. With an increasing interest in reducing overall health care costs and with the development of new biotechnologically derived compounds and improved and novel infusion-related technologies, parenteral products have become an important component in the care of patients in hospitals and the home health care setting. In the present article, information will be presented on history and the following: the use of parenterals in health care, the advantages and disadvantages of using parenterals, routes of administration, vascular access devices and infusion sets, types of parenteral products, components of parenteral products, parenteral packaging, convenience and needleless systems, needleless injection, extemporaneous compounding of parenteral products, infusion pumps and devices, and future parenteral dosage forms.

History and Use of parenterals

A detailed history of early parenteral medications can be found in the first edition of this encyclopedia. One of the first historical references to the parenteral administration of a compound was in the late 15th century when a blood transfusion from three young boys was given to Pope Innocent VIII, resulting in the death of all four individuals. These deaths led to a ban in the use of this type of medical treatment, namely an infusion, for several centuries. It was not until the 17th century that studies on the parenteral administration of compounds was first studied in animals. The development of the hypodermic needle and the use of parenterally injected drugs in humans is first reported in the mid-19th century. By the end of this century, there was an increased interest in the use of intravenous administration of glucose and normal saline solutions. Baxter produced the first commercially prepared intravenous solutions in 1931. However, parenteral products and their administration became acceptable and a mainstay in the treatment of patients in the mid 20th century. This could be attributed, in part, to our increased understanding of microbial and viral agents, increased recognition of the dangers associated with parenteral therapy, the development of antibiotics and other drug classes, and the availability of new systems or infusion technologies. In the mid 1960s, many hospitals introduced intravenous admixture services. In the last 20 years, the area of infusion pumps and systems and improved vascular access devices has enabled parenteral therapy to extend beyond the institutional setting to clinics, ambulatory infusion centers, and home health care. In addition, the administration of parenteral drugs is also frequently utilized in basic and clinical research in animals and humans.

In today's health care environment, parenteral products are a key component of therapy for hospitalized patients. Vascular access for parenteral infusion therapy is obtained in the vast majority of hospitalized patients at some point in their therapy. There are very little data as to the use of parenteral products in today's health care environment. It was suggested that 40% of all pharmaceutical dosage forms are administered as a type of injection and that over 350 million units of large volume parenterals and 100 million units of IV admixtures (piggybacks) were used annually in the late 1980s. These numbers have certainly increased since that time with the advent of new drugs and infusion methodologies. Infusion therapy in home health care continues to have a strong market in the United States. While the annual growth rate of home infusion therapy decreased between 1982 and 1993, 29% of acute care hospitals provided or were developing a home health care program. In the current market, home infusion therapy is being integrated into alternative sites, such as ambulatory infusion centers. Due to the rapid and increasing use of parenteral drugs, it is critical for health care providers and scientists to understand the various available dosage forms, specific products, routes of administration, catheter types, and various infusion devices. In addition, company websites are a valuable source of current information, including available parenteral products, infusion sets and ports, devices and infusion pumps.

Advantages and Disadvantages of Parenteral Products

Generally, parenterally administered drugs are advantageous because they can provide rapid and reliable drug systemic effects, long-term drug delivery, and targeted drug delivery. The disadvantages of parenteral products are predominately associated with safety issues related to infection and thrombosis, tissue damage and/or pain upon injection, and the use of requirements for specific equipment, devices, and techniques.

Routes of Administration

The most commonly used routes are intravenous, intramuscular, subcutaneous, and intradermal. Formulations intended for administration into the central nervous system should not include preservatives. For intramuscular, intradermal, and subcutaneous, a single needle and syringe is generally used to administer the drugs. For intravenous and intra-arterial, drugs are administered using vascular access or port devices. Other parenteral routes of administration (e.g., epidural, intra-articular, and intrathecal) usually require specialized delivery sets. In some cases, the specific drug requires a specialized delivery set be utilized due to the dose of the drug or the physicochemical properties of the drug (e.g., nitroglycerin).

Vascular Access Devices and Infusion Sets

Vascular access can be achieved through short peripheral, long dwell peripheral, central lines, and ports. These various devices differ in their insertion, characteristics, dwell time or time they should be in place, and usage and safety features. In peripheral access, the distal veins on the hand and arm are often used, with the basilic and cephalic veins in the arms being the most common site for peripheral infusions. Alternatively, the metacarpal veins can also be utilized. The basic devices are a winged infusion device or the over-the-catheter needle, with needle sizes ranging from 16 to 26 G (20- or 22-gauge being the most common size). These catheters are usually utilized only for 48 h. A midline catheter is usually inserted into a large vein and is intended to be used over a 2- to 4- week period (Richardson). Peripherally inserted central venous catheters (PICC) are designed for long-term infusion therapy up to a year. The devices are inserted into a peripheral vein and threaded so that the tip of the catheter is within the central vascular system. Central venous catheters (CVC) are inserted into the subclavian or jugular vein and threaded until the tip is located in the superior vena cava. The types of central venous catheter are a non-tunneled, Groshong, Hickman, and Brovaic. A non-tunneled CVC can be inserted at the bedside, whereas the Groshan, Hickman, and Brovaic require surgical insertion. Vascular access ports (VAP) are an alternative to central venous access. These devices are surgically implanted usually into the chest wall or arm subcutaneous tissue and are composed of a rigid reservoir with a self-sealing rubber septum, and the tip of the catheter is placed into a central vein. The drug is placed into the reservoir via an injection. A VAP allows repeated, intermittent access and drug delivery (in some cases up to 2000 times), depending upon the size of the needle. Examples of these types of ports include a P.A.S Port (SIMS Deltec), Vital-Port, and BardPort and CathLink.

There are three basic types of intravenous administration: (1) primary set; (2) secondary set; and (3) a volume control set. The basic components of all these sets include a piercing spike (to insert into the bag or bottle), drip chamber and drip orifice, tubing ranging in length from 160 to 250cm (63–

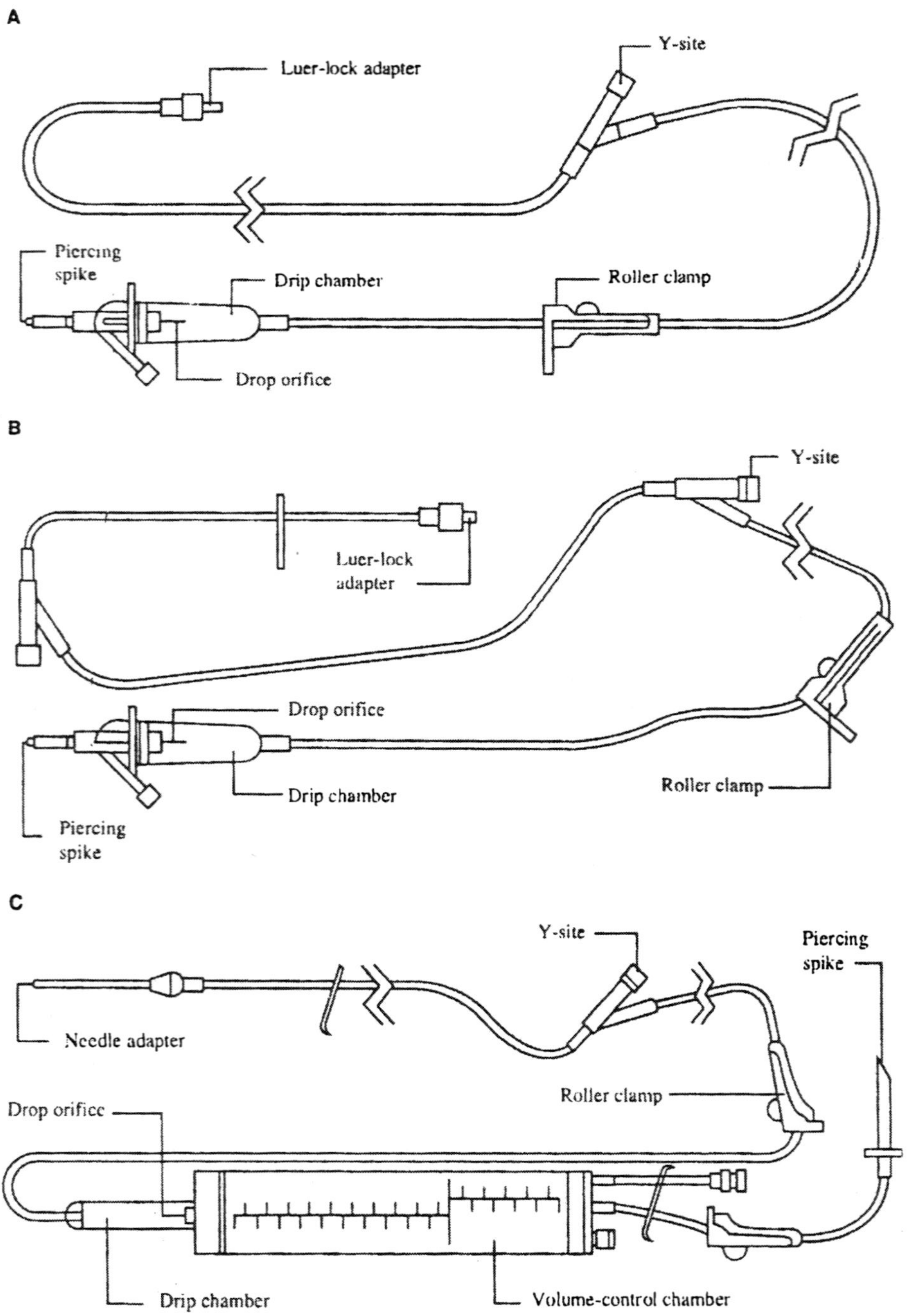

Fig. 5.7. Types of infusion sets used for parenteral therapy: A-primary; B-secondary; and C-volume-controlled infusion sets.

98.58 in.), a roller clamp or other flow control device on the tubing, a Y-site for infusion of other components, an in-line filter (ranging from 0.2 to 170 μm) and leuk-lok adapter to attach to the vascular access device. A primary infusion set is designed to deliver solutions from the parenteral container via gravity. If an additional infusion is needed, the secondary set can be connected to the primary set via one of the Y-sites. A volume control administration set is used to deliver a small amount of solution through the use of the volume chamber. In general, administration sets are classified into macrodrip sets that can deliver 10–20 drops/ml and a microdrip set that delivers drugs at a slower rate of 60 drops/ml.

Types of Parenteral Products

Parenteral products can be divided into two general classes according to the volume of the product. All parenteral products are sterilized and must meet all the requirements for sterility and particulate matter and must be pyrogen-free. They must be prepared using strict sanitation standards in environmentally controlled areas by individuals trained to meet these standards. The injections are overfilled with a small excess over the labeled volume to ensure that the required volume can be obtained from the product. *Small-volume parenterals* (SVP) or injections are 100 ml or less and can be provided as a single- or multidose product. In contrast, large-volume parenterals (LVP) are intended to be used intravenously as a single-dose injection and contain more than 100 ml of solution. SVPs and LVPs are often combined during the extemporaneous preparation of intravenous admixtures, to be discussed later in this article.

The U.S. Pharmacopoeia (USP) classifies injections into five different types. The dosage form selected for a particular drug product is dependent upon the characteristics of the drug molecule (e.g., stability in solution, solubility, and injectability), the desired therapeutic effect of the product (e.g., immediate vs. sustained release), and the desired route of administration. Solutions and some emulsions (e.g., miscible with blood) can be injected via most parenteral routes of administration. Suspensions and solutions that are not miscible with blood (e.g., injections employing oleaginous vehicles) can be administered via intramuscular or subcutaneous injection but should not be given intravenously.

Parenteral products contain excipients such as buffers, solvents, non-aqueous solvents, antimicrobial preservatives, antioxidants, and chelating agents. Coloring agents are prohibited in parenteral products. All excipients must meet compendial standards, and the excipients must not interfere with the efficacy of the product (to be discussed more in detail later in this article). Parenterals are packaged in airtight containers using specific, high quality materials so that they do not interact with the product and to maintain the sterility of the product. For example, the type of glass to be used in a specific parenteral drug product is indicated in the monograph. The types of packaging and containers for SVPs and LVPs will be discussed later in this article.

A SVP product is available for most of the major therapeutic classes of drug. It is often desirable for a manufacturer to provide both an oral and parenteral dosage form for a specific drug product. A "*drug injection*" is a liquid preparation that is composed of drug substances and or solutions. A "drug for injection" is a dry solid that upon the addition of a suitable vehicle (usually a vehicle in which the drug is stable and soluble) provides a solution that conforms to the requirements for an injection. Drugs for injection are often lyophilized or freeze-dried to assist in the reconstitution of the solid. A "*drug injectable emulsion*" is a liquid preparation of a drug or drug substances dissolved in a suitable emulsion vehicle. A "*drug injectable suspension*" is a liquid preparation of solids suspended in a suitable vehicle. A "drug for injectable suspension" is a dry solid (often lyophilized) that is intended, upon the addition of a suitable vehicle, to yield a preparation that in all aspects meets the requirements for an injectable suspension.

LVPs are often administered via intravenous infusion in a large single-dose container. The therapeutic goal of these products is to provide electrolytes, body fluids, and nutrition. These solutions may or may not be isotonic with blood depending upon the concentration of the components, which include sodium chloride, dextrose, mannitol, Ringers (sodium, potassium, calcium, and chloride) and Lactated Ringers (calcium, potassium, sodium, and lactate), sodium bicarbonate, ammonium chloride, sodium lactate, fructose, alcohol, dextran, and amino acids. Other drugs (small volume injectables) are often combined to these LVPs, provided that these two products are compatible during the extemporaneous preparation of intravenous admixtures.

Components of Parenteral Products

Parenteral products are optimized during their development to provide the requisite solubility (per the required dose), stability, and syringeability. In addition, these products must meet the desired requirements for the rate of drug release based upon the dosage form and biopharmaceutical properties. Finally, it is important that parenteral products also be evaluated for their potential to cause tissue damage and/or pain associated with the injection of the formulation. The adjuvants in parenteral products can include solvents, vehicles, cosolvents, buffers, preservatives, antioxidants, inert gases, surfactants, complexation agents, and chelating agents.

It is important to understand the various types of waters used in parenteral products. The most frequently used solvent in parenteral products is Water for Injection, USP, which is not required to be sterile but must be pyrogen-free. In contrast, Sterile Water for Injection, USP is water that has been sterilized, does not include a preservative or antimicrobial agent, is pyrogen-free, and is provided in single containers no larger than 1000 ml. The use of this product is for the reconstitution of other parenteral products, in most cases antibiotics. This product must not be given alone. Bacteriostatic Water for Injection, USP is sterile water that can contain one or more preservative or antimicrobial agent (specified on the label) and is packaged in prefilled syringes or vials that are no larger than 30 ml. It is also used in the reconstitution of SVPs. The limitation with Bacteriostatic Water for Injection, USP is the presence of the antimicrobial agent that is contraindicated in newborns. Other solvents used for parenteral formulations are Sodium Chloride Injection, USP and Bacteriostatic Sodium Chloride Injection, USP, Ringers Injection, USP, and Lactated Ringer's, USP.

Other vehicles may be added to parenteral products if the aqueous solubility is limited. However, these vehicles must be non-toxic, non-sensitizing, and non-irritating. In addition, these solvents must be compatible with the drug and other components in the formulation. Cosolvents often used in parenteral formulations include propylene glycol, ethanol, polyethylene glycols, glycerin, and dimethylacetamide. In addition, fixed vegetable oils, such as peanut, cottonseed, sesame and castor oil, can be used; however the USP provides clear restrictions on their use in parenteral products.

Buffers can also be provided in parenteral formulations to ensure the required pH needed for solubility and/or stability considerations. Other excipients included in parenteral products are preservatives (e.g., benzyl alcohol, ρ-hydroxybenzoate esters, and phenol), antioxidants (e.g., ascorbic acid, sodium bisulfite, sodium metabisulfite, cysteine, and butyl hydroxy anisole), surfactants (e.g., polyoxyethylene sorbitan monooleate), and emulsifying agents (e.g., polysorbates). An inert gas (such as nitrogen) can also be used to enhance drug stability. Stability and solubility can also be enhanced by the addition of complexation and chelating agents such as the ethylenediaminetetraacetic acid salts. For a more detailed list of approved excipients in parenteral products, the reader should consult the monographs within the USP.

Parenteral Packaging

In general, all parenteral products must be manufactured under strict, current good manufacturing processes (cGMP) to ensure the final product is sterile and pyrogen-free. Sterilization is defined as the complete destruction of all living organisms or their spores or the complete removal from the product. Pharmaceutical products can be sterilized by steam sterilization, dry-heat sterilization, filtration sterilization, gas sterilization, and ionizing-radiation sterilization. The USP provides monographs and standards for biological indicators required to test the validity of the sterilization process. These products must also be tested for pyrogens—fever-producing substances that arise from microbial contamination most likely thought to be endotoxins or lipopolysaccharide in the bacterial outer cell membrane.

Injections are provided in either multiple-dose containers or single-dose containers. A multiple-dose container is often a vial that will allow the withdrawal of successive portions of the contents without a change in the strength of the product and while maintaining the sterility. A single-dose product is intended for a single parenteral administration. These products can be an ampul, vial, or a syringe. For some drugs, there are specific double-chambered vials that contain the reconstitution solvent and the powdered drug (e.g., Mix-O-Vial—to be discussed later). Types I, II, and III glass are required for parenteral products and are specified in the individual monograph for a given drug.

Ampuls are utilized for a single dose and, as such, do not require a preservative. However, in many cases, the manufacturer will include a preservative, as the drug formulation is the same for both the ampul and multiple-dose vial. The disadvantages of ampuls are that these containers become contaminated with glass particles when opened and require the use of a syringe to remove the drug solution. A filter needle must be used sometime during the withdrawal of the solution or delivery of the drug solution to a flexible bag or other intravenous solution to ensure the glass is removed from the solution. Ampuls are opened via breaking the neck at a prescored position.

Vials can be used for single or multiple doses. The glass containers are sealed with rubber closures that permit the withdrawal of the drug solution via a syringe. The disadvantage of these systems is associated with ensuring that the drug solution is compatible with the rubber closure. Furthermore, when utilizing vials in the extemporaneous preparation of sterile intravenous admixtures, the health care practitioner must minimize the potential of coring during the introduction of the needle through the rubber seal. Furthermore, there is always the concern of contamination of the solution with repeated withdrawals. The potential for contamination can be minimized by the use of single-dose vials.

Parenteral solutions can also be packaged in syringe dosage forms for a single-dose use. As such, they can be considered a type of convenience container (to be discussed later). The syringe and needle are sterile until opened. They are ideal for emergency situations or the home health care environment.

LVPs are usually provided in glass containers, flexible plastic bags, or semirigid containers. These systems are also classified as open systems (non-vacuum) and closed systems (vacuum). The largest manufacturers of LVPs are Abbott Laboratories, Baxter Healthcare Corporation, and B. Braun.

Glass containers are sealed with a thick rubber disk and a target in the center for the piercing spike. Glass bottles can be either vented with a plastic venting tube or non-vented, thereby requiring either a non-vented administration set or a vented administration set, respectively. The advantages of glass containers for parenterals are that they are easy to sterilize, can be accurately read, and are generally inert and less susceptible to incompatibilities with drugs or leaching of components compared to the plastic flexible intravenous bags. The disadvantage of glass is associated with handling the glass bottles and the potential for breakage.

Plastic intravenous fluid containers were first introduced due to the need to start intravenous therapy while transporting soldiers from the battlefield or triage area to the hospitals. These containers are flexible due to the presence of plasticizers, with the bags being composed of polyvinyl chloride. In contrast, semirigid containers are often composed of polyolefin. The most common manufacturers of intravenous solutions are Abbott Laboratories— Lifecare, Baxter Healthcare—Viaflex, and B. Braun Medical—Excel. The major advantages of plastic flexible bag systems for parenterals are that they do not require the use of a vented administration set as they collapse when empty, and they are less susceptible to breakage. It is also easier to store and transport these bags. The difficulties with these flexible plastic bags for infusions solutions are the potential for incompatibilities of the drug substance with the components in the bag, the potential for the bag to get perforated during its use, thus compromising the sterility of the solution, and the difficulty in reading the volume remaining in the bag. One major concern with the use of flexible plastic bags is the potential for the drug compound to leach out the plasticizers from the systems. Semirigid containers are similar to flexible plastic containers in that they are lightweight and nonbreakable and can be easily transported and stored. These containers are less likely to be perforated during their use. More importantly, these containers do not contain plasticizers and, as such, may be more compatible with drug substances. The disadvantages are related to their similar properties to glass containers, in that they require venting, can be more susceptible to cracking upon extreme changes in temperature, should not be frozen, and do not adapt well for ambulatory care.

Convenience and Needleless Systems

Whereas the compounding and administration of parenteral products and intravenous admixtures continues to be a vital and important component in the care of hospitalized and home health care patients, there is continued interest in easing the preparation, storage, and administration of these products with respect to controlling contamination of the finished product and protecting the health care providers from needle-stick injuries. It is estimated that more than 750,000 needle-stick injuries occur every year. Commonly used convenience and/or needleless systems include premixes, bags, and vial systems, prefilled syringe systems and double-chambered vial systems.

For drugs with suitable stability in intravenous solutions, premixes provide an alternative to the extemporaneous compounding of admixtures. These products are ready to administer, reduce the chance for a medication error, reduce the potential for infection, and decrease the chance for needle-stick injuries. In addition, there is an advantage in using these products with respect to the shelf-life of the product. The stability and storage requirements for each product is provided by the manufacturer. For example, the FirstChoice Premix products (Abbott) in the over- wrap have a shelf-life of, typically, 18 months, whereas those products in which the overwrap has been removed and which are stored at room temperature can be stable for up to 30 days, provided no additional drugs or additives have been added to the product. The diluents in these premix products include 0.45 or 0.9% sodium chloride, 5% dextrose, water for injection, Lactated Ringers, and combinations of these diluents in volumes ranging from 50 to 1000 ml in plastic or glass containers. Drug classes that are currently formulated as premixes include amino acids, dextrans, electrolytes, cardiovascular, anti-infectives, analgesics, and gastrointestinal and respiratory compounds.

The Add-Vantage system and the Mini-Bag Plus system are needleless drug delivery systems composed of a drug-containing vial and a diluent in a flexible plastic intravenous bag. The drug in the vial comes in contact with the diluent, followed by the drug being transferred back into the bag with the vial still attached; this system can then be attached directly to the infusion equipment. In the Add-Vantage system, there are specialized vials and intravenous bags and it is necessary for the health care professional to activate the system by removing the vial stopper, thus allowing the diluent to enter the vial. The Mini-Bag Plus system is designed to allow the simple reconstitution of standard 20 mm powdered drug vials. The Monovial Safety Guard is an integrated, self-contained system that allows the transfer of a reconstitution solution from a flexible intravenous bag or vial into a drug-containing vial, and it is only available for a limited number of drugs.

As such, the advantages of these systems are that the product can be easily stored and quickly prepared without the need for calculations, specialized equipment (such as laminar airflow hoods) or needles and syringes. They also allow for a quicker turnaround time for the first dose. These products enhance safety for both the patient, by reducing the chance for medication errors (e.g., the wrong drug added to the vial, the incorrect amount of drug to be added to the bag, or a product being incorrectly labeled), and for the health care practitioner, by minimizing the chance for a needlestick injury. In addition, these products can help to reduce costs associated with unused doses because the unwrapped products can be redistributed for short periods of time. At present, a variety of therapeutic classes of drugs from anti-infectives to cardiovascular agents to pain management at various doses are available for reconstitution in bags containing 0.9 or 0.45% sodium chloride or 5% dextrose in 50 to 250 ml bags.

Prefilled syringes are composed of drug solutions placed in a syringe with a needle and needleless systems. The advantages of these systems are the convenience associated with a standard dose, less chance for medication error associated with extemporaneous compounding of these syringes, usefulness in emergency situations, and ease of storage. The needle and syringe are sterile until opened. Prefilled syringes are available for drugs ranging from anti-infectives, analgesics, and antipsychotics to antiemetics.

Doubled-chambered vials are advantageous in that the reconstitution solution is separated from the drug until desired by the health care practitioner. The Mix-O-Vial system is a combination of a powdered or lyophilized drug in a lower container and an appropriate diluent with a preservative and other active ingredients in an upper container. Following removal of the dust cover and upon pressure on the top plunger, the solution comes in contact with the drug and the vial is shaken until a solution is obtained. The upper plunger can then be swabbed with a disinfectant and the appropriate volume of drug removed with a needle as in the standard preparation of an intravenous admixture using a vial.

With an increased interest in eliminating needle-stick injuries associated with parenteral drug administration in health care workers, needleless systems are becoming more common in patient care. For example, the Interlink System is designed for needleless access during intravenous therapy. These types of products are available for injection sites, Y-sites, vial adapters, infusion and vein access, syringe products and catheter extension sets. Other needleless catheters and infusion sites include the Introcan Safety IV catheter and the Sifesite injection caps (B. Braun).

Needleless Injection

The concept of needleless injection is not a new one and has been thought about since the 1940s. Current products utilize either spring action or compressed gas (e.g., helium or carbon dioxide) as a propellant to deliver a drug through the skin. These needleless systems offer several advantages. The first potential advantage is reduced pain and anxiety, an advantage for use in children. The second advantage is that needleless injection causes less tissue damage than conventional needles. Finally, a needleless system results in a diffuse pattern of exposure and, therefore, increases surface area and absorption rate. The main disadvantage of this system is unreliability in reference to pain and discomfort and skin characteristics that can influence the amount of drug entering the body. This system has been used to administer vaccines, insulin, and drugs for topical applications (e.g., penile erectile dysfunction) and as a means to deliver DNA for gene therapy.

Extemporaneous Compounding of Parenteral Products

Whereas the presence of the various convenience parenteral products has assisted health care practitioners in safely and accurately delivering drugs to the patients, the extemporaneous compounding of parenteral products continues to be an important component in institutional settings and home health care. Parenteral intravenous admixtures include the withdrawing of the drug solution from an ampul(s) or vial(s) and placing it into various large volume solutions, syringe dosage forms for patients, total parenteral nutrition solutions and cassettes, or other delivery systems for home health care patients. The American Society of Health-System Pharmacists, the National Association of Boards of Pharmacy, and the USP provide practitioners with useful technical assistance bulletins, rules, and standards for the preparation of parenteral products. The concerns associated with the extemporaneous preparation of parenteral products are maintaining sterility of the products through proper aseptic techniques, calculating and providing the correct dosage, preventing or reducing drug–drug, drug–solution, or drug–container incompatibilities during the preparation or administration of the product, and maintaining and providing drug stability and quality control.

The majority of extemporaneous parenteral products are prepared by pharmacists working in hospitals, home health care, or long-term care facilities. These products must be prepared using aseptic technique and using the appropriate supplies (e.g., syringes, needles, and filter needles, and caps) and equipment (Class 100 laminar airflow hoods enclosed within a class 10,000 clean room). Aseptic technique which differs from sterilization, is a process by which an individual can manipulate sterile products and containers to prevent microbial contamination. Pharmacists and other personnel involved in the extemporaneous preparation of parenteral products require special knowledge and training and should receive additional training and education on a routine basis to ensure proper aseptic techniques are being followed consistently. In addition, these individuals must be able to perform the required calculations (e.g., dosing, milliequivalents, milliosmoles, and powder volume) needed to prepare intravenous admixtures. Equally important to the safe preparation of intravenous admixtures is an understanding of general principles and concepts related to drug and solution or container incompatibilities and to drug stability and also specific knowledge as to whether a specific drug is compatible or stable with another drug, solution, or container.

Infusion Pumps and Devices

Infusion pumps and devices are an essential component to the delivery of parenteral drugs, particularly those given by the intravenous route. For drugs that are administered via intravenous infusion, there are two forces that control fluid flow: (1) the pressure of an active force of the liquid that can be generated via gravity flow (viz., hydrostatic pressure) or mechanically via a positive pressure pump and (2) resistance, or an opposing force, that is generated via the infusion sets, a vascular access device and/or blood vessels. The maximum flow rate will depend upon the ratio of the change in pressure exerted by the liquid to that of the change in resistance.

An infusion control device (ICD) is a device that maintains a constant infusion rate in a gravity flow system (controller) or via a positive pressure pump. A positive pressure pump is a device that provides mechanical pressure (2–12 psi) to overcome the resistance to flow in the vessels. The types of positive pressure pumps are categorized according to how they deliver the solution and their degree of precision in the flow rate. Positive pressure pumps include peristaltic pumps, cassette pumps, syringe pumps, non-electric or disposable pumps, and patient-controlled analgesic pumps (PCA). Syringe pumps are usually the most accurate pumps, with flow variances at 2% or less. Non-electric or disposable syringe and PCA pumps are useful for ambulatory care. PCA pumps are very useful for the parenteral administration of analgesics (viz., morphine) and can be easily programmed to deliver bolus doses and provide a dosing history.

Non-electric or disposable pumps are lightweight, and the solution is delivered based upon a vacuum or through the generation of a gas in the system. A recent consensus development conference on the safety, cost, simplicity of use, and training of intravenous drug delivery systems, focusing on acute care and non-electronic devices, reviewed the use of manufacturer-prepared (e.g., premixed or frozen products), point-of-care activated systems (manufacturer-prepared products that require the drug and diluent to be mixed at the point of care), pharmacy-based intravenous admixture, intravenous push medications in prepared or premade syringes, augmented iv push systems (syringe pumps), and volume control chambers. Manufacturer-prepared products, point-of-care activated products, and pharmacy-based intravenous admixture programs were recommended as being superior intravenous drug delivery systems, with the manufactured products being considered the safest systems due to the quality assurance in the preparation of these products.

Future Parenteral Dosage Forms

Current research is leading to newer types of parenteral dosage forms that will be useful for both immediate and sustained drug delivery, for systemic and targeted drug delivery, and for the delivery of small molecules and macromolecules (e.g., proteins, peptides, and DNA). There has been an increased interest in developing a wide variety of particulate drug delivery systems for parenteral products, which have included liposomes or other phospholipid vesicles, microspheres, microcapsules, nanoparticles, or microemulsions. The development of new biomaterials, such as the linear and branched biodegradable polyesters, has increased the interest in the development of these systems for microsphere formulations for parenteral drugs. An advantage is that drug molecules can be incorporated into these particulate carriers, and, as such, the rate of drug release can be modified, cellular uptake can be facilitated, or the degree of tissue damage or pain can be reduced.

Microemulsions, defined as clear solutions obtained by tritrating normal coarse oil-in-water emulsions with a medium chain alcohol and composed of the non-polar phase, surfactant and cosurfactant, appear to be potentially useful for parenteral administration, as these are clear and stable formulations that are able to be filtered and might besuitable for intravenous administration. In addition, other researchers are investigating in situ forming gel or implants that can be easily injected intramuscularly or subcutaneously and that result in the formation of a depot at the site of injection with the potential to modify or extend the release of the drug or macromolecule.

Parenteral products will continue to play a vital role in the treatment of patients when the oral route is contraindicated, when it is necessary to carefully control drug blood levels in response to therapeutic effects, when a prolonged therapeutic effect is needed through a long-acting injectable, or when a drug effect is to be targeted to a specific tissue or organ, to name a few instances. Advances in the technology required for the administration of parenteral dosage forms in the last 100 years have expanded their clinical uses for in-patient and out-patient settings. In addition, there is improved convenience and safety for the health care providers who prepare and administer these products. It seems likely that more parenteral dosage forms will become available in the marketplace in response to the compounds being developed through biotechnology.

6

MOLECULAR GENE THERAPY

At the dawn of the twenty-first century, cancer and cardiovascular disease are the first causes of mortality and the focus of considerable attention and mobilization of financial and human resources. Increased understanding of pathogenesis and its underlying molecular processes has led to proven or investigational therapies, such as gene therapy. The concept of gene therapy (and gene transfer) first appeared in the 1960s when the structure of DNA was defined, and much effort has since been devoted to developing suitable strategies. Although gene therapy was initially considered primarily in terms of treatment of genetic disease, the concept has evolved, and now the two main fields of gene therapy are cancer and cardiovascular disease. Gene therapy consists of overexpressing a functional gene, replacing a mutated gene, or expressing an exogenous gene with the aim of correcting a malfunction, inducing an immune response, or stimulating angiogenesis. Currently, stem cell research is generating new hope in the field of cell therapy, with which gene transfer is increasingly associated. The first challenge was to transfer DNA into cells, and *in vitro* and *in vivo* gene transfer techniques were developed: mechanical (gene gun), physical (calcium phosphate precipitation), chemical (synthetic gene transfer agents), and biological (viruses). Some of these techniques are commonly used, at least *in vitro*, and have been evaluated in clinical trials, whereas others are currently under investigation. Clinical testing is contingent on technical quality and reproducibility and finding answers to a variety of questions.

- Does the vector or gene transfer procedure work as expected? Optimally?
- Is the preparation optimal?
- What about the route of transfer?
- What is the fate of the nucleic acid and of the vector (if any)?
- When do the vector and nucleic acid dissociate?
- Does the nucleic acid reach its target (and only its target)?
- Does the procedure have any deleterious effect?
- How long is it before expression occurs?
- How long does the transgene persist in the targeted cell or organ?
- How long is transgene expression effective?

Before addressing these questions, it is first essential to ensure that the nucleic acid is transferred into the cell (or organ) and is active. Transfer can be observed *in vitro* by means of microscopy or electron microscopy. Using nucleic acid probes tagged with gold particles, it is possible to observe the presence of a DNA sequence. Direct labeling is also possible using radionuclides, such as phosphorus 32, and is mostly applied *in vivo* in animal models because of its low resolution. Direct labeling is sometimes impractical, so indirect labeling has been developed. Staining techniques have been improved in parallel.

Although imaging approaches can be used to observe, understand, and document all phenomena involved in gene transfer, many are destructive or "*invasive*" and often require sacrifice of the animal, as in all histopathological, immunohistological, and immunofluorescent techniques. These techniques yield information that is valuable but that only offers a snapshot of a particular moment in time: Researchers are usually interested in a longer-term image of induced phenomena. The use of several groups of the same animal species to obtain this longer-term image is not really satisfying, and so noninvasive techniques tend to replace invasive or destructive ones. These noninvasive techniques can track processes in a single group of animals and have the ethical advantage that they reduce the number of animals used. Also, invasive approaches can be applied to *in vitro* and *in vivo* research experiments, but not to clinical studies, which may explain why we lack information on the fate of gene transfer agents and transgenes in humans. This technological drawback may be partially responsible for the slowness with which gene therapy is being transferred from the lab bench to the bedside.

The most studied imaging methods are positron emission tomography (PET), single-photon emission (computed) tomography (SPE (C)T), bioluminescence, magnetic resonance imaging (MRI), and gamma imaging. Whereas TEP, SPECT, MRI, and gamma imaging are easily performed on animals, bioluminescence is largely limited because of tissue absorption, with a 90% decrease in signal for each centimeter of tissue. Given this limitation, it is clear that better reporter proteins and reporter genes are needed. Optical imaging is usually performed with proteins that emit green light [luciferase or green fluorescent protein (GFP)], and a shift toward red or near-infrared emission is considered to restrict this absorption and allow the signal to leave the animal's body. Bioluminescence usually yields just planar information, but never devices give 3D information. One technique combines laser scanning, which defines the animal's topography, and filters to select the emitted photons (different wavelengths). Software is used to reconstruct a 3D image of the animal. In another, tomographic, approach, a charge-coupled device (CCD) camera rotates around the animal giving whole-body information on photon emission.

Improvments in molecular biology also exists in the MRI field. The ferritin reporter gene was developed for use with MRI. Overexpression of the transgene in the modified cells (various methods of gene transfer are possible) leads to intracellular ferritin excess and iron entrapment. Ferritin associates with iron, which accumulates (aggregates) in the cell as nanomagnets that can be imaged by MRI. Initially, the very common reporter gene beta-galactosidase was used for MRI The paramagnetic ion is "blocked" using a galactopyrannoside screen and so is not accessible to water. When the reporter gene beta-galactosidase is expressed, its enzymatic activity alters the galactopyrannoside structure and frees the paramagnetic ion, which can then be imaged by MRI. Another approach for MRI uses a reporter gene that encodes a membrane transferrin receptor. The transgene receptor is modified to be resistant to downregulation, so the receptor is largely overexpressed in comparison with untransfected cells. Internalization of super-paramagnetic structures (such as MION) conjugated to transferrin is increased in modified cells.

As noted above, gene transfer is increasingly associated with cell therapy. Imaging can provide information on the fate of the reinfused modified cells and also on the expression of the transgene or the corrected gene. By loading the cells of interest with contrast agents, it is possible to use MRI to track their movements through the animal's body. The exitation devoted to quantum dots also spreads to cell therapy. Indeed, recently the fate of cells reinjected to mice was studied after labeling those cells by means of self-illuminating quantum dots. It was then possible to image the cells migration by fluorescence imaging *in vivo*.

In vitro Imaging Studies

Characterization of Gene Transfer Agents

Structure

Unless DNA is transferred by a physical method, it is necessary to generate a structure able to carry the nucleic acid. When virus capsid or synthetic molecules are involved, they must be characterized physically to allow rational studies on how they ensure vectorization. The structures of gene transfer agents have to be defined to understand how they interact or associate with other components. Visualization of the structures alone is currently possible only by microscopy. Classically, transmission electron microscopy (TEM) is performed after negative staining with uranyl acetate. Vector characterization is frequently combined with characterization of the "*nucleic acid-vector*" association. TEM is also used, for example, to confirm that the DNA has intertwined with the polymer assembly. Atomic force microscopy is a relatively new tool that enables the visualization of nanostructures. It will probably give much information on the structures obtained according to the preparation way and also on the association of the nucleic acid with its vector.

Nucleic acid—Vector interaction and kinetics

One way to confirm that the vector interacts with or encapsulates the nucleic acid is to visualize the interaction. Scanning force microscopy has shown that polymers and cationic lipids interact with DNA in a similar way. TEM has been used to observed this kind of interaction between DNA and synthetic gene transfer agents. Although fluorescence resonance energy transfer (FRET) data are usually represented graphically, it is theoretically possible to obtain images of the fusion events using fluorescence microscopy, which shows how lipids used to prepare lipoplexes interact and mix and also gives information on the capacity of a structure to interact with a membrane model representing the cells.

Gene Transfer Agent Pathways: Localization and Persistence of the Transgene at its Target

To improve gene transfer agents, we need to know which hurdles they will have to overcome. Early studies of intracellular trafficking of the vectors were performed by means of electron microscopy.

Transmission electron microscopy

To observe polyplexes, thin cell sections are negatively stained using uranyl acetate and observed by TEM, which can track gene transfer agents. Existing structures can be observed, but when the polymer dissociates, nothing is visible any more. To observe the nucleic acid either free or associated with its vectors, a labeling using gold-labeled probes can be used. The nucleic acid sequence is recognized by a probe that has been tagged with gold particles. The intracellular progression of the nucleic acid can thus be visualized.

Fluorescence microscopy

This microscopic approach is used to study the trafficking of either the vector or the nucleic acid. By a fluorescent labeling of the structure of interest (with fluorochrome such as FITC or TRITC), it is possible to visualize the internalization and trafficking processes using fluorescence microscopy or confocal microscopy. Using this approach, Midoux's group studied the internalization of polyplexes in HepG2 cells. An interest of this last technique is that both the vector and the nucleic acid can be labeled. The complex evolution (and its disruption) can be observed.

Magnetic resonance imaging

MRI can be used to track complexes during transfection even at the cellular level. MRI microscopy achieves a resolution of about 1 μm. It is based on the co-complexation of the DNA and the contrast agents with a cationic polymer (theoretically, it is also possible with all cationic gene transfer agents). By adding selective molecules, it is possible to target specific cells. A gadolinium derivative is used to follow the fate of the complex (DNA polymer) within the cell. This real-time visualization reveals only the contrast agent aggregates. No information is given on the organization of the visualized structure, and it is not possible to say whether or when the complexes have been disrupted.

Evaluation of Gene Transfer Efficiency

Given how hard it is to demonstrate the functional activity of genes, a nucleic acid delivery system is usually developed using reporter genes encoding proteins that are easily detected through enzymatic reaction or their intrinsic fluorescence.

Fluorescence microscopy

To ensure that a delivery system or a vector efficiently transfers a nucleic acid into a cell, the easiest approach is to use a reporter gene encoding a protein that can be visualized directly. Reporter genes such as GFP or its new derivatives RFP (red) or BFP (blue) are satisfying because gene expression can be easily visualized by fluorescence microscopy. Moreover, by using a fusion protein, this approach not only reveals expres-sion but also defines cellular localization, particularly when using confocal microscopy. Indirect visualization can also be performed using a nucleic acid that encodes a tagged protein. By incubating the cells with a fluorescent ligand that specifically forms a covalent bond with the tagged protein, the transfected cells appears fluorescent.

Bioluminescence

The bioluminescence approach is not frequently used for *in vitro* studies because of the scarcity of the equipment required. The classic reporter gene luciferase can be used to visualize changes in cells, which is of particular interest when working with a nucleic acid that encodes both luciferase and its substrate, luciferin.

Magnetic resonance imaging

When used with MRI, classic contrast agents can track complexes but give no information on gene expression, which is why new reporter genes were developed to modify and hence activate contrast agents, including the gene-encoding ferritin, transfer agents, and enzymes that enable "smart" MRI contrast agent activation. These smart contrast agents are prepared in a weak relaxivity state. When they enter a cell genetically modified by gene transfer, they are transformed into a strong relaxivity state, which is the case of EGad, a gadolinium complex. When Egad interacts with â-galactosidase, a widely used reporter protein, the Egad chelate is disrupted and the relaxation properties of gadolinium can be imaged. All these MRI approaches applied to cells and to animal models are potentially applicable to humans. MRI is particularly interesting because it gives real-time information potentially at high resolution.

In Vivo Imaging Experiments

Imaging Biodistribution of Gene Transfer Agents

It is essential to study the biodistribution of components involved in gene transfer (virus, synthetic vector, or nucleic acid) to identify all *in vivo* barriers. This study indicates what proportion of the administered dose actually reaches the target, as well as any unexpected localizations (according to the quantity at each site) or blocking sites, which is of particular interest because it allows prediction of the dose that will produce a significant therapeutic effect. Biodistribution studies indicate the time when the nucleic acid is released from its vector. Using markers specific to each component (by labeling or conjugating), it is possible to follow both of them separately and also to observe their separation and fate (i.e., their elimination route and metabolism). The most frequently used approach is direct, in which a radionuclide (usually a β-emitter) is used to label the different components. Indirect studies are also possible, such as the use of markers that are supposed to mimic the behavior of the studied molecules. Invasive imaging methods are used less frequently. In some, the compounds involved are radiolabeled and administered before sacrifice of the animal. The animal's body is thinly sectioned using a cryomicrotome and visualization is done either by classic autoradiography or phosphorus imaging. Gene vectors may also be labeled with fluorescent markers and visualized on microsections. As a result of whole-body dilution, this approach is essentially used to pinpoint a component in the cells of a defined organ, after localization by scintigraphy or autoradiography. Although invasive approaches have been widely used, live imaging is now largely preferred, mainly using the methods described below.

Radioisotopic imaging

Radioisotopic imaging (using γ-emitters) efficiently tracks the distribution of viral and nonviral vectors. In these two cases, the adenovirus and the GLB43 lipid vector were labeled with ^{99m}Tc pertechnetate using a stannous tin procedure. Although most available devices give planar imaging, this approach is quantitative. Scintigraphic imaging can be applied to all kinds of animals and also to humans (depending on the radioactive dose). The method used to label the vector is not always suitable for the nucleic acid, as nucleic acid chelation may inhibit its expression. It is, therefore, necessary to choose between information on expression and on location.

Magnetic resonance imaging

MRI is a multivalent approach that also predicts gene transfer efficiency (i.e., whether the transgene actually reached the targeted site). The transgene pathway can be mimicked using a contrast agent, which is administered as the nucleic acid would have been (i.e., associated with a gene vector or directly injected into the targeted tissue). Thus, a gene transfer approach can also be validated by MRI. Moreover, as MRI visualizes tissues and organs, any deleterious effects after gene transfer can be monitored.

Imaging Gene Transfer Efficacy

The sites of gene transfer clearly must be defined whatever the animal model used or clinical application. For most applications, a specific target is considered. Different administration routes will result in particular expression levels and accuracy of targeting. Direct visualization on thin sections is a common approach in which immunofluorescent probes of the expressed protein are used to study transgene expression. For example, Bartoli et al. visualized the transgenic protein (α-sarcoglycan) by immunohistochemistry using a secondary antibody conjugated to the fluorochrome Alexa488 in animal models of muscular dystrophies. Animal care and ethical issues are of increasing importance even in research, and so when suitable technology is available, it is preferable to use noninvasive methods to study gene transfer. Tomography is useful in this regard as it gives information on gene expression in terms of time lag, duration, magnitude, and location.

Bioluminescence

Since a pioneering 1998 study of bioluminescence in living mammals, bioluminescence technology has advanced greatly and is probably now the most accessible and common approach to *in vivo* imaging. It is, however, limited by the data acquisition, as the most frequently used devices equipped with a CCD camera do not give tomographic information (because of the cost of the tomographic apparatus) and the main part of the emitted light is absorbed by the tissues. Moreover, this absorption depends on tissue type and depth, so it is difficult to extrapolate the results from one animal to another. Another limitation is the diffusion of the substrate. In most cases, the luciferase substrate is injected intraperitoneally. If the transfected site is less accessible because of disease or another cause, the substrate concentration is reduced locally, as is the luminescent signal. This bias can be prevented by using a genetic construction that simultaneously expresses both luciferase and its substrate.

New tomographic devices based on bioluminescence are able to generate a 3D reconstruction, using software to calculate photon absorption for the various tissues. Two advantages accrue from this ability: First, this approach is quantitative and, second, it more precisely localizes the source(s) of luminescence induced by the gene transfer procedure. Although bioluminescence techniques are evolving, they are still only applicable to small animals. The hurdles inherent to this imaging approach and to the use of such reporter genes prevent its application to humans.

Fluorescence

Most bioluminescence imaging devices are also equipped for fluorescence imaging. Fluorescent markers are less sensitive than bioluminescent ones and so are used less. Most of the frequently used reporters emit at a wavelength similar to that of natural molecules, particularly GFP and DsRed. The background is also high with these probes, so few markers are wholly satisfying. However, whole-body fluorescence imaging has been used to visualize gene expression.

Positron emission tomography

PET can be used to study gene transfer expression in living animals. It has a satisfactory resolution (around 1 mm) for definition of organ targeting and, above all, gives a quantitative signal. The most commonly used positron-emitting radioisotopes are ^{18}F, ^{15}O, ^{13}N, and ^{11}C. PET imaging is used diagnostically in humans to monitor function or localize tumors. Its potential has been progressively enhanced and the increased resolution of microPET methods enables imaging in small laboratory animals. The three main PET approaches to *in vivo* imaging involve an intracellular enzyme-encoding reporter gene, a membrane receptor-encoding reporter gene, or a membrane transporter-encoding reporter gene.

The enzyme approach consists of a genetic modification using an enzyme-encoding reporter gene, usually encoding an HSV-tk mutant (HSV1-sr39tk). When the genetic modification is performed, the neo-synthesized enzyme is able to phosphorylate uracil derivatives such as [^{124}I]FIAU and acycloguanosine derivatives such as [^{18}F]FHBG. The phosphorylated substrate is unable to leave the cell and the intracellular accumulation of radiolabeled molecules generates a detectable signal. Using the reporter gene HSV-tk, a significant correlation has been demonstrated in rats (after adenovirus gene transfer) between the transgene expression and tissue accumulation of the reporter probe [^{18}F] FGCV.

The receptor approach consists of a genetic modification using a reporter gene encoding a receptor, usually the dopamine D2 receptor or the SSTr2 receptor. Using positron-emitting labeled probes that specifically target the receptor, it is possible to identify the sites where the genetic modification occurred. The transporter PET strategy consists of modifying the cells of interest with a gene that encodes a transporter able to generate intracellular accumulation of a radiolabeled reporter probe. The sodium iodide symporter (NIS) is one of the most used transporters in this application. Using sequences that enable simultaneous expression of two genes (such as IRES), it is theoretically possible to define expression of the gene of interest in terms of location, magnitude, and duration by studying reporter gene expression.

Magnetic resonance imaging

MRI can be used to assess gene transfer expression, which is visualized and localized in the animal's body through planar or spatial (2D or 3D) images. *In vivo* transgene expression can be observed in real time, thereby giving information on the time lag between gene transfer and gene expression. MRI has the great advantage of visualizing surrounding tissues. It is therefore possible not only to assess gene transfer efficiency but also any deleterious (inflammation, necrosis, and so on) or beneficial (such as tumor regression) effects. Any effects of gene transfer are defined early and at high resolution and sensitivity, whatever the gene transfer process adopted. MRI can be used for whole- body imaging of gene expression. In mouse brain, gene expression can be monitored after stereotaxic injection of recombinant adenovirus that encodes ferritin. The relevance of gene transfer to rat muscle by electrotransfer has also been documented by MRI. Expression of the reporter gene luciferase was well correlated with contrast agent entrapment (Gd-DOTA) when administered by the same procedure. Coadministration of the contrast agent and the reporter gene does not modify reporter gene expression. So, once the experimental parameters have been optimized, MRI can be used to indirectly evaluate gene transfer expression and location.

Advantages and Drawbacks of Imaging Approaches

Gene transfer approaches are not only used to study gene transfer agents. Some reporter genes introduce tags into *ex vivo* modified cells, thereby allowing imaging of their fate (migration, homing, and so on). To complete the gene transfer studies, safety can be studied in animal models by using ultrasound or X-ray computed tomography to document any tissue or organ alteration. Planar imaging is valuable and easy to perform, but does not really reflect the true situation, as photon emission depends on tissue type and depth. Moreover, emission is multidirectional, whereas collection is planar, which leads to a large loss of information. PET is currently only used to characterize gene expression (time lag, level, and duration), which may seem quite limiting with regard to the questions initially posed. Biodistribution studies using PET can be imagined in which a positron emitter is used to label vectors (either viral or nonviral) or the nucleic acid. Such an approach will be contingent on efficient labeling that does not alter the various components.

MRI of cells or small biological samples requires high magnetic fields (often up to 11.7 T), and the requisite equipment is limited in availability because of its prohibitive cost. Experimentally, MRI is very satisfying because the signal obtained not only yields an image but also provides information on sample content (MR spectroscopy). This twofold analysis will become increasingly powerful as higher magnetic field strengths are used. MRI will soon be able to give information simultaneously on changes in structure (by imaging) and in chemical composition (by spectroscopy) of the targeted site.

Bioluminescence devices are also able to give 3D images, but quantification is indirect and based on mathematical treatment that involves considerable extrapolation. Advances in gene transfer have gone hand in hand with developments in the imaging technologies used to assess transfer efficiency. In gene expression studies, the most frequently used imaging methods are optical (particularly bioluminescence) and nuclear (PET). Whereas optical approaches are limited by the tissue absorption of the signal, the nuclear approach suffers from insufficient resolution. Magnetic resonance offers high resolution, but higher magnetic fields and more relevant and sensitive probes are needed.

No single imaging method can fulfill all research requirements. For large-scale screening or preliminary validation of a new approach, the least expensive method is to be preferred. More costly methods can be applied once the gene transfer approach has been shown to be feasible for gene therapy. Some molecular systems enable two imaging strategies. Using a fusion protein encoding both luciferase and an HSVtk enzyme, gene transfer has been documented using optical bioluminescence and PET. Such fusion proteins are very promising and current improvements might be of great value in gene transfer imaging. An alternative to these fusion proteins is to use two reporter genes (delivered by the same route) to enable a combination of methods, such as PET and fluorescence imaging. Reporter genes may also be coupled with a therapeutic gene through an IRES sequence to monitor modified cells after subcutaneous injection in the mouse. This approach visualizes where expression occurs and its therapeutic effects. But what of functional changes induced by the reporter gene? In the case of PET, three approaches can be envisioned, involving enzymes, receptors, or transporters. How might these proteins impact on cell function? Is therapeutic gene expression really representative of the effects in normal conditions? And how reliable a picture of reality is given by imaging techniques? Proposed solutions to such outstanding questions may be interesting in research terms but are not always appropriate in a clinical setting. It seems best to tackle these problems by comparing and combining data from various imaging approaches.

7

ANTIBACTERIAL DRUG DISCOVERY

More than half a century ago, a revolution in the field of modern medicine was ushered in by the discovery of penicillin, the first in a series of antibiotics that fought bacterial infections with unprecedented success. Over the following decades, numerous drugs with progressively higher potency and broader spectrum of antibacterial activity were introduced, leading to the belief that infectious diseases caused by bacteria no longer posed a major threat to human health, especially in the developed world. However, there have been several recent developments that call for a more cautious view. First, it is increasingly clear that bacteria are remarkably adept at becoming resistant, not only to currently utilized antibacterial drugs, but also to many of their structural analogs. Second, certain bacterial species with intrinsic resistance to multiple drugs are causing infections with an increasing frequency. Third, changes in demographics are leading to an increase in the number of people with impaired immunity to bacterial infections. Together, these factors are encouraging renewed efforts toward the discovery and development of new antibacterial drugs.

In light of the fact that effective inhibition of bacterial enzymes is a well- known mechanism by which several currently available drugs elicit their antibacterial activity, enzymes continue to draw attention as potential targets for new antibacterial compounds. Currently, several approaches are being pursued to study and utilize enzymes for the purpose of antibacterial drug discovery. First, genomic approaches are being used to discover previously unknown enzymes that could serve as potential targets. Second, known enzymes, yet to be utilized as targets, are being studied with the goal of identifying inhibitors that could be developed into potential antibacterial drugs. Third, enzyme targets for known classes of drugs are being studied with renewed interest to gain further insight into their molecular mechanisms of action and structure–activity relationships (SAR) in order to develop newer inhibitors with higher potency, altered spectrum of activity, superior pharmacokinetic properties, or lower toxicity profiles. Finally, enzymes involved in the development of resistance to currently available antibacterial agents are being studied to develop inhibitors that could help existing drugs circumvent bacterial resistance. To focus on the approaches discussed above, the following two sections of this chapter will discuss specific examples without attempting to include all the enzymes that are, or could be, potential targets of antibacterial drug discovery. The first section will focus on examples to discuss the biochemical background that forms the rationale for choosing certain enzymes as targets. The next section will then focus on examples of the methodologies used and recent progress made toward discovering inhibitors and antibacterial leads. Although enzymes also play important roles in down-stream drug development issues such as toxicity, metabolism, and drug–drug interactions, this chapter will be limited to the study of enzymes in antibacterial drug discovery efforts

Bacterial Enzyme Tagets: Biochemical Background

Unknown Enzymes as New Targets

With the advent of genomic and proteomic technologies, it is now possible to simultaneously identify numerous genes and their protein and enzyme products that could be potential targets for new antibacterial compounds. With the DNA sequence of a number of bacterial genomes being known, it is possible to identify proteins and enzymes that could serve as targets for new antibacterial agents with different goals. Enzymes that are ubiquitous in bacteria could be targeted to identify potential inhibitors with broad-spectrum applications, while enzymes that are specific to particular pathogens could be targeted for inhibitors with narrow-spectrum applications. In many cases, enzyme functions can be predicted from homology analyses. In fact, DNA sequence sampling has been effectively used to identify new enzymes as potential targets in *Streptococcus pneumoniae*. While several genomics-based approaches have been described and reviewed elsewhere, it is particularly interesting to note that certain functional genomic approaches combine molecular genetics with whole-cell inhibition of enzymes that lead to cell growth inhibition. These approaches could not only identify potential targets, but also their potential inhibitors. The advantages of this approach include identifying those enzymes whose inhibition results in bacterial cell growth inhibition. Bacterial enzymes and protein factors that are specifically expressed *in vivo* during infection are also drawing special attention. The *in vivo* expression technology (IVET) and similar approaches have the potential advantage of identifying enzymes whose inhibitors could lead to drugs that interfere with the molecular events involved in bacterial pathogenesis and virulence, thereby leading to potentially novel antibacterial agents with unique mechanism(s) of action.

Known Enzymes as New Targets

Several enzymes in this category are of significant interest. Many of these enzymes have been cloned, overexpressed, purified, and biochemically characterized. This facilitates the development of high-throughput screens as well as structure-function-based drug design efforts. In most cases, the enzymes catalyze biochemical reactions involved in pathways that are known to be essential for bacterial survival. For example, lipid A is an essential component of the outer membrane of Gram-negative bacteria and is essential for bacterial growth. Recently, inhibition of a deacetylase, involved in the biosynthesis of lipid A, has been exploited to discover potent inhibitors with *in vitro* and *in vivo* antibacterial activity. Removal of N-formyl groups from nascent bacterial polypeptides is an essential step in bacterial protein synthesis. Bacterial peptide deformylases are responsible for this activity and are being studied to identify inhibitors. Bacterial signal peptidases are members of the serine protease class of enzymes and are responsible for the proteolytic removal of N-terminal signal peptides from pre-proteins that are secreted. Recently, the *spsB* gene, coding for the type I signal peptidase in *Staphylococcus aureus*, has been shown to be essential for bacterial growth. Signal peptidases are ubiquitous in Gram-positive and Gram-negative bacteria and appear to be significantly different from their eukaryotic counterparts, based on DNA sequences. Thus, bacterial signal peptidases are considered attractive targets for new antibacterial agents.

While there are several known inhibitors of bacterial cell wall biosynthesis with antibacterial activity, it is important to point out that numerous enzymes are involved in this pathway. For example, the *murA*, *murB*, *murG*, and *mraY* gene products are enzymes involved in peptidoglycan synthesis in *Escherichia coli* and are being studied as potential targets for new antibacterial agents. Other enzymes involved in bacterial cell wall synthesis, such as the D-alanine-D-alanine ligase and glucosamine 6-phosphate synthase, are also being studied.

Known classes of enzymes that are involved in regulating sensory signal transduction and virulence in bacteria have drawn attention as targets for novel antibacterial agents that might be especially effective in combating bacterial virulence. Bacterial two-component kinases are the best-known class of enzymes in this category. These histidine protein kinases undergo ATP-dependent autophosphorylation at a conserved histidine residue. The phosphate is subsequently transferred to an aspartate residue of the "*response regulator*" (the second component), which is usually a DNA-binding protein that regulates transcription of specific genes. The phosphorylation status of the "*response regulator*" modulates its DNA-binding activity, thereby regulating bacterial gene expression. Numerous pairs of these two-component systems are widespread in bacteria and are essential for cell differentiation and virulence as well as response to environmental changes. Recently, a new type of two-component system (encoded by the *yycFG* genes) that regulates bacterial cell division in *S. aureus* has been found to be essential for bacterial growth. The two-component kinase VanS is known to regulate vancomycin resistance in enterococci. VncS, another two-component kinase, has been linked to vancomycin tolerance in *S. pneumoniae*. In addition, inhibitors of a fungal two-component system are being studied as potential antifungal agents. Inhibitors of bacterial two- component kinases could therefore represent a novel class of agents with multiple modes of antimicrobial activity.

Table 7.1. Additional examples of enzymes as antibacterial drug targets

Enzyme	*Function*
t-RNA Synthetase	Translation
ppGpp Degradase	Metabolism of bacterial stress signal
ppGpp	
Dihydroneopterin aldolase	Folate biosynthesis
RNAse P	RNA processing
SecA	Protein secretion
MurA-F	Peptidoglycan synthesis
Mur ligases	Peptidoglycan synthesis
Coenzyme A reductase	Oxidative stress and redox balance

Known Enzymes as Known Targets

Enzymes that are established targets of known antibacterial agents are also being studied with the goal of identifying superior inhibitors. The advantage of enzyme targets in this category is their demonstrated essentiality for bacterial growth and survival. Several of these enzymes are being studied with renewed interest for two reasons. On the one hand, a better understanding of the structure-function and biochemical properties of these enzymes could lead to the discovery of new inhibitors that may not be susceptible to existing and emerging mechanisms of resistance. On the other hand, by studying enzyme targets, a better understanding of the mechanisms of action of known inhibitors at the molecular level could be developed and used to design new members of known classes of inhibitors.

Bacterial dihydropteroate synthase, an enzyme involved in folate biosynthesis, is the target for sulfonamides, which were among the earliest antibacterial agents. Sulfonamides are structural analogs of *para*-aminobenzoic acid, one of the substrates of dihydropteroate synthase. The biochemical mechanism involved in the inhibition of this enzyme is being studied with renewed interest. Dihydrofolate reductase is the second enzyme involved in folate biosynthesis to be a target for known antibacterial agents such as trimethoprim. Newer analogs of trimethoprim are being developed. A combination of sulfonamides and trimethoprims is commonly used to treat a variety of infections. This example shows that in certain cases it is advantageous to target two enzymes, such as the synthase and the reductase in this case, in a biosynthetic pathway to accomplish a successful clinical outcome. Bacterial DNA gyrase is a type II topoisomerase involved in regulating the level of DNA supercoiling. The activity of this enzyme, a target for the quinolone class of antibacterial agents, is essential for bacterial DNA replication and, consequently, for growth and survival. Understanding the molecular aspects of how quinolones inhibit DNA gyrase has played an important role in the design of new-generation quinolones with improved potency and spectrum of antibacterial activity. In addition, during the process of understanding the quinolone mechanism of action, topoisomerase IV, an enzyme involved in bacterial chromosome segregation, was discovered as a second target for the quinolones. Generation of multistep point mutations in the genes of DNA gyrase and topoisomerase IV has been shown to incrementally increase the level of quinolone resistance in several pathogens. Thus, quinolones with comparable potencies toward both of the targets are now believed to be more desirable because of the lower probability of stepwise resistance development. Additional classes of bacterial DNA gyrase inhibitors, such as coumarins and cyclothialidines, have been identified, although they have yet to be developed as successful antibacterial agents. Unlike quinolones, these inhibitors interact with the *gyrB* subunit of DNA gyrase and therefore have a different mechanism of action relative to quinolones.

Bacterial RNA polymerase, the target for the rifamycin class of antibacterial agents, is the enzyme responsible for transcription of genomic DNA in bacteria. Like DNA gyrase, RNA polymerase is a multifunctional, multisubunit enzyme with multiple active conformations. This increases the number of possible mechanisms of inhibition of RNA polymerase. For example, in addition to the β subunit, which is the apparent target for rifamycin, bacterial transcription initiation is a unique process in which the σ subunit plays a unique role in the recognition of bacterial promoter sequences. Alternative σ subunits, such as σ^S and σ^E, have been implicated in the transcription of virulence genes in pathogens such as *Salmonella typhimurium* and *Pseudomonas aeruginosa*. These alternative σ subunits associate with the core RNA polymerase to activate transcription of specific genes that are essential for pathogenic bacteria to cause infection in humans and animals. As part of the bacterial RNA polymerase holoenzyme, the σ subunits therefore represent an as yet unexploited, but attractive set of targets for antibacterial drug discovery.

Enzymes involved in bacterial cell wall biosynthesis are well-known targets of several classes of antibacterial agents including β-lactams, which are among the most commonly used drugs to treat bacterial infections. The targets of β-lactams are the so-called penicillin-binding proteins, which are transpeptidases involved in the cross-linking of peptidogylcans. Enzymes involved in bacterial fatty acid synthesis are also being studied as targets of known antibacterial agents. The enoyl-acyl carrier protein reductase, the *inhA* gene product, is the target utilized by isoniazid, an antibacterial agent used against *Mycobacterium tuberculosis*. Recently, the enoyl-acyl carrier protein reductase, the*fabI* gene product in *E. coli*, has been identified as the molecular target for the 2-hydroxydiphenyl ether class of agents which include triclosan, a broad-spectrum antibacterial agent that is widely used in a variety of consumer products. Therefore, further studies of bacterial fatty acid biosynthetic enzymes could lead to new antibacterial agents.

Resistance-Determining Enzymes as Targets

As mentioned in the Introduction, bacterial resistance to currently used antibacterial agents poses a major threat to their continued effectiveness. Interestingly, a number of enzymes are involved in the development of antibacterial resistance via several mechanisms. For example, there are enzymes that catalyze the inactivation of antibacterial agents. β-Lactamases are the best-known examples of this class of enzymes and have been studied extensively as targets for new inhibitors that are used in combination with β-lactams to prevent their inactivation. Several β-lactamase inhibitors have been developed and are used in combination with β-lactams (e.g., amoxicillin/clavulanic acid, piperacillin/tazobactam, and others). Bacterial resistance to the macrolide class of antibacterial agents is mediated by the *erm* class of gene products, which function as ribosomal RNA methyltransferases. Numerous members of this class of enzymes have been identified. These enzymes methylate the 23S rRNA component of the 50S subunit of bacterial ribosomes, thereby reducing the affinity of macrolides for ribosomes. Attempts at identifying inhibitors of methyltransferases have been made, and potent inhibitors have been identified using high-throughput screening. Some of these inhibitors inhibited bacterial cell growth *in vitro*, although their true mechanism of action against bacterial whole cells remain unclear. More recently, a series of triazine-containing compounds that inhibit Erm methyltransferases have been identified using an NMR-based screen followed by a parallel synthesis approach to optimize inhibition potency. Further investigation of these various classes of Erm methyltransferase inhibitors could lead to therapeutic agents that reverse macrolide resistance in bacteria.

Bacterial resistance to vancomycin is another example of enzymes playing a key role at the molecular level. Vancomycin is a well-known antibiotic that inhibits bacterial peptidoglycan synthesis and is used to treat infections by multiple-drug-resistant Gram-positive pathogens such as methicillin-resistant *S. aureus* (MRSA). Resistance to vancomycin has now emerged as a significant problem in hospital-acquired infections caused by *Enterococcusfaecium* and *Enterococcusfaecalis*, pathogens that are resistant to multiple antibacterial agents. Studies on the molecular basis for this resistance revealed the involvement of several enzymes. At least three enzymes, encoded by the *vanH*, *vanA*, and *vanX* genes, are involved in converting the D-alanyl-D-alanine dipeptide, the target for vancomycin, to D-alanyl-D-lactate, which is still capable of transpeptidation but insensitive to vancomycin. First, the *vanX* gene product, a dipeptidase cleaves the terminal D-alanine of the D-alanyl-D-alanine dipeptide. Next, the *vanH* gene product, a dehydrogenase reduces D-pyruvate to D-lactate, which is then used to replace the D-alanine of the dipeptide by the *vanA* gene product, a ligase. Recently, the VanX peptidase and the VanA ligase have been the targets for discovery of new inhibitors that could potentially inhibit vancomycin resistance in enterococci and prolong the use of this antibiotic.

Methodologies: Antibacterial Drug Discovery

While identification of a target is very important in antibacterial drug discovery, it is only the first in a series of steps leading to the identification of a lead compound. As far as enzyme targets are concerned, certain follow-up steps are common to all of these targets, regardless of their role in bacterial growth and physiology.

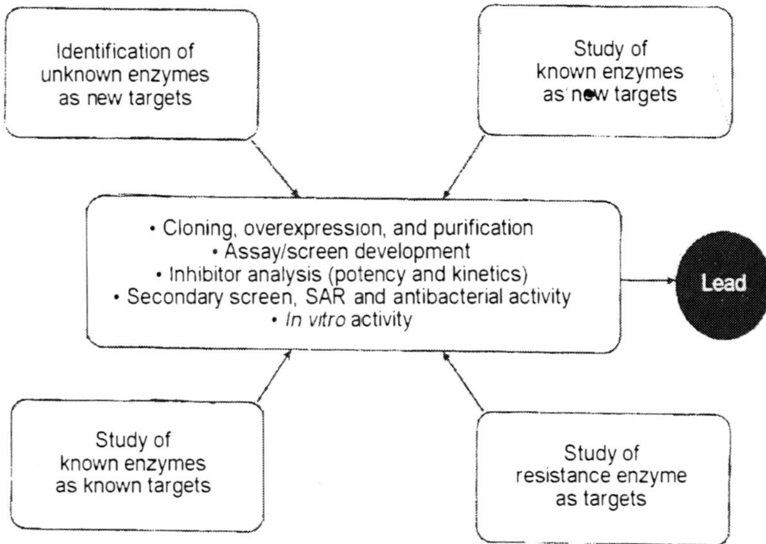

Fig. 7.1. A summary of enzymology-based approaches in antibacterial drug discovery.

Overexpression and Purification of the Enzyme Target: The *murG* Gene Product

As mentioned in the previous section, enzymes involved in bacterial cell wall biosynthesis are being studied by renewed interest. Among these enzymes is the *murG* gene product that catalyzes the formation of lipid II, a precursor of peptidoglycan, which is a primary component of the bacterial cell wall. As the first step toward studying this enzyme as a target for new antibacterial agents, the *murG* gene from *E. coli* has been cloned and expressed from a plasmid. To facilitate purification of the enzyme product, the *murG* gene was tagged with multiple histidine residues. This is a popular technique that usually retains the activity of the enzyme while allowing its efficient purification using metal affinity (nickel) chromatography. Plasmids expressing the cloned gene were used to complement the *murG* mutation in *E. coli*, indicating that the cloned enzyme retained its biological activity. Affinity chromatography (nickel) was then used to purify the enzyme, which demonstrated activity in a peptidoglycan polymerization assay.

Development of a Functional Assay: The *vanHAX* Gene Products

Once the role of a gene product as a potential enzyme target is identified via genetic techniques, such as cloning and complementation, the next step involves its biochemical characterization including the development of a quantitative assay. Once the vancomycin-resistance genes in enterococci were characterized genetically, suitable enzymatic assays were developed. Three distinct enzymatic activities were linked to the products of *vanA*, *vanX*, and *vanH*. Enzymatic characterization of these gene products not only helped elucidate the biochemical mechanism of vancomycin resistance in enterococci, but also provided the biochemical basis for screen development.

Elucidation of the Enzyme Structure via X-Ray Crystallography

β-lactamases

The β-lactamases, a group of resistance-determining enzymes, has been studied extensively via structural analysis. Use of β-lactamase inactivators, such as clavulanate, sulbactam, and tazobactam (as discussed in the previous section), has led to the selection of inhibitor-resistant β-lactmases. Recently, X-ray crystallographic studies have been used to elucidate the mechanism of inhibitor insensitivity of an inhibitor-resistant β-lactamase from *E. coli* at the atomic level. Using a high-resolution X-ray structure (2.3 Å), it has been shown that the Asn276-Asp point mutation results in facilitating the turnover of clavulanate, thereby treating it as another β-lactam substrate, rather than a mechanistic inactivator. This finding could facilitate the design of newer β-lactamase inactivators capable of evading the effect of the Asn276-Asp mutation. In a separate study, potent (K_i = 27 nM), non-β-lactam inhibitors were designed using the X-ray crystal structure of AmpC, an intrinsically resistant β-lactamase that was complexed with *m*-aminophenylboronic acid. These inhibitors were also able to potentiate the antibacterial activity of β-lactams.

Bacterial signal peptidase

Bacterial signal peptidase is an example of a known enzyme that could serve as a target for new antibacterial agents. Recently, a catalytically active, soluble fragment of signal peptidase from *E. coli* has been crystallized as a complex with a β-lactam inhibitor. This represents a major step in the efforts toward the rational design of inhibitors that can be readily tested for their enzyme inhibition and bacterial growth-inhibition activities.

Development of High-Throughput Screening

Even though a biochemical assay for an enzyme target might be available, development of a high-throughput screen can still pose significant challenges. First, the assay has to be miniaturized to a microtiter format (e.g., 96- or 384-well format). Second, steps involving liquid handling, such as the addition of substrate, cofactor, reaction termination buffer, etc., and detection of the reaction product have to be simplified to facilitate automation. Third, the assay has to have adequate detection sensitivity to be quantitatively reliable with acceptable levels of well-to-well, plate-to-plate, and day-to-day variations.

Bacterial RNA polymerase

A high-throughput assay for bacterial RNA polymerase has been successfully developed and validated using a 96-well, automated format. The reaction mixture contained a DNA template, nucleotide substrates

(NTPs), supplemented with α-^{33}P-labeled CTP in Tris-acetate buffer (pH 6.8). The polymerase reaction was carried out at 34°C for 40 min (providing linear kinetics). The effect of dimethylsulfoxide (DMSO), the usual solvent for test compounds used in a screen, was taken into consideration. The radiolabeled RNA transcripts were allowed to bind diethyl aminoethyl (DEAE) beads, which were then separated via filtration, and radioactivity associated with the wells was quantitated to measure the RNA polymerase activity. The standard deviation of the measured activity was typically <15% of the average. Use of this assay to screen for RNA polymerase inhibitors from chemical libraries and natural products led to the identification of DNA intercalators (known to inhibit RNA polymerase activity), rifampicin (a known inhibitors of RNA polymerase), and several derivatives of rifampicin from Actinomycetes extracts. Therefore this assay can be reliably utilized to detect novel inhibitors of bacterial RNA polymerase.

Bacterial two-component kinase

By virtue of their prevalence and importance, eukaryotic tyrosine, threonine, and serine protein kinases continue to be targets of intense research. As a result, reliable and quantitative assays to monitor their activity have been developed. However, in the case of bacterial two-component kinases, which are autophosphorylating enzymes with no known low-molecular-weight substrates or reaction products, traditional assays are limited in terms of their throughput. Recently, a high-throughput autophosphorylation assay was developed using CheA, the two-component kinase that regulates chemotaxis in *E. coli*. Cell extracts from an *E. coli* strain, containing a recombinant plasmid to overexpress the *cheA* gene, were used as the source of the enzyme. Partially purified (~50%) enzyme preparations, with no contaminating autophosphorylation activity, were used for the assay. The autophosphorylation assay was performed in a 96-well format using DEAE or nitrocellulose filter plates. [γ-^{33}P]ATP was used as a phosphate-donating substrate and ^{33}P-labeled, phosphorylated CheA was detected as the reaction product. Following a 30-min reaction at room temperature, free [γ-^{33}P]ATP was removed by washing the filter wells with high-salt buffer under vacuum. Radioactivity associated with the washed and dried wells was measured by scintillation counting. Using this screen, several inhibitors of CheA have been identified from combinatorial libraries. Other members of the two-component kinase family, such as NtrB (NRII) and KinA have also been used to screen for inhibitors.

Coupled VanA/VanX screen

To screen for inhibitors of both VanA and VanX enzymes, a coupled high- throughput assay was developed by linking the two reactions catalyzed by these two enzymes. The coupling of the two reactions was facilitated by the fact that the product of the VanX dipeptidase reaction is D-alanine, a substrate utilized by the VanA ligase, along with D-lactate. Since the VanA reaction hydrolyzes ATP, the resulting inorganic phosphate was used for measuring the coupled enzyme activity. The assay was validated using D-cycloserine, a known inhibitor of VanA, and was used in a high-throughput format to screen approximately 250,000 synthetic compounds. While none of the inhibitors detected by this screen was able to reverse vancomycin resistance in *E. faecium (vanA)*, one compound, VAN32, showed synergistic activity with vancomycin against *E. faecalis (vanB)*

Analysis of Inhibitors

Regardless of the properties of a particular enzyme target, numerous preliminary inhibitors are usually identified as a result of a high-throughput screen. However, the number of compounds identified at this step as inhibitors usually depends on the minimum potency deemed necessary for further investigation. A variety of approaches are subsequently used to verify the potency and specificity of the inhibitors. A few of these approaches are discussed below, using the examples of efforts following high-throughput screening for bacterial two-component kinases. Screening of KinA as a prototypical two-component kinase led to the identification of several classes of inhibitors, such as cyclohexanes, benzimidazoles, bis-phenols, salicylanilides, trityls, and benzoxazines. Several members of these inhibitor classes showed significant antibacterial activity against Gram-positive pathogens, including methicillin-resistant *S. aureus* (MRSA) and vancomycin-resistant *E. faecium* (VRE). In addition, a correlation between the KinA inhibition potency (IC_{50}) and antibacterial activity against *S. aureus* was observed. RWJ-4981 5, a lead compound identified in this study, also showed bactericidal activity against MRSA. In serial passage experiments, MRSA isolates showed a lower tendency to develop resistance to RWJ-49815 than to ciprofloxacin, a known fluoroquinolone. These findings were followed with a series of whole-cell analyses designed to establish a link between the two-component kinase inhibition activity of these compounds and their antibacterial activity. Using assays to determine membrane damage, bacterial viability, hemolysis, and macromolecular synthesis, this study found that the leads with potent enzyme inhibition activity either damaged *S. aureus* membrane or caused hemolysis of equine erythrocytes. Most of these compounds also caused a generalized inhibition of macromolecular (DNA, RNA, and protein) synthesis in bacteria. The authors therefore concluded that the antibacterial activity of the leads identified by the KinA screen was most likely attributable to a nonspecific effect, rather than to the inhibition of two-component kinases.

Whole-Cell Screening of Enzyme Inhibitors: Lipid A Biosynthesis

It is important to note that potent enzyme inhibitors can be identified by screening for whole-cell inhibitors of biosynthetic pathways. A successful example of this strategy is the discovery of L-573,655, a member of the carboxyamido-oxazolidines. This compound was identified using a whole-cell screen to identify inhibitors of lipid A biosynthesis, an essential pathway for Gram-negative bacteria. Unlike the two-component kinase inhibitors discussed above, the specificity of L-573,655 was demonstrated by its inability to inhibit bacterial DNA, RNA, protein, and phospholipid synthesis. Secondary screening of the nine enzymes involved in *E. coli* lipid A biosynthesis identified the second enzyme in the pathway, UDP-3-O-[*R*-3-hydroxymyristoyl]-GlcNAc deacetylase, as the molecular target for this inhibitor. Subsequent SAR studies of over 200 analogs of L573,655 led to the identification of L-161,240, which had a *K* of 50 nM for the enzyme target and significant antibacterial activity against several Gram-negative pathogens, such as *E. coli*, *Enterobacter cloacae*, and *Klebsiella pneumoniae*. In addition, this compound demonstrated *in vivo* efficacy by protecting mice from lethal bacterial infection.

Using specific examples, this chapter attempted to provide a broad overview of the roles of enzymes as targets of antibacterial drug discovery. On the one hand, more detailed knowledge of bacterial pathogenesis and physiology, together with genomics, will lead to the identification of additional enzymes as potential targets for new drugs. On the other hand, advances in high-throughput screening, combinatorial chemistry, parallel synthesis, and automated data processing will undoubtedly enrich the field of antibacterial drug discovery. Developments in molecular diagnostics might also open up new possibilities for targeted, narrow- spectrum therapies based on specific inhibition of enzymes. While the area of antibacterial drugs is a mature one, with numerous potent and effective enzyme inhibitors, the targets were usually identified following the discovery of the inhibitors. Use of enzyme targets for *de novo* discovery, design, and development of antibacterial agents is a field that is still in its early days.

8

Vectors for Gene

Gene therapy is a conceptually simple and attractive process, which consists of the introduction of one or more functional genes in a human/non-human receptor (*in vivo*, *in situ*, or *ex vivo*). It constitutes a promising alternative for the treatment, diagnosis, or cure of genetic defects such as cystic fibrosis or acquired diseases like cancer and AIDS. DNA vaccines can also be developed on the basis of genes to provide immunity against infectious agents (e.g., malaria) or treat noninfectious diseases such as tumors and allergies.

Gene Therapy

Milestones

Although gene therapy is a recent endeavor of the human mind, it has nevertheless come a long way since the early, nonauthorized administration of Shope papilloma virus to argininemia-suffering patients by Stanfield Rogers et al. Despite the flawed design and consequent failure of this clinical trial, Rogers was one of the first scientists to anticipate the therapeutic potential of viruses as carriers of genetic information. The first federally approved gene therapy clinical trials took place in 1990 when an adenosine deaminase (ADA)-deficient patient was given her own T cells engineered with a retroviral vector carrying a normal ADA gene. This experiment paved the way for further clinical trials. In 1993 an adenovirus vector (AdV) was first used in a clinical trial designed to evaluate the potential of direct transfer of cystic fibrosis transmembrane conductance regulator (CFTR) cDNA in the treatment of cystic fibrosis (CF).

The first setback faced by gene therapy came in 1999 when a patient suffering from ornithine transcarbamylase (OTC) deficiency died after administration of an adenovirus vector encoding OTC. The year 2000 saw gene therapy's first major success: A gene therapy protocol could correct the phenotype of an X-linked severe combined immunodeficiency (SCID-X1) syndrome in two patients who had been re-infused with autologous CD34 bone marrow cells transduced *ex vivo* with a retrovirus vector encoding the γC receptor gene. These successes were later shadowed by the development of leukemia-like syndrome in recipients of the treatment as a consequence of retrovirus integration in proximity to the LMO2 proto-oncogene promoter. In October 16, 2003, a recombinant adenovirus vector expressing the tumor-suppressor gene p53 was approved by the State Food and Drug Administration (SFDA) of China for the treatment of head and neck squamous celi carcinoma. Developed and manufactured by Shenzen SiBiono GeneTech (China) and trademarked under the name Gendicine, it became the first human gene therapy product to reach the market in April 2004. As of September 2005, 2600 patients had been treated with Gendicine, with projections estimating 50,000 patients to receive the product by 2006.

Vectors

The transport of the therapeutic transgenes toward the nuclei of the target cells can be carried out both by viral and nonviral vectors such as plasmid DNA. Plasmid DNA molecules are extra-chromosomal carriers of genetic information that have the ability to replicate autonomously. These vectors constitute an attractive gene transfer system because they are safer and easier to produce when compared with viral vectors. However, plasmid DNA vectors are less effective in transfecting cells when compared with viral vectors, which have a natural ability to deliver and express their genes in a wide variety of cell types and tissues.

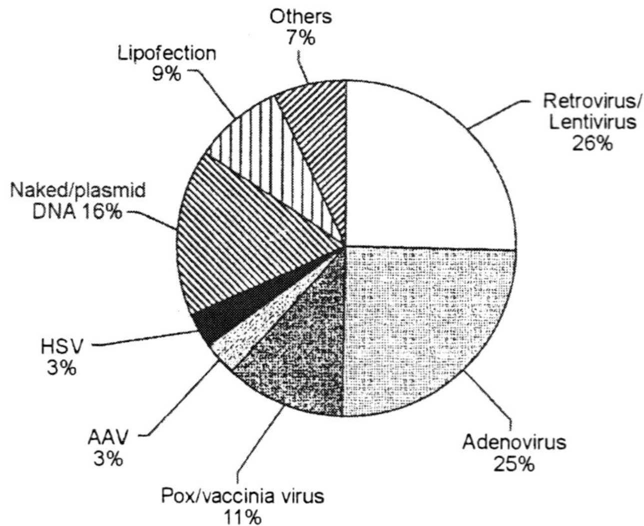

Fig. 8.1. Breakdown of gene therapy clinical trials in terms of vector type (N = 1076).

The major drawback of viral vectors is undoubtedly related to safety aspects. When confronted with viral vector particles, the human immune system, which has evolved to tackle wild-type infections, will likewise generate an immune response. The potency and severity of this response can ultimately lead to death, as occurred in the 1999 OTC gene therapy clinical trial. Thus, a safe and effective use of viral vectors in gene therapy requires the modification of natural viruses to impair replication and expression of viral proteins and thus minimize toxicity and immunogenicity. The infection pathway of these recombinant viral vectors should of course remain unaltered. Further goals of virus modification are to provide room in the viral genome for transgenes, to modulate transgene expression, and to improve the selectivity of infection. Most recombinant viral vectors used in gene therapy clinical trials belong to one of the following categories: (1) adenovirus, (2) retrovirus/lentivirus, (3) pox/vaccinia virus, (4) adeno-associated virus (AAV), and (5) herpes simplex-1 virus (HSV-1). According to the data provided in the *Journal of Gene Medicine Database* and updated in July 2005, 25% of the total 1076 gene therapy clinical trials were using AdVs. The popularity and high expectations generated toward AdVs is well expressed by the fact that both the first gene therapy tragedy and success used adenovirus to deliver transgenes.

Adenovirus in Gene Therapy

Adenoviruses were discovered in cultures of human adenoids in 1953 by Rowe et al. and have since then been implicated in several respiratory, ocular, and gastrointestinal human diseases. Nonhuman adenoviruses have also been found in many other mammalian (dogs, horses. sheeps, chimpanzees, etc.) and non-mammalian (ducks, fowl, geese, etc.) species. Overall, more than 100 members have been included in the *Adenoviridae* family. This section will only give a brief description of the major characteristics of the adenovirus and its vectors.

The extensive studies that followed the discovery of adenoviruses unveiled many features that make them a popular gene delivery vector. For instance, adenoviruses are extremely efficient in the transduction of both quiescent and actively dividing cells in most tissues and their genome can be manipulated easily to generate recombinant adenoviruses with improved properties. It is also possible to propagate them to high titers, and thus, it becomes relatively easy to generate sufficient amounts for research purposes and small-scale clinical trials. On the down side, adenoviruses can generate potent immunogenic reactions in human recipients, although in some instances this immunogenicity may enhance antitumor effects and vaccination efficiency. Furthermore, and because adenoviruses persist in the nucleus of transduced cells as extra-chromosomal episomes, the expression of transgenes is transient.

Biology and Properties

The 51 distinct serotypes of human adenovirus (Ad1 to Ad51) are classified into six groups (A to F) on the basis of sequence homology and hemagglutination properties. Most AdVs used in gene therapy are derived from serotype 2 (Ad2) and 5 (Ad5) of the subgroup C. The efficacy of Ad2 and Ad5 derived vectors, however, may be limited by the preexistence of humoral and/or cellular immunity to these serotypes in most human populations. Thus, other serotypes such as Ad11 and Ad35 to which most humans do not have neutralizing antibodies may be clinically useful. The antivector immunity may also be circumvented by the physical shielding of the adenovirus coat and the use of nonhuman adenovirus serotypes. Adenoviruses are nonenveloped viruses with 26- to 45-kbp-long linear genomes of double-stranded DNA (the genome of human Ad2 comprises 35,937 base pairs). The genome is encapsidated in an icosahedral protein coat (12 vertices, 20 surfaces) made essentially of 240 nonvertex hexons and 12 vertex pentons, each with one or two protruding fibers. Each hexon protein is a trimer of the identical polypeptide II (pII), and each penton protein is formed by the interaction of five polypeptides (pIII). These pentons are tightly associated with one or two fibers made of three polypeptides (pIVs) each. Overall, the fiber protein is composed of an N-terminal tail for penton binding, a rigid shaft, and a distal globular knob domain responsible for interaction with host cell receptors. The net charge of each hexon monomer in the Ad5 serotype is −23.8. This makes adenoviral capsids highly negative with an overall surface charge of over −17,000. Other minor protein components can be found in the capsid, including protein IIIa, VI, VIII, and IX. The size of the adenovirus particle is around 70–110 nm, and its molecular weight falls within the range 150–180 × 10^6. The buoyant density of an adenoviral particle in CsCl is 1.32–1.35 g cm^{-3}. Assuming a 170 × 10^6 MW and a 35,937-bp-long genome, the protein and DNA content of one Ad2 viral particle (VP) can be estimated to be 24 × 10^{-5} (86% of dry weight) and 4 × 10^{-5} (14% of dry weight) pg/VP, respectively. The corresponding water content, if a 100-nm viral particle is assumed, is approximately 60%.

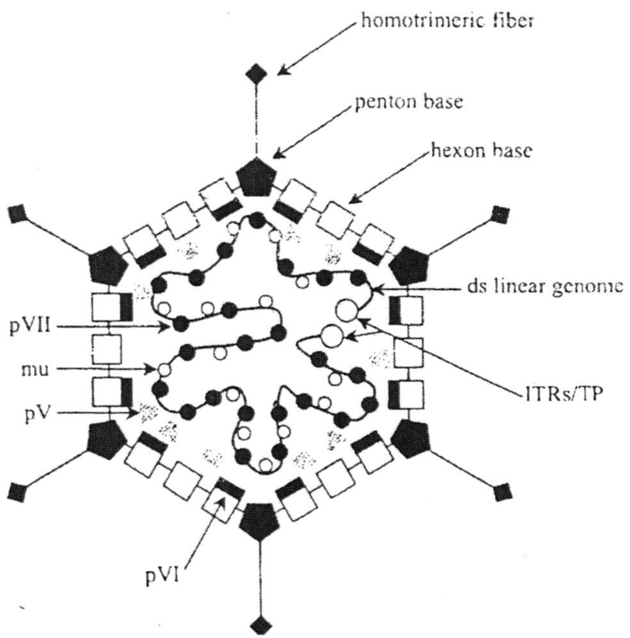

Fig. 8.2. Schematic structure of an adenovirus particle. Major capsid (hexon, penton, fiber) and core (pV, pVII, Mu) proteins are shown.

The core of an adenoviral particle consists of the DNA genome complexed with four polypeptides (pV, pVII, mu, TP). The extremities contain inverted terminal repeat (ITR) sequences (100–140 bp) covalently linked to terminal proteins (TPs), which function as replication origins. The nearby ψ sequence at the left end of the genome consists of a series of seven repeats and is required for efficient packaging. The genes in both strands are grouped into early and late transcriptional units. The basis of this classification is the two-phase infectious cycle (30–40 h), which is characteristic of adenoviruses. In the "early" phase, the virus particles enter the host cell through binding of the homotrimeric protruding fibers to the coxsackievirus B and adenovirus receptor (CAR). After endosomal uptake, release, and capsid dismantling, the viral genome is transported and delivered to the nucleus. The early genes E1 to E5 are then selectively transcribed and translated to modulate functions of the host cell and thus create an optimal environment for virus replication. Specifically, this involves driving the host cell into S-phase (E1A gene), suppressing the host's cell apoptotic machinery (E1B gene), modifying the host's immunological environment (E3 gene), encoding proteins for viral DNA replication (E2 gene), and blocking cellular protein synthesis.

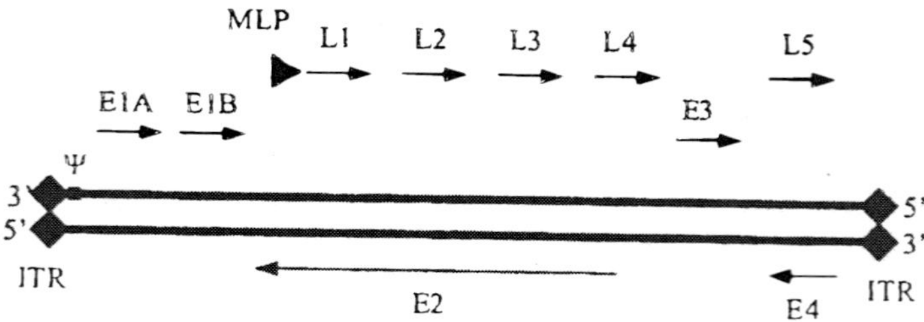

Fig. 8.3. The adenovirus genome.

The "late" phase of the infectious cycle involves the synthesis of structural proteins of the virus, capsid assembly, genome encapsidation, and maturation of fully infectious viral particles. These events are associated with the transcription and translation of the "late" genes L1 to L5. A key player in the transcription of the late genes is the major late promoter (MLP), which is activated early on via the E2 gene.

Recombinant Adenovirus Vectors

A safe and effective use of AdVs requires the engineering of natural viruses into useful recombinant adenovirus vectors by using molecular biology tools. These modifications are essentially designed to: (1) impair replication and expression of viral proteins and thus minimize toxicity and immunogenicity, (2) provide room in the viral genome for the therapeutic transgenes, and (3) modulate trans- gene expression. Once these recombinant vectors are available, transgenes can be inserted in their genome. In many cases, tissue- and cell-specific heterologous promoters are inserted along side to provide better expression.

First-generation vectors

Most first-generation AdVs have been constructed by deleting the viral early gene E1. The goal underlying this deletion is to impair viral replication and production of capsid proteins and thus prevent the vectors from causing disease in the gene therapy recipient. Simultaneously, room is made for transgenes up to 6.5 kb, which are usually expressed under the control of an heterologous promoter. The propagation of these E1 replication defective vectors can only be accomplished in complementing cells lines such as the human embryonic kidney 293 (HEK-293) or the human retinoblast (PER. C6).These cells are transformed with the E1 gene and therefore trans-complement its deficiency in the recombinant vectors. First-generation AdVs are characterized by several problems. For instance, recombination between the replication-defective virus and the E1 sequences in the

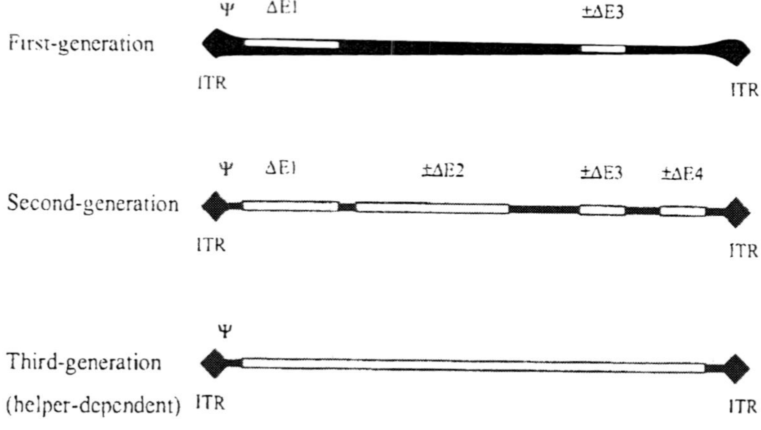

Fig. 8.4. The three generations of adenovirus vectors.

complementing HEK-293 cell line can occur during propagation, giving rise to replication-competent adenoviruses (RCA) that will contaminate the recombinant virus being produced. This problem has been circumvented in the PER.C6 cell line in which a rational design of the El transgene prevents generation of RCAs. Another problem with first-generation vectors is that despite the deletion of the El gene, viral protein expression is not completely shut off. The concomitant low level of viral replication taking place in the transduced host cells, thus, can generate a cytotoxic-T lymphocyte (CTL) immune response that in the end will destroy the transgene-expressing cells and contribute to gene silencing. Despite this residual immunogenicity, first-generation vectors may find application in cases such as cancer therapy and vaccination where a short-term transgene expression is desirable. It is worth mentioning that the transgene product itself, depending on its own intrinsic immunogenicity, can also trigger a cellular immune response capable of destroying the transduced cells. However, the magnitude and nature of this immune response seems to vary considerably depending on the specific transgene product being expressed.

Second-generation vectors

Second-generation AdVs have been constructed by additionally deleting the viral regulatory E2 and/or E4 coding sequences, on the expectation that progressive deletions should reduce viral antigen expression, increase *in vivo* persistence, and reduce antiviral immune response. The E2 gene encodes proteins that are required for initiation and elongation of viral DNA synthesis and the activation of the MLP, whereas E4 encodes proteins involved in the accumulation, splicing, and transport of early and late viral mRNA and in DNA replication and virus particle assembly. As in the first generation, complementing cell lines able to express the missing functions must be generated and isolated to ensure propagation of the recombinant viruses. The HEK-293 cell line can be conveniently adapted to this end. A first advantage of these doubly deleted vectors is the reduced probability of the emergence of RCAs, because this would require simultaneous reversions in the El and E2 or E4 regions. Several studies with El/E2 and El/E4 deleted vectors have shown reduced synthesis of viral proteins, extended transgene expression, and reduced toxicity.

Third-generation vectors

A third generation of AdVs has been further developed by deleting most or virtually all viral genes in the genome. These gutless or helper-dependent vectors can accommodate inserts up to 30 kbp and have shown reduced immunogenicity and prolonged transgene expression in mice. The reduced immunogenicity still observed should be attributed either to the injected viral proteins or to the transgene product. Growth of helper- dependent vectors depends on coinfection of an El-complementing cell line such as HEK-293 by an El-deleted helper virus (hence, the name helper-dependent) that provides missing replication and assembly functions *in trans*. The simultaneous propagation of the helper virus can be limited by resorting to a Cre-lox mechanism that allows the packaging sequence to be deleted. In short, the helper genome is provided with loxP-sites that flank the ψ signal, whereas complementing 293 cells are engineered to stably express the enzyme Cre-recombinase. During infection, Cre-recombinase excises the loxP-flanked signal rendering the helper genome unpackable. Nevertheless, the two types of viral particles (helper-dependent and helper) must be separated after propagation, a task that is difficult to accomplish.

Oncolytic adenoviruses

A class of AdVs has been developed to specifically kill cancer cells, an approach that has been termed virotherapy. Contrary to the approach pursued with first-, second-, and third-generation adenovirus vectors, these oncolytic or conditionally replicating adenoviruses (CRAds) are engineered in such a way that they retain the ability to replicate. This replication however, is tumor selective—the virus will only infect and proliferate in malignant cells with mutations in specific tumor suppressor genes. Thus, a transgene is actually not required for the therapeutic effect to take place.

Targeting Strategies

Several therapeutically relevant human cells (e.g., skeletal and smooth muscle cells, endothelial cells, hematopoietic cells, and some tumor cells) are not easily transduced by adenovirus vectors due to low or inexistent levels of expression of the CAR receptor. On the other hand, the broad tropism of adenoviruses may lead to the undesirable expression of the transgene in nontarget cells. Thus, an improvement in the transduction selectivity of existing adenovirus vectors is crucial to circumvent these limitations and improve efficacy in many clinical applications. The following strategies have been devised to meet this end: (1) structural retargeting, (2) tropism ablation, and (3) transcriptional targeting.

Structural targeting relies on the structural modification of the adenoviral capsid by genetic incorporation of peptides, IgG-binding domains, and fiber proteins from other serotypes, metabolic biotinylation, and PEGylation. These ligands are selected or designed to direct vector attachment to alternative cell receptors in CAR-deficient cells. The goal of tropism ablation, on the other hand, is to reduce transduction of nontarget, CAR-expressing cells. This "*de-targeting*" strategy can be accomplished by constructing "*knobless*" vectors or by introducing point mutations in the fiber protein knob. The capsid of these mutant vectors is then modified with ligands (e.g., peptides) adequate for transduction of the target cells (retargeting).

In transcriptional targeting, cell-type-specific promoters are used to restrict transgene expression to specific tissues. The adenoviral particles may infect different cells, but the transgene is expressed only in those cells that actively express transcription factors required to drive expression from the cell-specific promoter. For instance, this approach has been used in the context of adenoviral-mediated treatment of gastrointestinal cancer. This application has been limited by the undesirable expression of the transgene (which codes for HSVtk-herpes simplex virus thymidine kinase) in the liver due to the vector hepatotropism. Thus, the transgene was placed under the control of the cyclooxygenase-2 (cox-2) promoter, which is inactive in liver cells but active in many gastrointestinal cancers. Experiments showed that the cox-2 promoter could confine the cytocidal effect of HSVtk specifically to cyclooxygenase-2-positive gastrointestinal cancer, while mitigating the otherwise fatal hepatotoxicity.

Applications

Most adenovirus vector applications and clinical trials described and reported in the literature have targeted genetic diseases and cancer. This section will briefly mention the most significant applications.

Genetic diseases

In the case of genetic diseases, the transgene encodes a protein that is missing or is defective in the host organism. A typical and well-studied example is cystic fibrosis, the first human disease targeted in an adenovirus gene therapy clinical trial. Cystic fibrosis is an inherited, recessive disease caused by a variety of mutations in the gene encoding the CFTR protein. Although multiple organs are affected, the lung is the life-threatening organ. The virus-vector mediated shuttling of a normal copy of the CFTR gene toward the affected lung cells could potentially prevent the onset, or halt the progression, of the disease. The choice of adenoviruses as CFTR gene delivery vectors is logical given their natural ability to infect lung cells. Nevertheless, barriers such as the lack of CARs in airway epithelial cells and alveolar macrophages, and the specific pulmonary-associated T-helper cell response, have prevented a successful transgene expression. Significantly, all clinical trials currently under way involving AdVs and directed toward genetic diseases target cystic fibrosis.

Adenoviral gene therapy has also targeted muscular dystrophy, a genetic disease characterized by progressive muscle weakness. Muscular dystrophy is caused by mutations in the X-linked dystrophin gene (DMD), which lead to prematurely aborted dystrophin synthesis. The lack of this important structural protein in muscle cells causes fiber damage and membrane leakage. In this context, gene therapy attempts to deliver a dystrophin expression vector to the nuclei of striated muscle cells. Given the huge size of the DMD gene (2.6 Mb), minigene cassettes (14 kb) have been generated that are capable of expressing therapeutic levels of a functional dystrophin protein. Nevertheless, vectors with a capacity large enough to accommodate the 14-kb dystrophin cDNA are still required. Unlike first- and second-generation AdVs that are limited to 7–8-kb transgenes, third-generation adenovirus vectors adequately meet this requirement. The use of such vectors has resulted in a prolonged expression of the transgene in mice muscle cells. Despite these promising results, barriers such as the lack of adenovirus receptors in the target muscle cells and potent immune response have to be overcome before a therapeutic use is developed. Further examples of the application of AdVs to treat genetic diseases include OTC deficiency, factor VIII deficiency, Tay-Sachs disease, and glycogen storage disease II.

Cancer

Different strategies have been pursued in an attempt to treat cancer via gene therapy, by taking advantage of molecular differences between normal and tumor cells. Once transferred to the target cells, expression of the transgene delivers the antitumor effect. Clinical data suggest excellent safety when AdVs are injected locally. Synergistic effects with treatment options such as radiotherapy and chemotherapy have further improved the efficacy of cancer gene therapy. Most efforts have relied on one of the following approaches: (1) tumor suppression, (2) suicide therapy, (3) cancer vaccination, and (4) virotherapy. The tumor suppression approach attempts to induce apoptosis by delivering a tumor suppressor gene that is missing or defective in the tumor cells. On the contrary, normal cells infected by the tumor suppressor delivery vector will not be detrimentally affected. The approach is perfectly illustrated with p53, a gene whose mutations have been associated with several tumors. The delivery of wild-type p53 gene efficiently induces apoptosis in cells of different tumors, as demonstrated in several phase I and II clinical trials. Additionally, this toxic effect can extend to neighbor, uninfected tumor cells, a phenomenon known as the "*bystander effect*". This effect has been attributed to the ability of p53 to block angiogenesis. Combination of p53 with immunomodulatory genes, cytotoxic drugs, or radiotherapy may further improve efficacy. Recombinant adenoviruses encoding the p53 gene have been used to treat more than 20 kinds of cancer indications, including head and neck squamous cell carcinoma, lung cancer, breast cancer, and liver cancer. Studies have focused both on the effect of adenoviral gene therapy alone or in combination with conventional therapies such as chemotherapy, radiotherapy, and surgery. The efficiency of the adenovirus/p53 strategy is well illustrated with the results of a phase II/III clinical trial using the commercial product Gendicine. In this study, 135 patients with head and neck squamous cell carcinoma were divided into two groups. The first group received Gendicine in combination with radiotherapy, whereas the second group received radiotherapy alone. Significant difference in terms of complete or partial tumor regression was shown between the two groups, with 93% of the patients responding in the Gendicine/radiotherapy group *versus* 79% in the radiotherapy group.

The second approach used to kill tumor cells is suicide gene therapy, which combines the delivery of suicide transgenes with the separate administration of a harmless prodrug. Once reaching the target cancer cells, the suicide gene expresses an enzyme that metabolizes the prodrug into a cytotoxic agent that kills cells. The diffusion of the cytotoxic agent into neighbor cells further generates a "bystander" effect that increases the efficacy of the strategy. An example of such a transgene/prodrug combination that has been tested in the clinic is herpes simplex virus thymidine kinase (HSVtk)/ganciclovir. The suicide HSVtk transgene is first delivered to cancer cells, for example, via AdVs. The administered ganciclovir is then metabolized by the expressed HSVtk into ganciclovir triphosphate, a nucleotide analoge that blocks DNA synthesis. When a DNA strand incorporates this analoge, chain termination results and cells die upon induction of apoptosis. This effect is, of course, more pronounced in tumor cells, which divide much more actively when compared with native cells. Another feature that contributes to the attractiveness of the approach is the use of a drug such as Ganciclovir that is widely used clinically. Another example of suicide cancer therapy is the combined use of *Escherichia coli* cytosine deaminase (CD) with the prodrug 5-fluorocytosine. In this case, 5-fluorocytosine is metabolized by the expressed CD into 5-fluorouracil, a pyrimidine antagonist that blocks DNA and RNA synthesis. The subsequent direct and bystander inhibitory effect can be enhanced further by combination with radiotherapy.

Cancer can also be treated by the adenovirus-mediated delivery of transgenes to tumor cells with the goal of boosting antitumor immunity. These adenoviral "*cancer vaccines*" can harbor either immunomodulatory genes (e.g., IL2 or IL12) and/or tumor antigens (e.g., MART 1 or gp 100 melanoma antigens), which once expressed should induce tumor regression. Human dendritic cells isolated from patients have also been transduced with AdVs designed to express tumor antigens. The therapeutic effect is achieved after reinfusion of the transformed cells.

Virotherapy constitutes a fourth approach that has been attempted clinically to treat cancer. The oncolytic vector Onyx-015 is a characteristic example of virotherapy. The mode of action can be explained as follows. Both adenoviruses and tumor cells need to block the p53 function to replicate. In normal cells the intact p53 function blocks replication of the Onyx-015 vector. In tumor cells, however, and because the p53 gene is mutated, infection with the adenovirus vector Onyx-015 is followed by replication and cell destruction. Furthermore, because after cell destruction an increased number of viral particles is released, the infection/propagation/cell death process can continue in neighbor cells. In one phase II study, the intratumoural injection of Onyx-015 combined with chemotherapy resulted in an 83% tumor response in head and neck cancer patients. The efficacy of oncolytic vectors can be further improved by resorting to transductional targeting, such has the genetic insertion of an integrin binding RGD-4C motif in the fiber proteins of the vector. This modification resulted in enhanced infectivity in ovarian cancer cells, which suggests improvements in clinical efficacy.

Safety Aspects

Adenovirus infection triggers both cellular and humoral responses. Viral pro teins (either synthesized *de novo* or not) are processed by antigen-presenting cells and presented to CD8+ T cells (by means of MHC class I molecules) and CD4+ T- helper cells (by means of MHC class II molecules). This induces proliferation of cytotoxic T lymphocytes that specifically destroy the infected cells. CD4+ T-helper cells are also involved in the production of adenovirus-specific neutralizing antibodies directed toward the virus capsid. The risks associated with this immunogenicity have been vividly demonstrated by the death of a patient in the 1999 OTC clinical trial. After the direct administration of a high dose of the adenoviral vector (3.8×10^{13} viral particles) to the liver, wide dissemination into the circulation triggered a massive activation of innate immunity followed by systemic inflammation that led to fever, intravascular coagulation, and multiorgan failure. Responsibility for eliciting the immune response was attributed to viral capsid proteins rather than the transgene. In subsequent years, a wealth of evidence accumulated confirming that AdVs may induce harmful immune and inflammatory responses, especially when large doses are administered systemically. Adverse effects to adenovirus administration, however, may vary from individual to individual and depend on predisposing and underlying conditions.

The improvement of safety through minimization of toxicity and immunogenicity has been one of the major drivers in the development of recombinant AdVs. Nevertheless, even when third-generation "*gutless*" vectors are used, reduced immunogenicity due to the injected viral capsid proteins or to the transgene product is still observed. Thus, a need exists for the development of safe and effective methods capable of downregulating the host immune response against both adenoviral capsid proteins and transgene products. For instance, conventional immunosuppressive agents such as cyclosporine and FK506 may partially reduce immune responses and thus increase transduction and long-term transgene expression. However, low doses of these agents must be used to prevent substantial organ toxicity. Improved results have been obtained by combining the use of immunomodulatory immunoglobulins and immunosuppressive agents. With this strategy, the immune response against adenovirus proteins and the transgene product dystrophin has been abrogated to a degree not achievable with the use of either agent alone.

Another problem associated with immunity to AdVs is the generation of memory cells. Upon subsequent administration of the same vector, the immune response is boosted by these cells, effectively reducing the efficacy of the repeated dosing.

Adenovirus Manufacturing

The increasing number of adenoviral gene therapy applications that are moving from the laboratory to the clinic is creating a need for large amounts of highly purified recombinant AdVs. This demand is expected to increase as the first products reach the market. Thus, there is a clear need for a parallel development of efficient, scalable, and reproducible adenovirus manufacturing processes capable of delivering high amounts of infective AdV particles.

GMPs and Validation

Recombinant AdVs, such as all products that are to be administered to humans or animals, must be manufactured in accordance with a set of regulations issued by regulatory authorities such as the U.S. Food and Drug Administration (FDA) or the European Medicines Agency (EMEA) in the European Union. These regulations are known as current Good Manufacturing Practices (cGMPs) and cover all aspects of the production, from choosing and testing raw materials, to utilities, packaging, shipping, and transferring of final products to the clinic. If these items are not in conformity with GMPs, the product is deemed to be adulterated and cannot be legally approved. In the specific case of AdVs, the facilities and processes used in manufacturing should be designed carefully to guarantee maximum protection to the product, to personnel, and to the environment. For instance, dedicated facilities should be used to prevent cross-contamination from previous or parallel batches of other bioproducts. Confinement of production operations to class C clean rooms is also advisable to avoid dissemination of recombinant adenoviruses into the air.

One cornerstone provision of cGMPs is validation, a concept introduced to assure product consistency. The validation of downstream processing operations aims to prove that they are capable of consistently removing impurities (e.g., host cell components, process-related materials, adventitious agents) to acceptable levels. Additionally, acceptance limits and operating ranges for each step must be determined. Validation studies usually lead to optimized processes with reduced variability and, as a consequence, to a decrease in the number of failed batches. Thus, the development of adenovirus manufacturing processes (and associated facility) should be undertaken with validation in mind, not only to improve quality assurance and accelerate approval, but also to reduce costs.

Product Specifications and Quality Control

One core concept hovering GMPs is quality assurance (QA). Among other attributes, QA is a means of guaranteeing the excellence, security, and dependability of the manufacturing process or its product. QA is a key issue in process development, validation, and product approval, as well as on the assessment of the endproduct quality in comparison with product specifications. The characterization of recombinant AdVs thus constitutes a crucial aspect in all steps of product development, from basic research to clinical trials. As it is the case for other biologics, adenovirus products have an inherent variability in their composition, stability, and potency. They are also subject to the variability inherent to the biological nature of some of the methods used to test them. An AdV should be well characterized to demonstrate that it is consistent in composition, exhibits long-term physico-chemical and biological stability, and is free of adventitious agents (micro-organisms, adeno-associated viruses), contaminants, and impurities. This requires the development and setup of a range of "*validatable*" analytical methodologies capable of fully characterizing the product during processing and in its final formulation, while ensuring the production of a consistent product. The molecular structure of AdVs, hence their biological activity (potency), may be sensitive to factors such as temperature (labile for $T > 40°C$), pH (labile for $pH < 6$), and freeze/thawing cycles. Thus, a correct evaluation of product stability requires the use of conventional analytical techniques (e.g., circular dichroism and light scattering). Analytical techniques also play an important role in the analysis of source materials, in the assessment of the impact of changes in manufacturing processes, and in the validation of processes and cleaning.

The exact final specifications (identity, efficacy, safety, potency, and purity) for an adenovirus vector product will usually depend on the intended therapeutic use, and thus, they are defined during clinical trials. However, regulatory agencies such as the FDA, the EMEA, or the SFDA provide guidelines and quality standards that are helpful during product and process development.

Environmental and Safety Issues

An assessment of the environmental impact of a process is an essential part of the design. The costs associated with the treatment and disposal of the waste generated by a particular process solution should be estimated beforehand. This information is one key element in the final decision on which process to select. Environmentally unfriendly operations such as those that generate large amounts of hazardous solvents and materials, which are usually costly to dispose of, should definitely be avoided. Additionally, adequate systems should be in place to provide an efficient decontamination of solid (e.g., autoclaving and incineration) and liquid wastes (e.g., heat or caustic inactivation) before release from the manufacturing area. Once inactivated, these wastes should pose limited risk to the environment. Nevertheless, process optimization should always be geared toward minimization of waste generation. The formation of aerosols during processing should be minimized because adenovirus can spread via airborne transmission and contribute to dissemination within the manufacturing rooms and facility. Unit operations that need special safety precautions (e.g., explosion-proof tanks, blow-out walls, emission containment, personnel protection, etc.) to operate should also be carefully considered, because these requirements can dramatically increase the cost of equipment, building design, and construction. Overall, environmental and safety issues require an intimate knowledge of the process technology solutions available.

Process Considerations

A process for the manufacture of an AdV consists of several activities aimed at the production of a certain amount (measured as number of viral particle [VP] units or infectious viral particle [IVP] units) of the target product at an acceptable cost and quality. The generation of fully qualified cell banks and virus seeds is at the forefront of these activities. These banks should be extensively tested for contaminants, including RCAs. A rigorous screening of raw materials, especially those of biological origin, is also mandatory to guarantee that extraneous organisms and contaminants are not introduced into the process. Upstream and downstream processing unit operations are selected, arranged, designed, and operated to manufacture a bulk product. After filling and finishing, the product can be distributed and shipped. These activities should be GMP-compliant and thoroughly scrutinized under a quality control program, as discussed in the previous sections. Flowsheets for the recovery and purification of biologicals are usually established with several rules of thumb and on the basis of accumulated experience with the target product. Simulation tools can also be used to rapidly evaluate bioprocess alternatives

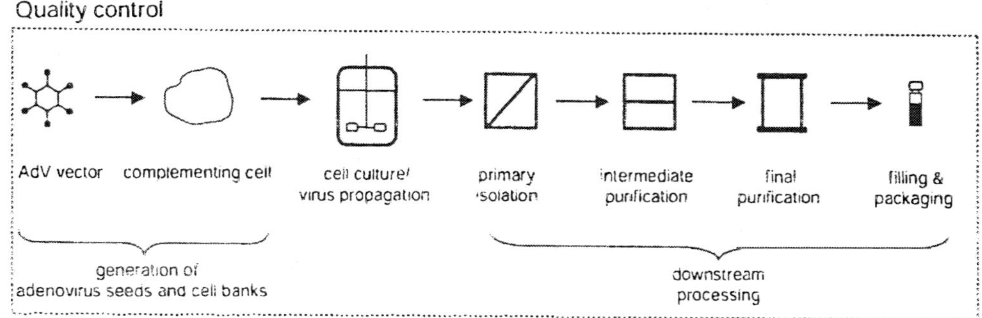

Fig. 8.5. Outline of the activities involved in a typical AdV production process.

and speed up development. The specifics of adenovirus purification were first addressed by researchers that have developed a range of efficient lab-scale protocols, most of them based on CsCl density-gradient ultra- centrifugation. Unfortunately, many of these protocols use reagents (e.g., CsCl is toxic) that are not acceptable for the manufacturing of a biological pharmaceutical. Furthermore, ultra-centrifugation is not amenable to scale-up due to the limited capacity of commercial ultra-centrifuges. Nevertheless, many published adenovirus production processes include modifications or adaptations of specific steps used in these laboratory procedures.

Cell culture is usually optimized to obtain high cell densities (cells/mL) and specific titers of infectious viral particles (IVPs/cell). The final goal is of course to maximize overall mass production (specific titer × cell density = IVP/mL). Next, a sequence of unit operations must be set up to recover the viral particles and eliminate host cell impurities (genomic DNA, RNA, proteins, RCAs, etc.) until the desired level of purity is met. For a product with an intended use in humans, this removal of impurities is mandatory to avoid side effects upon administration to patients. The downstream processing unit operations can be grouped into three different stages: primary isolation, intermediate purification, and final purification. Ideally, the overall process should have a limited number of high-recovery steps, so that processing costs are reduced and acceptable yields are obtained. The process should also use Generally Regarded As Safe (GRAS) reagents. Furthermore, lengthy operations and processes should be avoided to cut costs from overhead, amortization of equipment, and direct labor charges. Processes with overall adenoviral particle yields of 32%, 50%, 60%, and 71% have been reported in the literature.

Production

Most E1-deficient recombinant adenoviruses are propagated in the HEK-293 and PER.C6 cell lines (and derivatives thereof) as discussed above. The generation of RCAs is minimal in PER.C6 but remains a concern for HEK-293. Both cell lines have been documented for GMP manufacturing. The production of these cells can be accomplished by a variety of methods, which depend on whether adherent or suspension cell lines are being used.

An adenoviral production process with HEK-293 and PER.C6 is a two-phase process. In the first phase, cultures are started at an appropriate seeding density (e.g., 0.3×10^6 cells/mL) and allowed to grow until a cell density around $0.5–1 \times 10^6$ cells/mL is reached. The second phase starts at this point with the infection of the culture at a ratio of virus titer to cell density (known as multiplicity of infection—MOI) adequately chosen (e.g., MOI = 10). An exchange of medium is usual, but not mandatory, before infection. The cell density at the time of infection is a crucial parameter, with specific viral particle productivity (IVP/cell) usually dropping for cell densities higher than 0.5×10^6 cells/mL. After infection, viral particles propagate and accumulate in the cells with maximum titers ($\sim 10^{10}–10^{11}$ VP/mL) typically obtained 48 hours postinfection (hpi). Maximum cell densities of 1×10^7 cells/mL have been reported. Loss of viability and cell death ensue thereafter.

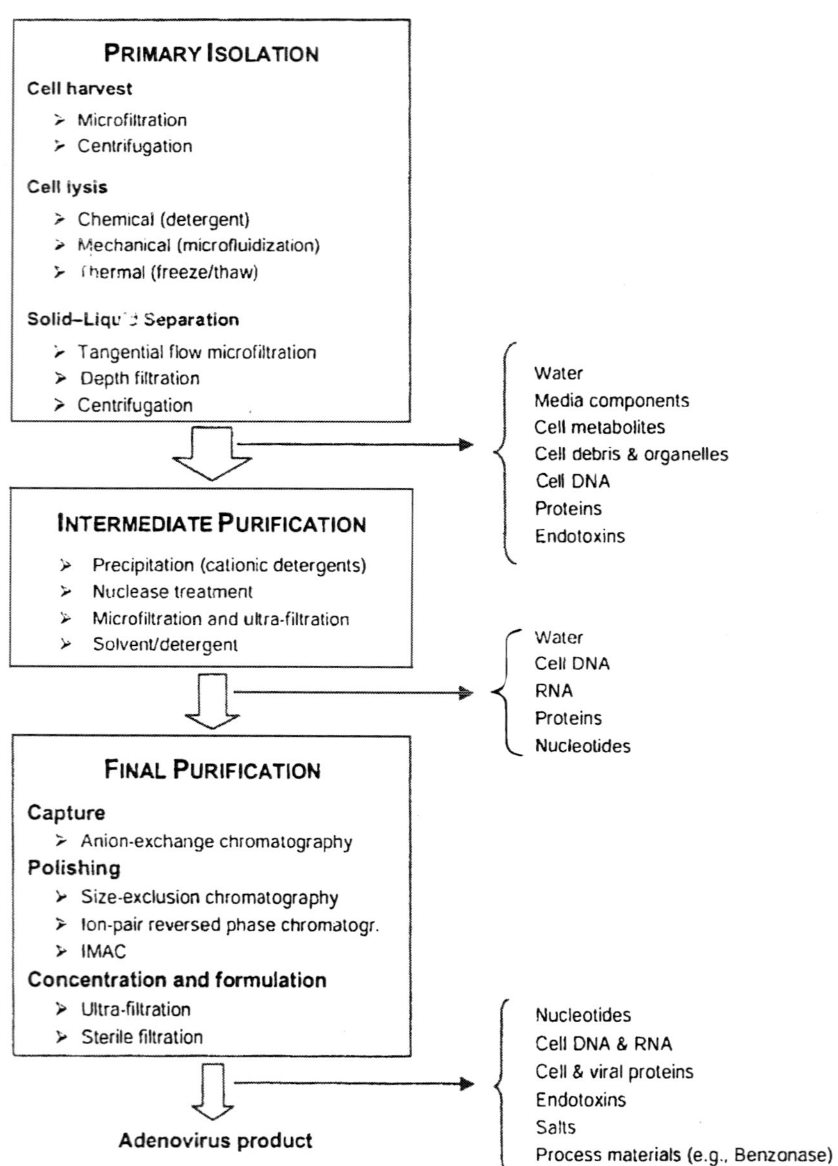

Fig. 8.6. Generic block of downstream processing of AdV vectors showing unit operation options in each section.

Adherent cell culture

Adherent or anchorage-dependent cell line require attachment to a surface for their survival and replication. These cultures are labor intensive, require both a large amount of space and specific equipment handling, and have a limited potential for scale-up. Thus, they are more adequate during the early stages of product and process development.

Adherent cells can be grown in stationary or microcarrier cultures. Stationary cultures use devices such as flasks, roller bottles, and cell factories that provide wall surface area for cell attachment. Microcarrier cultures, on the other hand, can be implemented in agitated bioreactors. These microcarriers are small porous particles (0.2 mm) that provide large surface areas for cell attachment and can be suspended in the culture medium by gentle agitation. The culture environment is thus easily controlled and the scale-up is done by increasing the bioreactor volume. In comparative studies, stationary cultures usually yield higher adenovirus titers (up to 1.1×10^4 VP/cell) than microcarrier cultures (up to 8.5×10^3 VP/cell).

Suspension cell culture

Suspension cell lines are more convenient for large-scale manufacturing. A further advantage is that they can be grown in serum- free media, without the addition of bovine-derived components. This advantage reduces costs and batch-to-batch variability and facilitates downstream processing and validation. Conveniently, both the HEK-293 and the PER.C6 cell lines can be adapted to grow on suspension cultures. When grown in serum-free media, these cell lines allow high growth rates and cell densities as well as high yields of adenoviral particles. The tendency of cell derivatives to aggregate, however, is usually a recurrent concern with suspension cultures, especially at high cell densities.

The cultivation of cells and adenovirus propagation in suspension bioreactors has been performed in batch, fed-batch, and perfusion modes. In batch operation, no nutrients are added during the course of growth or infection. Although batch cultures are simple to perform and contamination risks are low, essential nutrients are rapidly depleted from the medium and cell viability decreases.

The fed-batch mode is used to maintain cell viability after infection by supplementing limiting nutrients (e.g., glucose, glutamine, and amino acids) or reducing the accumulation of toxic metabolites (e.g., ammonia and lactate). It also improves viral titers by increasing the cell density at which cells can be infected up to 2×10^6 cells/mL, without reducing the per-cell yield of product. Both the medium composition as well as the feeding strategy are important parameters. Nutrient depletion and the buildup of toxic metabolites cannot be completely alleviated by fed-batch cultures. Operation under perfusion mode can overcome this limitation by ensuring a constant renewal of medium in the bioreactor. Briefly, cells are retained at high concentrations inside the bioreactor by using devices such as hollow fibers and membrane units, whereas fresh medium is continuously supplemented. Consequently, the cell density at which cells can be infected can be increased. With this strategy, HEK-293 cell densities of 8×10^6 cells/mL could be achieved at the time of infection, and viral titers of 7.8×10^9 IVP/mL were obtained at 60 hpi.

Downstream Processing

Primary isolation and intermediate purification

The suspension generated during cell culture constitutes the starting point for downstream processing. In the primary isolation stage, cells are harvested and viral particles are released from the cells together with other impurities. A significant reduction in volume occurs, and the most plentiful impurities such as extracellular liquid, proteins, genomic DNA, and cell debris are removed. Cells are typically harvested by centrifugation or microfiltration. The resulting cell slurry is then resuspended in an adequate volume (1/10 to 1/20 of the culture volume) of a suitable buffer or of the culture medium itself. The subsequent cell lysis operation is typically performed using freeze/thaw cycles, osmotic shock, sonication, microfluidization, or by the addition of detergents such as Triton X-100 or Tween-20. Unlike lysis by freeze/thawing and sonication, cell shearing by microfluidization is more rapid, reproducible, and easy to scale-up.

After lysis, cleared lysates are obtained by removing cell debris and larger unruptured organelles with centrifugation, depth filtration, or tangential flow microfiltration operations. Treatment with nucleases (e. g., Benzonase, Pulmozyme, DNase, RNase T1, and RNase I) is usually performed before or after clarification, to reduce the cellular DNA and RNA load. This step not only improves purity, hence the safety of the viral product, but also it reduces agglomeration of viral particles, which is usually induced by adhesion of nucleic acids. In some cases, nuclease treatment can be carried out at the end of the process, after chromatographic purification. As an alternative to nuclease digestion, cationic detergents can be added during lysis to selectively precipitate cellular DNA. Recent experiments with the detergent domiphen bromide have shown that it is possible to obtain three logs of DNA clearance without losses in the infectivity of purified viral particles. Thus, the use of DNA removal operations such as nuclease treatment and anion exchange chromatography may be eliminated or reduced.

The viral particle-containing solutions resulting from nuclease treatment and cationic detergent precipitation are typically filtered, concentrated, and conditioned before chromatographic purification. The inclusion of a solvent/detergent step at this stage may be included to inactivate potential enveloped viruses that could have been coamplified.

Final purification

A pharmaceutical product such as an AdV requires a high degree of purity. This level of purity is usually achieved with a combination of chromatography and filtration operations. The goal is to separate the viral particles from the most recalcitrant impurities thatpersistin the streams. The chromatographic operations described in the literature for virus purification explore properties such as size, charge, hydrophobicity, and metal affinity.

Anion-exchange (AEX) chromatography is widely used as a viral particle capture step. It explores the interaction between the negatively charged hexons in viral capsids and the stationary phases bearing positively charged ligands such as quaternary amines. Impurities (media components, low-molecular-weight DNA, penton, hexon, and fiber proteins are eluted at low salt (<0.25-M NaCl), whereas bound capsids are displaced with a salt gradient. A recent study shows that the NaCl concentration required to elute viral capsids from the anion exchange column is a function of the serotype being purified (ranging from 0.27 to 0.45 M), and it correlates very well to the electrostatic properties of the hexon protein in each serotype. Tentacular, perfusion, and soft gel in rigid shell materials have all been used for AEX purification of adenovirus particles. The reported AEX viral particle yields range from 63% to 80%.

AEX can also be performed in expanded-bed adsorption (EBA) mode. Under this mode of operation, cell lysates can be applied directly to the column from below. Large debris and unlysed cells that can move freely around the anion-exchanger beads eventually leave through the top of the column, whereas adenoviral particles bind to the anion-exchange matrix. Extensive washing from below limits nonspecific interactions between the particulates and the resin. Finally, the flow is reversed, the anion-exchanger beads are allowed to pack, and the viral particles are eluted under a salt gradient. Due to its early use in the downstream processing, EBA can be considered as an intermediate purification unit operation.

Adenovirus particles have also been purified by affinity chromatography by taking advantage of an ingenious targeting approach. Briefly, the fiber capsid protein of adenovirus 5 vectors was genetically fused to a biotin acceptor peptide (BAP). These BAP-modified fibers were then metabolically biotinylated during virus propagation in the HEK-293 cell line. The resulting covalently biotinylated viral particles could then be purified from crude lysates by avidin-affinity chromatography.

AEX alone is unlikely to be sufficient to produce an adenovirus product with the required purity. The inclusion of a chromatographic polishing step may thus be necessary as a means to remove traces of DNA and protein impurities. Size-exclusion, ion-pair reversed phase, and metal affinity chromatography have all been used toward this end. In the case of size-exclusion, if an adequate matrix is selected, virus elute in the flowthrough because of its large size, whereas low-molecular-weight impurities are retarded. The column loading volume can be increased up to 20% of the bed volume, because a group separation is achieved. An extra advantage of size exclusion as a polishing step is that it can also be used to exchange buffer. This enables formulation to be carried out simultaneously with polishing. In the case of ion-pair reverse phase chromatography, elution conditions are carefully selected to retain impurities in a PolyFlo matrix and to allow the viral particles not to bind. Under this negative chromatography operation mode, viral particles are recovered in the flowthrough with an 87% recovery yield. This leads to some dilution of the adenovirus stream, as is always the case when products are recovered in the flowthrough. Processes for adenovirus purification typically end with concentration, formulation, and sterile filtration operations. Concentration and formulation are usually carried out in ultra-filtration units equipped with 100–300-kDA membranes. The exact composition of the formulation buffer will depend on the intended application, mode of administration (injectable, aerosol), and required short-term and shelf stability. A typical liquid formulation may include an aqueous buffer supplemented with cryoprotectants (e.g., sucrose) and stabilizers such as the nonionic-surfactant polysorbate-80, the chelating agent EDTA, and the oxidation inhibitors ethanol and histidine. Filtration under sterile conditions is typically performed with 0.22-μm membranes.

Analysis and Evaluation of an Adenovirus Production Process

In this section, a pilot-scale process that has been developed specifically for the production and purification of AdVs for gene therapy is analyzed and evaluated for large-scale manufacturing with the use of the process simulator software SuperPro Designer. The major objective of the analysis presented here is to estimate the cost of the production of an adenovirus therapeutic product. Results further provide insights into process weaknesses and strengths, effectively directing bioprocess engineers toward better processes.

Process Description

As a design basis we have assumed a plant capacity of around 1×10^{18} viral particles of purified recombinant adenovirus produced per year. This amount of product is sufficient to treat 125,000 patients per year on the basis of 1×10^{12} VP doses given weekly for a total of 8 weeks, as described in a Gendicine clinical trial. The plant is designed to operate 330 days a year, with a new batch initiated every 11 days—this corresponds to 30 batches at 33.3×10^{15} VP/batch. The total batch time is around 17 days. Guidelines and quality standards issued by regulatory agencies have been used to set up product specifications in terms of final purity. Finally, we have assumed that, at the end of the process, the bulk adenoviral product will be distributed in vials, each containing a 1×10^{12} VP dose of 0.6 mL of sterile formulation buffer. This corresponds to a viral titer of 167×10^{11} VP/mL, which is higher that the specified value of 6.7×10^{11} VP/mL. The entire flowsheet for the production of adenovirus is divided into cell culture and virus propagation and downstream processing sections. The overall adenovirus particle recovery yield per batch is around 67% (33.3×10^{15} VP are recovered out of the 5×10^{16} VP that are present in the whole cell lysate). This figure is within yields reported in the literature for similar processes. Input data used in the simulation software SuperPro Designer were taken from the reference publication and supplemented with information from other published processes. Educated guesses were made to provide for missing data.

Cell culture section

The activities in this section include media sterilization, inoculum preparation, cell growth, and virus propagation. Serum- free (SF) medium is sterilized by 0.2-μm filtration and used for both inoculum preparation and cell growth/virus propagation. The culture is assumed to take place in fed-batch mode (with a single nutrient addition), in a bioreactor with a working volume of 1000 L. This size is a reasonable assumption, given that cultures with volumes as high as 10,000 L are currently being developed for production of HIV adenoviral vaccines. The inoculum is added to 500 L of culture medium at a seeding density of 3×10^5 cell/mL, and cells are allowed to grow for 6 days. Then, 500 L of fresh SF medium are added, and cells at a concentration of 0.5×10^6 cell/mL are infected at a

MOI of 10. Cell growth and virus propagation are conducted at 37°C and pH 7.2, with constant addition of a gaseous mixture (80% air, 10% CO_2, 10% O_2) at 0.05 vvm. Harvest is performed 48 hpi, with typical values assumed for the final cell concentration (1×10^6 cells/mL), adenovirus titer (5×10^4 VP/cell), and ratio of infectious viral particle to total viral particles (1 : 10).

Downstream processing section

The activities in this section include cell harvest and cell lysis, nuclease digestion, and chromatographic purifications. Cells from the suspension culture (1 m^3) are harvested by continuous centrifugation, resuspended in SF medium (1/10 of the original volume), and lysed by microfluidization (e.g., 2000 psi and 1 pass). Cell DNA is then drastically reduced (≈4.5 logs) by adding Benzonase up to a final concentration of 150 IU/mL. After removal of debris by centrifugation, the supernatant is clarified in a 0.2-μm dead-end filtration unit. Adenovirus capture and purification is performed by AEX chromatography column (Fractogel EMD-DEAE, 0.4-m bed height, 0.6-m bed diameter) according to the instructions presented by Tang et al. Briefly, each cycle comprises six distinct operations: (1) equilibration with 22 bed volumes (BVs) of buffer J1 (50-mM sodium phosphate pH 7.5, 265-mM NaCl, 2-mM $MgCl_2$, 2% (w/v) sucrose) at 4 cm/min, (2) loading of 106 L of feed at 1 cm/min, (3) washing with 4 BVs of buffer J1 at 2 cm/min, (4) washing with 8 BVs of 94% buffer J1 and 6% buffer J2 (50-mM sodium phosphate pH 7.5, 600-mM NaCl, 2-mM $MgCl_2$, 2% (w/v) sucrose), (5) elution of bound adenovirus particles with 10 BVs of linear gradient from 6% to 100% buffer J2 at 2 cm/min, and (6) column cleaning with 4 BVs of 1-M NaCl at 4 cm/min. The total cycle time is 12.26 h. The bound viral particles are eluted with an overall yield of 89%. The adenovirus pool is then concentrated 10 times by ultra-filtration using a 100-kDa membrane. A step yield of 96% is assumed based on data published for ultrafiltration of different viral particles. A size exclusion chromatography column (Superdex 200, 0.8-m bed height, 0.4-m bed diameter) is included as a polishing step (95% step yield). The column is loaded with the totality of the viral solution (12% of the bed volume), and upon elution with an adequate buffer (e.g., 20-mM sodium phosphate pH 8.0, 100-mM NaCl, 2-mM $MgCl_2$, 2% (w/v) at 0.43 cm/min), a pool of adenoviral particles is obtained that is five times diluted relatively to the feed. The total cycle time is 18.3 h. Concentration and formulation into an adequate buffer (2.5% glycerol, 25-mM NaCl, 20-mM Tris, pH) is subsequently carried out in an ultra-filtration unit equipped with a 100- kDA membrane. Finally, the adenovirus product is sterile filtered into glass vials (1×10^{12} VP in 0.6 mL).

Process scheduling

The plant batch time is approximately 405 hours, with a new batch (i.e., inoculum preparation) initiated every 264 hours. This batch start time roughly corresponds to the fourth day of the cell culture in the previous batch. The inoculum preparation, cell culture, and virus propagation procedures, with a duration of approximately 367 hours, are clearly identified in the chart as the time bottleneck. Comparatively, the downstream processing is complete within a mere 38 hours. The time bottleneck in this section is the size-exclusion chromatography polishing step, which takes about 18 hours.

Inventory Analysis

Remarkably, the annual mass production of purified adenovirus vector constitutes a minor fraction (~0.3 ppm) of the total amount of materials required for its production. Apart from the adenovirus vector, cell debris, and gases, all output materials end up in liquid waste streams, which are disposed of after adequate treatment (e.g., heat or caustic inactivation) to minimize environmental impacts. Water is the major raw material used (~97%), most of it for equipment cleaning. This is typical in the production of biopharmaceuticals as can be seen by checking IgG, recombinant β-glucuronidase, and plasmid DNA production examples. Serum-free medium (~0.2%) and gases (~1%) are used in the cell culture and virus propagation steps. Large amounts of sodium chloride, sodium phosphate, and sucrose (~0.8%) are required as buffer components in the chromatographic operations. A substantial amount of sodium hydroxide (~0.5%) is also used for equipment cleaning.

Cost Analysis and Economic Assessment

Economic evaluations were based on the following assumptions: (1) the entire direct fixed capital is depreciated linearly over a period of 10 years assuming a 10% salvage value for the entire plant, (2) the project lifetime is 15 years, and (3) 1×10^{18} VP of adenoviral product will be produced per year. For a plant of this capacity, the total capital investment is around \$17.8 million. The unit production cost is ~\$7.2/dose (10^{12} VP) or \$24,715/g. This figure is considerably higher when compared with production costs of other biopharmaceuticals such as β-glucuronidase (\$43.0/g), insulin (\$42.2/g), IgG (\$908/g), and plasmid DNA (\$375/g). The total equipment purchase cost was estimated to be around \$2.8 million. The most expensive piece of equipment is the bioreactor used for cell culture and virus propagation, priced at \$506,000. The cost of unlisted equipment (including the equipment used in the inoculum preparation section) was assumed to represent 20% of the total equipment cost.

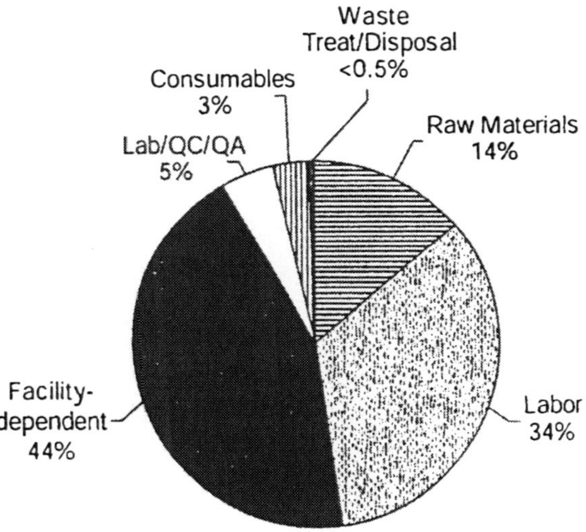

Fig. 8.7. Breakdown of the annual operating cost.

Facility-dependent cost (44% of the AOC) is the principal operating cost in this process, as is typical for high-value products that are produced in small quantities. Labor-related costs come next, accounting for 34% of the AOC. The annual cost of raw materials is around \$1.0 million, 92% of which are associated with the culture SF medium (priced at \$28/L). The cost of consumables is around \$193,000, representing approximately 3% of the AOC. The chromatographic resins in the AEX and size-exclusion chromatographic steps represent 84% of this value. The cost of utilities (electricity, steam, and cooling agents) is minimal, representing less than 0.1% of the AOC.

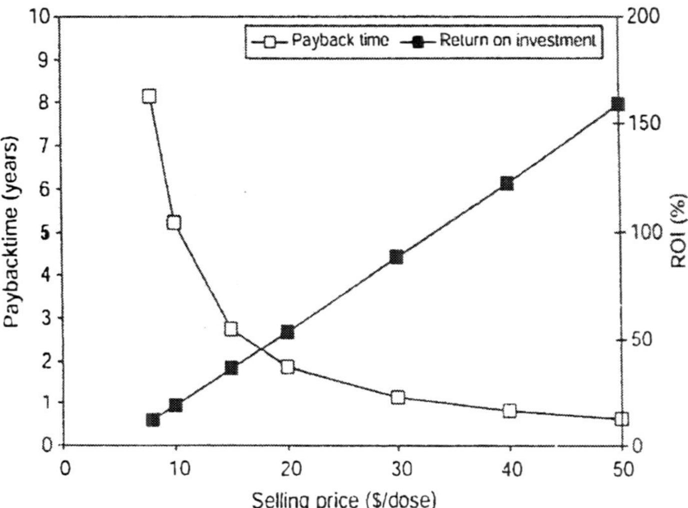

Fig. 8.8. Return on investment and payback time at different AdV selling prices.

The ROI increases around 3.5% for every \$1 increase in the selling price of each AdV dose, whereas the payback time declines for every \$1 increase. If one assumes that a dose of product is sold at \$30, the annual revenue will amount to \$30,662,000 for an annual production of 1×10^{18} VP. This corresponds to a gross profit (i.e., revenue-operating cost) of \$23,513,000. At this selling price, the payback time is 1.14 years with an ROI of 88%. This economic picture could change slightly by the inclusion of costs that were not accounted for in this case study. Adenoviral gene therapy has matured to the point where several products should be hitting the market in the wake of Gendicine. Many of the initial drawbacks and barriers (e.g., immunogenicity, lack of specificity, and transient expression of transgenes) have been tackled with innovative solutions and strategies (targeting, gutless vectors) that have proved valuable in some cases. To provide sufficient material for the ongoing gene therapy clinical trials, production and purification processes must be developed and optimized in parallel to deliver the required selectivity, yield, efficiency, and productivity. The design of these processes under cGMPs should be based on a profound knowledge of the target molecule and associated impurities and on the performance of the available unit operations. Although several well-established processes have been documented in the literature, new developments are likely to surface within the coming years because of increased investments from academia and industry in the area. The analysis presented in this chapter indicates that the production and purification of a therapeutic adenovirus product is economically viable, even with a suboptimized process. Process improvements will certainly reduce costs. As an educated guess, we may estimate selling prices to be in the range \$20–\$50/10^{12} VP.

9

AUTOXIDATION AND ANTIOXIDANTS

By definition, oxygen is an absolute requirement for aerobic life, but it may also be viewed as toxic under certain conditions. A chemical reaction that usually takes place at ambient temperature between atmospheric oxygen and an organic compound is generally defined as autoxidation. The phenomena of autoxidation are commonly observed in everyday life. For example, the browning of fruit, deterioration of edible oils, and degeneration of old rubber bands are the results of autoxidation. In the human body, *reactive oxygen species* (ROS) produced during autoxidation processes are also commonly encountered. This is a normal part of human physiology, as long as defense systems are effective, but overproduction or failure to scavenge free radicals can result in toxic biological responses that can yield deterioration and degeneration of cells, tissues, or organisms.

There are numerous reports suggesting that free radicals are involved in various human disease states. Pathological phenomena related to autoxidation are due to reactive oxygen species, and most age-related diseases can be explained through reactions of free radicals with biological substances. A notable case is cancer or, more specifically, carcinogenesis. Free radicals play a critical role in the initiation of carcinogenesis by damaging nucleic acids and producing a variety of lesions. For example, 8-hydroxyguanine, 5-hydroxymethyluracil, and thymine glycol are formed by the attack of hydroxyl free radicals on deoxyribonucleic acid (DNA), and these mutations may be viewed as a cause of carcinogenesis. Another free radical- related disease state is stroke. Damage to the brain due to central nervous system (CNS) ischemia is caused by injury resulting from the interruption of blood flow (i.e., lack of oxygenation) which is then followed by reoxygenation of the brain (ischemia/ reperfusion). It appears that all or most aerobic tissue suffers damage once it undergoes an ischemia/ reperfusion insult. The severity depends on many factors, one of which is the length of the ischemic period. Considerable evidence is now accumulating that injury occurs almost exclusively during the reperfusion phase, and that the injury is due to oxygen free radical-mediated oxidative stress. Furthermore, some neuronal pathologies, such as Alzheimer's disease, may relate to lipid peroxidation of cell membranes by free radicals.

Autoxidation phenomena could be completely prevented by total exclusion of oxygen or other oxidizing substances from a biological system. This is generally not practical, but changes in endogenous factors, such as addition of inhibitors, may decrease the reaction rate or prolong the induction period. However complete prevention of autoxidation is unlikely. Substances that can suppress autoxidation are termed inhibitors or antioxidants. Preventive inhibitors decrease the rate of autoxidation by suppressing the rate of initiation reactions. Antioxidants in the true sense are substances that can inhibit propagation steps; that is, they interrupt autoxidation chain reactions. Other types of inhibitors, for instance, antiozonants, are not biologically relevant but may be important in industry (e.g., protective coatings). Antioxidants are known to inhibit *carcinogenesis* or *atherosclerosis*. For example, vitamins and phenolic compounds can function as chemopreventive agents. The mechanism of action and the biological role of autoxidation and antioxidants are discussed in this article.

AUTOXIDATION

Autoxidation Reactions

The majority of compounds that are subject to autoxidation are unsaturated substances or highly condensed polymers, and the target of ROS is commonly the diene functionality—or double bonds. Autoxidation of unsaturated lipids is a good model to demonstrate this mechanism. The initial reaction between molecular oxygen and a polyunsaturated fatty acid (PUFA) occurs as $RH + O_2 \rightarrow ROOH$, which involves the movement of a double bond as well as the insertion of oxygen. In general, there is a "*spin barrier*" that prevents the direct addition of ground-state molecular oxygen in a single step to an organic compound. In the case of autoxidation, since direct addition is eliminated by the spin barrier, the alternatives are: (i) electron transfer (i.e., redox reactions) involving, for example, a transition metal ion or (ii) the participation of free radicals, whereby the addition of a radical to molecular oxygen can give rise to another radical.

The important features of autoxidation are auto-catalytic and free radical chain reactions. The rate of oxidation is initially slow and increases as the reaction progresses. However, once autoxidation is initiated, the reaction continues until the reaction substrate or catalytic factor becomes extinct. In short, unsaturated lipids undergo three reaction phases: initiation, propagation, and termination. The participation of reactive oxygen radicals in autoxidation reactions is summarized in the following reaction steps.

Initiation : $X^\bullet + RH \rightarrow R^\bullet + XH$

Propagation : $R^\bullet + O_2 \rightarrow RO_2^\bullet$

$RO_2^\bullet + RH \rightarrow ROOH + R^\bullet$

Termination : $RO_2^\bullet + RO_2^\bullet \rightarrow$ Stable product

$RO_2^\bullet + R^\bullet \rightarrow$ Stable product

$R^\bullet + R^\bullet \rightarrow$ Stable product

Initiation is perhaps the process most difficult to define. This is because of the very low concentration of radicals and the likelihood of there being more than one process, since a large number of different radicals can abstract hydrogen from RH to form $R^\bullet$. For example, $X^\bullet$ may be a transition-metal ion, a radical generated by photolysis or high-energy irradiation, a radical obtained by decomposition of a hydroperoxide (e.g., $RO^\bullet$), or a radical formed from an exogenous initiator. The two propagation reactions form the basis of the chain-reaction process. The autoxidation reaction is generally assumed to be a very fast reaction with almost no activation energy. A major consequence of this phase is that the concentration of $R^\bullet$ is much smaller than that of $RO_2^\bullet$. Like initiation processes, termination reactions may also be divided into those involving organic free radicals exclusively, and those in which metal ions participate. Of the termination processes involving $R^\bullet$ or $RO_2^\bullet$, the biomolecular reaction

$$RO_2^\bullet + RO_2^\bullet \rightarrow \text{inert products}$$

has received the most attention since this is likely to be the most important termination reaction under physiological conditions.

Autoxidation of unsaturated lipids is affected by many factors, so that none can be considered exclusively prooxidative or antioxidative. The rate of autoxidation is increased with reactivity of the autoxidizing substrate, concentration of reactants (the number of active sites and the concentration of oxygen), modified physical factors (e.g., a rise in temperature or by irradiation), and especially with an increase in the rate of initiation reactions. The rate of chain initiation reactions is increased mainly by factors that increase free radical function in autoxidizing systems, for example, ultraviolet, X-Ray, or ionizing radiation. In various reactant systems, such as fats, oils, and biological membranes, heavy metals and their derivatives are important initiators of autoxidation reactions. The reaction rate, however, is suppressed by factors such as a reduction in the number of active sites, a decrease in the partial pressure of oxygen by a suitable selection of physical factors, and a decrease in the reaction temperature. The most important, however, is the reduction of initiation rate (i.e., the level of free radicals capable of chain initiation). Substances actively suppressing the concentration of the free radicals are antioxidants. Other substances are also very effective in suppressing autoxidation, particularly those eliminating free radical precursors (e.g., sulfur compounds that cause reduction of lipid hydroperoxide). Substances deactivating ozone (antiozonants) or singlet oxygen, which protect against irradiation, or heavy metals (metal scavengers), also act as inhibitors of lipid autoxidation.

Lipid Peroxidation

Oxidative damage to membrane lipids (i.e., lipid per- oxidation in biological systems) has been studied for many years. Lipid peroxidation is a primary event produced by oxidative stress or as a consequence of tissue damage, which can exacerbate tissue injury, due to the potential cytotoxicity and genotoxicity of the end products of lipid peroxidation. Membrane lipids with double bonds are most susceptible to oxidation. Lipid peroxidation can reduce membrane fluidity, leading to increased rigidity throughout the hydrophobic space of membranes, decreased permeability, osmotic fragility, and altered activity of certain membrane-bound enzymes and transport systems.

Membrane lipid peroxidation can change the activity of essential membrane proteins such as Na^+/K^+-ATPase. As a consequence, rates of ion pumping may be altered. Two well-characterized products of lipid peroxidation, malondialdehyde and 4-hydroxynonenal, have been shown to react with critical biomolecules that may have a key role in the development of certain pathological states. Microsomal lipid peroxidation forms mainly 4-hydroxy-2-nonenal with minor amounts of 4-hydroxy-2-octeal, 4-hydroxy-2-decenal, and 4-hydroxy-2-undecenal. α,β-Unsaturated aldehydes, such as 4-hydroxynonenal, are highly reactive electrophilic reagents that react easily with thiols by Michael addition to the CH=CH double bond. Aldehyde adducts of lipid peroxidation have been shown to induce glutathione depletion in hepatocytes, and corresponding abnormal liver function. Free hemoglobin, in the presence of xanthine/xanthine oxidase, will also promote the peroxidation of arachidonic acid and unsaturated fatty acids within normal cellular membranes. Furthermore, hemoglobin or red cell lysates cause brisk peroxidation of crude murine brain homogenates. This hemoglobin-driven peroxidation is blocked by an iron chelator (i.e., desferrioxamine) which indicates that iron released from heme is responsible.

Peroxides can play a physiological role in the cell but also mediate processes leading to heart disease and carcinogenesis. Fatty acid peroxidation may also be related to free radical-mediated metabolic activation of carcinogens or drugs, which lead to the initiation of carcinogenesis or cytotoxicity. Modification of membrane function as a consequence of lipid peroxidation includes uncoupling of oxidative phosphorylation in mitochondria, alteration of liver endoplasmic reticulum functions, and modification of the ionic permeability of phospholipid membranes. Radiation-catalyzed lipid peroxidation of erythrocyte membranes increases permeability to Na^+, K^+, and Ca^{++}. Ultimately, peroxidation leads to gross destruction of membranes, as demonstrated by release of lysosomal enzymes in irradiated lysosomes, hemolysis in irradiated erythrocytes, and release of various enzymes by disruption of the liver plasma membrane.

Free Radicals and Defense Systems

Free Radicals and Defense Systems

A free radical may be broadly defined as a molecule or ion containing an unpaired electron. Although most radicals are reactive and undergo dimerization or other reactions in which the unpaired electron becomes paired some radicals such as nitroxide radicals ($R_2NO^•$) are relatively stable. A major source of radicals in biological systems is molecular oxygen. This very reactive molecule is essential to the life of higher organisms, but nevertheless can be considered dangerous in excess.

Superoxide anion ($O_2^{•-}$) and hydrogen peroxide (H_2O_2) are normal metabolites in mammalian cells produced during the biological reduction of oxygen. The occurrence of oxidative radical reactions in biological systems is usually associated with cellular electron transfer chains of the mitochondria and certain enzyme activities. Free radicals are further generated during the course of specialized physiological reactions, such as the release of $O_2^{•-}$ and H_2O_2 by endothelium non-inflammatory cells, which might serve as cell signals promoting growth responses. Furthermore, environmental factors as well as the metabolism of xenobiotics are significant sources of free radicals, although their actual contribution to the redox state of the cell is difficult to assess.

Although of modest chemical reactivity, $O_2^{•-}$ and H_2O_2 contribute to the formation of more reactive species via various redox reactions. It is currently accepted that the reaction of both $O_2^{•-}$ and H_2O_2 with suitable metal complexes yields HO . Fenton-type reactions requires both $O_2^{•-}$ and H_2O_2 as precursors of $HO^•$. This proceeds via an intermediate catalyst, such as a transition metal chelate, which reacts to produce $HO^•$. $HO^•$ may account for some aspects of mitochondrial damage, such as oxidative impairment of mitochondrial DNA. The requisite conditions for $HO^•$ formation by mitochondria are met during mitochondrial electron transfer: mitochondria are a major source of $HO^•$ generated by H_2O_2 cleavage.

Haber-Weiss reactions : $Fe^{3+} + O_2^{•-} \rightarrow Fe^{2+} + H_2O_2$

Fenton reaction : $Fe^{2+} + H_2O_2 \rightarrow Fe^{3+} + HO^• + HO^-$

Another type of one-electron transfer reaction that contributes to the formation of oxyradicals involves the quenching of carbon center radicals ($R^•$) by molecular oxygen. This reaction leads to the formation of peroxyl radicals ($R\text{-}OO^•$), which generally have quite different reactivities from those of the parent $R^•$ species. As a result of the reactivity of these species toward unsaturated fatty acids, the propagation steps of lipid peroxidation follow the initiation step. These propagation steps occur at membrane hydrophobic sites, and the length of the chain reaction is determined by the availability of reactants, PUFA and O_2, and of chain-breaking antioxidants such as octocopherol, carotenoids, and ubiquinone.

In cells, the first line of defense against these reactive species is represented by primary antioxidant defenses involving enzymes that specifically remove free radicals or oxidants, such as superoxide dismutase, glutathione peroxidase, and catalase. In general, aerobes do not express an excess of antioxidant defenses, although these systems are often inducible by elevated O_2 if sufficient time for adaptation is allowed. Moreover, endogenous antioxidants may not prevent damage by ROS at ambient O_2. Thus, animals rely on a second line of defense in the form of repair systems, the most important of which removes mutagenic lesions in DNA induced by ROS. Superimposed on such defenses are inducible proteins such as heme oxygenase-1. Heme oxygenases remove the prooxidant heme and produce the antioxidant bilirubin in the process. Additional protection is provided by dietary antioxidants. The physiological role of some of these is well established (e.g., vitamin E and ascorbate), whereas the role of others (e.g., flavonoids, carotenoids) is currently uncertain. However, dietary antioxidants appear to be important in delaying/preventing certain human diseases, especially cardiovascular disease and some types of cancer.

Antioxidants

Natural antioxidants such as non-enzymatic dietary components are not specific but can scavenge organic and inorganic radicals. These agents are found in numerous plant materials and commonly include an aromatic ring as part of their molecular structure. There are a variety of cyclic ring structures that are generally associated with one or more hydroxyl groups to provide a labile hydrogen and a basis for free radical formation. These antioxidants can be classified as water soluble or lipid-soluble, depending on whether they act primarily in the aqueous phase or in the lipophilic region of cell membranes. Hydrophilic anti-oxidants include ascorbic acid and urate. Ubiquinols, retinoids, carotenoids, flavonoids, and tocopherol are representative lipid-soluble antioxidants. Plasma proteins, glutathione, and urate are endogenous, whereas ascorbic acid, carotenoids, retinoids, flavonoids, and tocopherols constitute some of the dietary antioxidants. These compounds possess the potential to scavenge and quench various radicals and ROS. Certain radical scavengers are not recyclable, however, others are recycled through the intervention of a series of enzyme systems or other non-enzymic antioxidant systems.

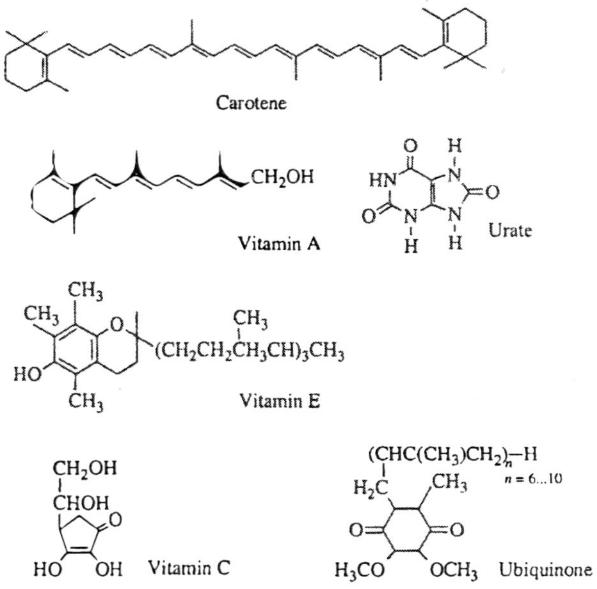

Carotene

CH_2OH

Vitamin A

Urate

CH_3 CH_3 HO CH_3 CH_3 $(CH_2CH_2CH_3CH)_3CH_3$

Vitamin E

CH_2OH CHOH HO OH Vitamin C

$(CHC(CH_3)CH_2)_n$–H H_2C CH_3 $n = 6...10$ H_3CO OCH_3 Ubiquinone

Fig. 9.1. Natural antioxidants.

Based on safety and other pragmatic reasons, the number of active substances used as antioxidants is restricted to a few phenolic substances. The flavonoids are an unusually large group of naturally occurring phenolic compounds ubiquitously distributed in the plant kingdom. These aromatic compounds are formed in plants from the aromatic amino acids, phenylalanine, tyrosine, and acetate units. Phenylalanine and tyrosine are converted to cinnamic acid and *p*-coumaric acid that condense with acetate units to form the cinnamoyl structure of the flavonoid. Flavonoids are generally known to be plant, flower, leaf, and fruit pigments. They are responsible for the brilliant shades of blue, scarlet, orange, etc., in flowers, fruits, and leaves. They are found in various fruits, vegetables, nuts, seeds, grains, spices, and herbs, as well as in beverages such as tea, cocoa, and wine. Dietary exposure to flavonoids is significant. The average diet in the United Kingdom and United States may contain up to 1 g of mixed flavonoids per day. Their dietary intake far exceeds that of vitamin E (a monophenolic antioxidant) and β-*carotene*.

Flavonoids act as potent metal chelators and free radical scavengers. They are powerful chain-breaking antioxidants. Moreover, flavonoids are known to possess vitamin C stabilizing and antioxidant-dependent vitamin C sparing activities. They are also known to increase the absorption of vitamin C. In addition, flavonoids are known to modify the activities of a host of enzyme systems including protein kinase C, protein tyrosine kinase and various other kinases, aldose reductase, myeloperoxidase, NADPH oxidase, xanthine oxidase, phospholipase, reverse transcriptases, ornithine decarboxylase, lipoxygenase, cyclooxygenase, and so on. Some of these enzyme systems are critically involved in immune function, carcinogenesis, cellular transformation, and tumor growth and metastasis. The physiologic and pathologic processes affected by flavonoids are diverse and numerous, and include secretion, mitogenesis, platelet aggregation and adhesion to endothelial surface, cell motility and malignant cell proliferation, cancer metastasis, and function/expression of adhesion molecules in various mammalian cell types. The antioxidant function and enzyme-modifying actions of flavonoids could account for many of their pharmacological activities.

Quercetin and other flavonoids are effective inhibitors of $O_2^{\cdot-}$-production by cells. Quercetin is a potent inhibitor of human neutrophil degranulation and $O_2^{\cdot-}$-production, and also inhibits the phosphorylation of neutrophil proteins accompanying neutrophil activation by phorbol myristate acetate.

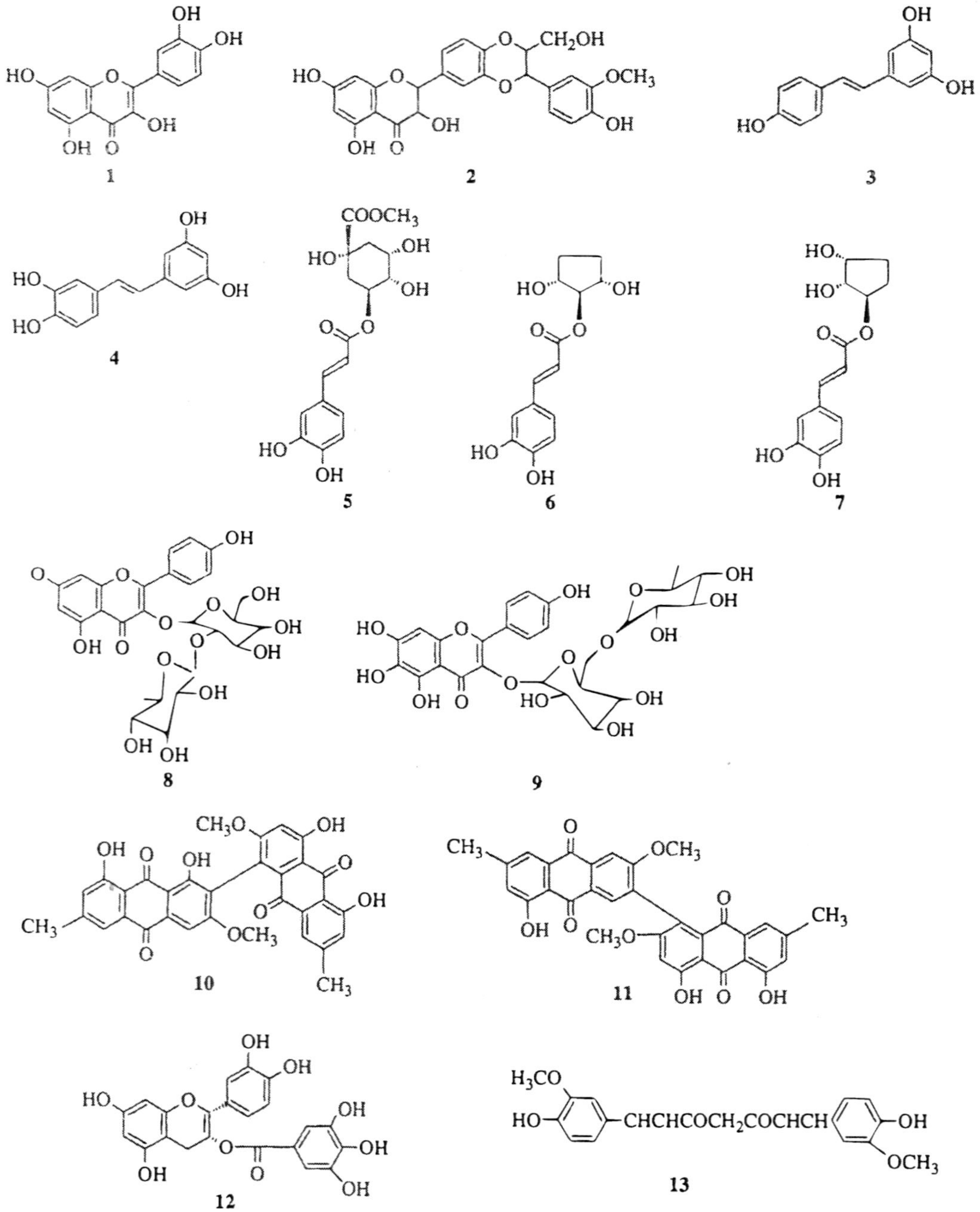

Fig. 9.2. Phenolic antioxidant isolated from plants; 1. quercetin; 2. silymarin; 3. trans-resveratrol; 4. piceatannol; 5. chlorogenic acid methyl ester; 6. 1-3′,4′-Dihydroxycinnamoyl)-cyclopenta-2,5-Diol; 7. 1-(3′,4′-Dihydroxycinnamoy)-cyclopenta-2,3-Diol; 8. kaempferol-3-O-neohespheridoside; 9. 5,6,7,4′-Tetrahydroxyflavonol-3-O-rutinoside; 10. floribundones I; 11. floribundones II; 12. (-)-epicatechin-3-O-gallate; and 13. curcumine.

Quercetin can also suppress lipid peroxidation in several biological systems, such as mitochondria, microsomes, chloroplasts, and erythrocytes. Silymarin, a 3-OH flavone present in *Silybum marianum* (the European milk thistle), protects rat liver mitochondria and microsomes from lipid peroxide formation induced by Fe^{2+}-ascorbate and NADPH-Fe^{3+}-ADP systems. Soybean isoflavonoids have shown antioxidative potency and prevent peroxidative hemolysis of sheep, rat, and rabbit erythrocytes. Quercetin and silybin were reported to exert a protective effect by the decrease in the xanthine dehydrogenase/oxygenase ratio observed during ischemia/reperfusion in the rat. The enzyme (xanthine oxidase) implicated in tissue oxidative injury after ischemia/reperfusion is a source of ROS that is formed from a dehydrogenase during ischemia. The protective effect of quercetin and silybin on the xanthine dehydrogenase/oxidase ratio is due to inhibition of the dehydrogenase.

Prooxidants

A prooxidant is an agent that can induce oxidative stress, which is defined as a shift 'in the prooxidant– antioxidant balance toward oxidant activity. Oxidative stress induced by a prooxidant in a biological system manifests itself as increased production of bioactive free radical species, a decrease or modulation of antioxidant defenses, and/or an increase in oxidative damage. The fine balance between the oxygen center radicals and antioxidants may be dependent on the concentration of prooxidant, oxygen tension, and interactions with other antioxidants.

Vitamins

Carotenoids

Carotenoids are a well-characterized class of pigments widely distributed in nature and responsible for the bright colors of various fruits and vegetables. Some of the more than 600 different carotenoids are well known, such as β-carotene, which is widely used as a precursor of vitamin A, a food colorant, and a food additive. These compounds have been shown to function as enhancers of gap–junction communication, stimulants of immune responses, and quenchers of electronically excited species, such as singlet oxygen and triplet sensitizers. The action of β-carotene and other carotenoids as antioxidants has recently attracted widespread attention. Carotenoids are thought to scavenge free radicals, and the antioxidant action of β-carotene and other carotenoids has been observed with in vitro andin vivo systems. However, carotenoids do not have structural features commonly associated with chain-breaking antioxidants. The extensive system of conjugated double bonds in their molecules imparts a prooxidant character and makes them very susceptible to attack by free radical species.

The development of either a harmful or beneficial cellular response by carotenoids will depend on their antioxidant or prooxidant characteristics, which are determined by various factors in the intra- and extra- cellular environments such as oxygen tension and β-carotene concentration. When an inappropriate prooxidant activity of carotenoids develops in normal cells, the reactive oxygen metabolites generated could induce damage to lipids, proteins, and DNA. This effect alters normal regulatory functions and can damage cellular integrity or induce neoplastic transformation. Some human intervention trials indicate that carotenoid supplements are of little or no value in preventing chronic disease, such as cardiovascular disease and cancer, and may actually increase lung cancer incidence in smokers. In contrast, when carotenoids act as prooxidants in already transformed cells, they could induce beneficial effects, such as inhibiting the growth and development of malignant lesions and/or producing tumor cytotoxic effects.

Although it has been reported that carotenoids may prevent normal cells from becoming transformed through their antioxidant activity, there is much evidence indicating that they may also block the growth of cells already transformed through their prooxidant action. Carotenoid autoxidation has been suggested to occur at a higher level in tumor cells than in normal cells. In tumor cells, therefore, it can be hypothesized that the prooxidant properties of carotenoids prevail over the antioxidant properties. In addition, some studies have shown that carotenoids act as prooxidant agents selectively in tumor cells by increasing the expression of heat-shock proteins and enhancing the formation of lipid peroxidation products, further reducing the levels of oxygen-protective enzymes and stimulating the expression of tumor necrosis α-factor.

Ascorbates

Ascorbate is an essential vitamin that must be taken from external sources. It is marketed as a dietary supplement because of its antioxidant properties. Several epidemiologic studies suggest that antioxidant vitamins in sufficient concentrations inhibit heart disease and cancer. However, there is considerable uncertainty about the optimal level of intake. Substantial evidence shows that ascorbate can also act as an oxidant, depending on the environment in which the molecule is present. It can induce cell death, nuclear fragmentation, and internucleosomal DNA cleavage in human myelogenous leukemic cell lines. More recently, it was reported that dietary supplementation of 500 mg/day of vitamin C to healthy volunteers for 6 weeks results in significant prooxidant effects. This is exemplified by an increase in lymphocytes with typical markers of DNA damage, mediated by oxygen radicals such as 8-oxoguanine and 8-oxoadenine.

Vitamin C supplementation is able to significantly affect CYP2E1-catalyzed drug metabolism in the rat and is linked to an overgeneration of the superoxide anion in hepatic microsomes. Generation of a superoxide anion induced by vitamin C supplementation provides a plausible explanation for the observed damage to DNA in peripheral blood lymphocytes. Ascorbate is a reducing agent in brain tissue homogenate but has an oxidizing effect in brain slices. A hypothesis put forth to explain the oxidative effects of ascorbate in cortical slices proposes that extracellular ascorbate is oxidized to dehydroascorbate which is rapidly carried into cells via a glucose transporter. The dehydroascorbate in cytosol is then reduced back to ascorbate, and, during the reduction process, cellular components are oxidized.

Tocopherols

Vitamin E, the major lipophilic antioxidant of exogenous origin in tissues, is the collective name for the eight major naturally occurring molecules, four tocopherols and four tocotrienols, that qualitatively exhibit the biological activity of α-tocopherol. α-Tocopherol is generally regarded as the most important lipid-soluble antioxidant in plasma, circulating lipoproteins, and tissues, whereas γ-tocopherol and tocotrienols are present in these tissues at much lower concentrations.

In an investigation of the antitumor activities of α-tocopherol acid succinate and acetate, the acid succinate form inhibited the growth of oral carcinoma cells, while stimulating the growth and differentiation of normal keratinocytes. The acetate form increased thymidine incorporation and mutant p53 expression in cancer cells, thereby increasing proliferation and expression of the cyclin regulator p34cdc. Vitamin E treatment reduced the time required for wound healing in the oral cavity and increased the in vitro growth of endothelial cells. Platelet adhesion was also inhibited, resulting in a possible reduction in thrombosis. The mechanism of action for this response appears to be blockage of the prostaglandin pathway at the site of cyclooxygenase activity, and it is a plausible mechanism that supports the use of vitamin E in periodontal disease.

The antioxidative activity of vitamin E is converted to prooxidant activity when mild conditions were used to initiate oxidation. A prooxidant effect of α-tocopherol on lipid peroxidation was found only when the samples were virtually free of ascorbate, or if the final concentration of ascorbate in the samples was physiologically low. Adding ascorbate to a near-physiological final concentration restored the antioxidant activity of α-tocopherol under mild oxidative conditions.

Retinoids

Retinoids, metabolic and synthetic derivatives of vitamin A, have been shown to function as effective antioxidants and inhibit the peroxidation of PUFA in lipid bilayers. For example, several retinoids

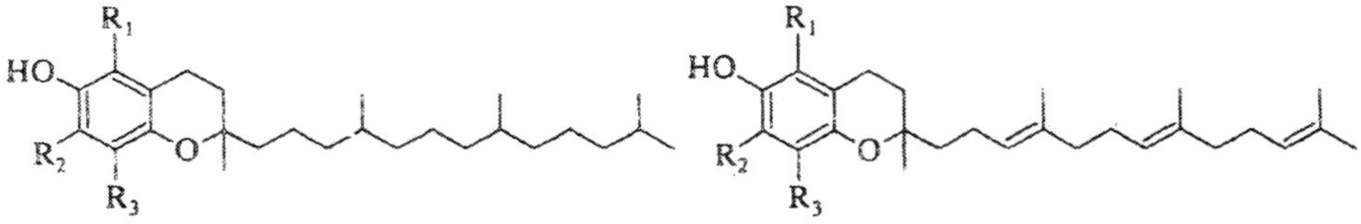

	R_1	R_2	R_3		R_1	R_2	R_3
α-Tocopherol	CH_3	CH_3	CH_3	α-Tocotrienol	CH_3	CH_3	CH_3
β-Tocopherol	CH_3	H	CH_3	β-Tocotrienol	CH_3	H	CH_3
δ-Tocopherol	H	CH_3	CH_3	δ-Tocotrienol	H	CH_3	CH_3
γ-Tocopherol	H	H	CH_3	γ-Tocotrienol	H	H	CH_3
Tocol	H	H	H	Tocotrienol	H	H	H

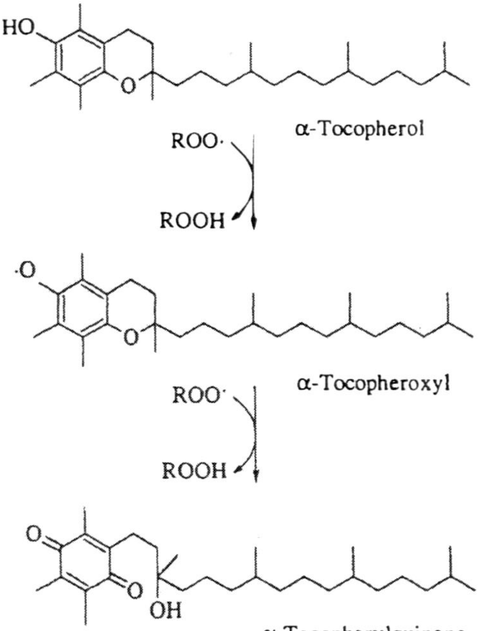

α-Tocopherol

ROO· → ROOH

α-Tocopheroxyl

ROO· → ROOH

α-Tocopherylquinone

Fig. 9.3. Chemical structures of the vitamin E groups and meabolic pathway of α-tocopherol.

inhibit ascorbate-dependent, iron-catalyzed lipid peroxidation in rat liver microsomes and brain mitochondria. Retinol palmitate was shown to function as an antioxidant in rat heart and brain tissues. However, retinoic acid was shown to stimulate the rate of 2,2'-Azobis(2-Amidinopropane)-initiated autoxidation of linoleic acid in sodium dodecyl sulfate micelles, and this observation may account for the prooxidant effect of retinoic acid in this system. In addition, possible detrimental effects of retinoids (e.g., promotion of tumor growth), increase in low-density lipoproteins (LDL) and triglyceride, and exacerbation of preexisting autoimmune disease have all been reported.

Phenolics

Phenolics are one of the major groups of non-essential dietary components that have been associated with the inhibition of atherosclerosis and cancer. The bioactivity of phenolics may be related to their antioxidant behavior, which is attributed to their ability to chelate metals, inhibit lipoxygenase, and scavenge free radicals. However, phenolics can also function as prooxidants by chelating metals in a manner that maintains or increases their catalytic activity. Also, poly-phenolics reduce metals, thereby increasing their ability to form free radicals from peroxide.

Flavonoids

Flavonoids, especially those with catechol or phyrogallol groups, obviously are prone to autoxidation reactions. In a recent paper by Morgan et al., the prooxidative and antioxidative properties of phenolics from soybeans and other legumes were documented. The primary phenolics (phenolic acids) and flavonoids were able to reduce ferric to ferrous ions and were able to chelate and alter the catalytic activity of iron. Most of the phenolics tested were also able to inhibit oxidation of linoleic acid micelles and ferrous ion-catalyzed oxidation of glutamine synthase, presumably through free radical scavenging and removal of iron from catalytic sites via chelation. Although flavonoids inhibited oxidation in certain systems, they did not protect against all forms of oxidative damage. The phenolics chelated iron, but this metal ion was still catalytically active and able to oxidize both deoxyribose and DNA. Prooxidant activity of phenolics has also been observed for carnosol, carnosic acid, quercetin, rutin, and luteolin.

It was also found that pH was essential in determining the oxidative role of phenolics. In general, a decrease in pH increased iron-reducing activity and reduced the ability of phenolics to chelate and inhibit the catalytic activity of iron. Increasing pH increased deoxyribose and DNA oxidation. Inhibition of lipid oxidation was also influenced by pH, with γ-resorcyclic acid being antioxidative at pH 5.8 and prooxidative at pH 7.4. Hydrobenzoic acid was antioxidative, and apigenin-7-glucoside was prooxidative at pH 7.4, yet neither had an effect on lipid oxidation at pH 5.8. These results suggest that the pH of biological tissues could also influence the antioxidative/prooxidative activity of phenolics.

A possible mechanism of cytotoxicity in polyphenols may be related to their prooxidant properties. Flavonoids autoxidize in an aqueous medium and may form highly reactive $HO^•$ radicals in the presence of transition metals. In addition, polyphenols and flavonoids may act as substrates for peroxidase and other metalloenzymes, yielding quinone- or quinomethide-type prooxidant and/or alkylating products. The prooxidant character of polyphenol cytotoxicity is supported by the formation of activated oxygen species during gallic acid induced apoptosis, and by the enhancement of gallic and caffeic acid induced apoptosis by non-toxic concentrations of copper ions.

Catechins, such as (–)-epicatechin and (–)-epigallocatechin abundant in green tea, possess the antioxidative and prooxidative characteristics of Cu^{2+}-induced LDL oxidation. In the initiation phase, LDL oxidation was inhibited by addition of catechin. In contrast, during the propagation phase of LDL oxidation, catechins served as accelerators of oxidation. Depending on redox status, they might form reactive oxidation products such as semiquinones and quinones and function to stimulate oxidative reactions.

Quercetin, a highly studied antioxidant flavonoid has the potential to inhibit free radical processes in cells by: (a) scavenging $O_2^{•-}$; (b) blocking lipid peroxidation; (c) reacting with peroxyl or lipid peroxyl radicals; d) inhibiting formation of $HO^•$; and (e) chelating iron ions. The biological effects of quercetin are believed to result from its antioxidant properties. Recently, it was clearly demonstrated that quercetin could function both as an antioxidant and a prooxidant, depending on concentration and free radical sources and their location in the cell. Also, quercetin was observed to be cytotoxic in a dose-dependent manner. Although the exact mechanism of cytotoxicity has not yet been fully elucidated, it may involve formation of $O_2^{•-}$ or its metabolite *o*-quinone. Such species are known to be toxic and

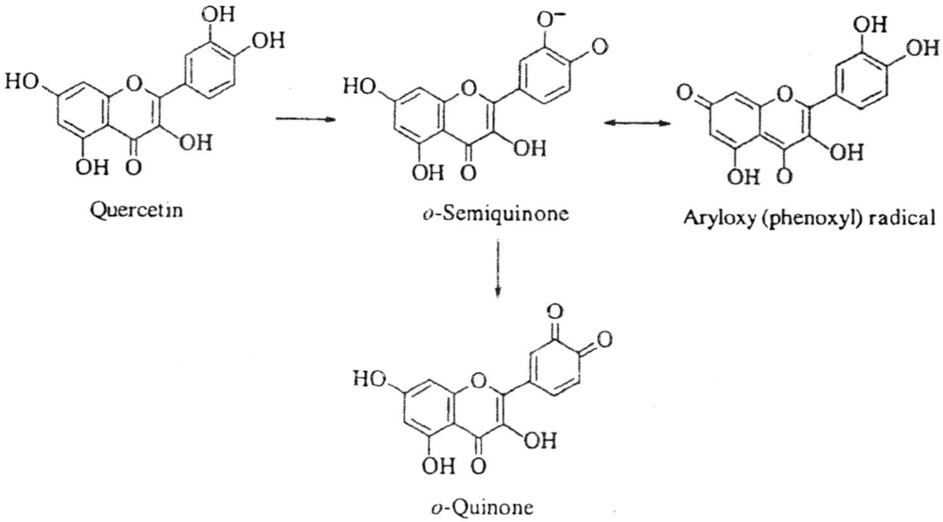

Quercetin → *o*-Semiquinone ↔ Aryloxy (phenoxyl) radical

↓

o-Quinone

Fig. 9.4. A simple scheme of quercetin oxidoreductive activation.

to bind irreversibly to various cell constituents by covalent binding with sulfhydryl groups or other essential groups.

Catecholestrogens

The antioxidant properties of estrogens have been demonstrated in many in vitro and in vivo studies. For instance, estrogens inhibit the oxidation of LDL, the peroxidation of lipids, and the oxidation of cholesterol. The administration of 17β-estradiol to ovariectomized pigs inhibits the oxidation of LDL. This effect has also been observed in postmenopausal women after administration of 17β-estradiol. These antioxidant activities of estrogens are believed to explain the lower rate of heart disease in premenopausal women, or postmenopausal women treated with estrogen, compared to that of men.

In contrast, prooxidant effects of estrogens have been established in other model systems. 17β-estradiol or other estrogens induce single-strand breaks or 8-hydroxylation of guanine bases of DNA in Syrian hamsters treated with these hormones. Moreover, metabolites of estrogen or diethylstilbestrol in the presence of peroxidase and DNA induce 8-hydroxylation of guanine bases. In addition to oxidant-induced damage of DNA, estrogens have also been shown to generate lipid peroxidation and oxygen-radicalmediated oxidation of amino acid residues of proteins, resulting in carbonyl-containing moieties.

Estrogens may exhibit either pro- or antioxidant activities depending on the nature of their metabolites and concentrations. Pharmacological concentrations of parent hormones or their metabolites clearly have antioxidant properties. This inhibitory mechanism may be based on the free radical scavenging action of the phenol moiety of estrogen. In contrast, 2- or 4-hydroxyestradiol enhances the oxidation of LDL by decreasing lag times of lipid peroxidation by 40–50% compared to control values in the absence of estrogen.

The catechol structure of catecholestrogens appears to be necessary for this prooxidant activity, as the parent hormones and other estrogen metabolites do not possess any detectable oxidant activity. Therefore, the in vivo prooxidant activity of estrogens may be dependent on their conversion to catecholestrogen metabolites in a specific organ or species. The mechanism of prooxidant activity of catecholestrogens is likely based on the reduction of metal ions, specifically Cu^{2+} to Cu^{+}, by the catecholestrogen metabolites. The lipid oxidation of LDL by Cu^{+} generated hydroxyl radicals, which further initiate oxidation of lipids.

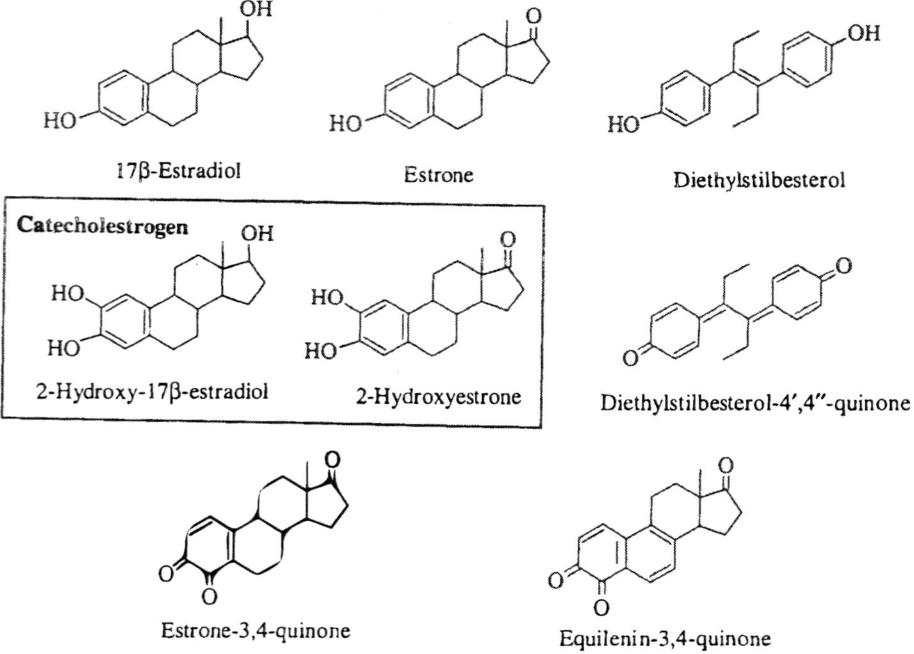

Fig. 9.5. The metabolites of estrogen.

Diseases Associated with Free Radicals

Ischemia/Reperfusion Injury

The syndrome of ischemia/reperfusion (I/R) injury has been characterized in recent years for the heart, brain, intestine, kidney, and other organs. This phenomenon consists of a paradoxical increase in tissue injury during the reperfusion period in an organ that has sustained relatively minor damage during a period of ischemia. It is now evident that reperfusion tissue injury is mediated through oxidant mechanisms associated with the generation of oxygen-based radicals. ROS have been implicated in both the myocardial dysfunctions that are observed during reperfusion following short periods of ischemia (the stunned myocarium) and the irreversible injury to cardiac myocytes that occurs during reperfusion after longer periods of ischemia.

Infusions of high concentrations of the catecholamines, epinephrine, or norepinephrine into experimental animals are known to produce myocellular mitochondrial swelling, myofibrillar disruption, plasma membrane blebbing, and myocardial necrosis. It has been suggested that these cardiotoxic effects result not from the catecholamines themselves but from the production of $O_2^{\cdot -}$ and H_2O_2 formed by a complicated series of reactions during the autoxidation of catecholamines. It was observed that vitamin E deficient rats were more sensitive to the cardiotoxic effects of isoproterenol, whereas myocardial damage induced by this synthetic catecholamine was reduced when the diet was supplemented with vitamin E. However, the results of studies demonstrating protection by antioxidants against catecholamine-induced myocardial necrosis must be interpreted with caution since accumulation of neutrophils, a major source of oxygen radicals, has been observed in such model.

Carvedilol, a potent antioxidant, prevents the lipoperoxidation of mitochondrial membranes, which suggests a strong contribution to the known cardioprotective activity of this compound through protection of mitochondrial function. A similar cardioprotective benefit is achieved by agents and antioxidant enzymes that scavenge hydroxyl radicals (or reduce their formation), but not by agents that reduce superoxide anion production. Some compounds of plant origin that have been shown to protect against ischemic injury are procyanidine from Vitis vinifera, resveratrol from red wine, and ginseng extract.

Cancer Carcinogenesis

The progression of tumor formation may be slow, often taking 10 years or more. It is important that carcinogenesis can be viewed as a multistage, micro- evolutionary process. It is generally agreed that cancer can be derived from a single abnormal cell, and work with experimental systems shows that carcinogenesis is divisible into three major stages: initiation, promotion, and progression. Initiation is a heritable aberration of a cell. Such initiated cells can undergo transformation to malignancy if promotion and progression follow. Initiation appears to be irreversible and can result from DNA damage. Promotion, however, is affected by factors that do not alter DNA sequences; it involves the selection and clonal expansion of initiated cells. This process is partly reversible and accounts for a major portion of the lengthy latent period of carcinogenesis. The final stage of tumor formation is the progression of a benign growth to a malignant neoplasm. There is loss of growth control, an escape from the host defense mechanism, and metastasis.

Certain initiators, such as radiation or chemical carcinogens, can induce the production of various free radicals and subsequent DNA base sequence alteration. In addition, cells of the immune system (e.g., neutrophils and macrophages) produce O_2^- and H_2O_2, which have been associated with the induction of experimental cancers. Oxygen free radicals and methyl radicals are known to damage DNA. In some cases, such free radicals may arise in reactions catalyzed by ferric and cupric ions localized in the vicinity of cellular DNA. Free radical mediated DNA damage can have serious consequences on an organism unless the damage is repaired. Although oxygen free radical effects can lead to DNA damage, they may also directly affect the protein components of the DNA repair apparatus. Unrepaired DNA alterations are inherited as mutations.

Oxygen radicals and related species may also be involved in tumor-promotion. Tumor-promoting phorbol esters not only can induce changes in cellular genes leading to some of the phenotypic characteristics of tumor cells, but they also can stimulate inflammatory leukocytes to release superoxide. The release of superoxide by phagocytic cells following stimulation with phorbol esters is proportional to their tumor- promoting activity. Low levels of both $O_2^{\cdot-}$ and H_2O_2, products of the "*respiratory burst*," can promote fibroblast growth, possibly fibroblasts that harbor an oncogene or a mutated protooncogene. Also, low levels of superoxide can stimulate growth or growth responses in a variety of cell types when added exogenously to culture medium. In particular, these species stimulate the activation and translocation of protein kinase C, as well as the expression of early growth- regulated genes such as the protooncogenes *c*-fos and *c*-myc. Superoxide and/or hydrogen peroxides might function as mitogenic stimuli through biochemical processes common to natural growth factors. Thus, signaling of growth responses involving released superoxide or hydrogen peroxide may be mediated through the oxidative modification of components of the signal transduction pathway. It is also possible that oxidative inactivation of serum protein inhibitors allows proteases to remodel the cell surface, thereby facilitating (modulating) the action of normal growth factors.

A final and decisive step in carcinogenesis is the invasion and metastatic spread of the tumor to various body spaces and cavities. This appears to be facilitated by the activation of genes for the release of proteolytic enzymes. Although high levels of immune cells appear to favor cell killing, lower numbers of immune cells can favor metastasis. Again, the released superoxide may serve to promote metastatic growth. Alternatively, superoxide could inactivate serum antiproteases, some of which are extremely sensitive to oxidative inactivation.

In addition, lipid peroxidation is associated with some phases of carcinogenesis. There is increasing evidence that covalent binding of carcinogens or toxic substances to cellular macromolecules, particularly those carrying genetic information, is the primary event in the initiation of carcinogenesis. Thus, covalent binding to macromolecules could be the basis of many pathological changes induced by toxic substances. The ultimate forms of xenobiotics are believed to be reactive electrophilic metabolites, which combine with nucleophilic groups of macromolecules. It is also possible that miscoding or mutagenesis may be of minor importance in the initial events of chemical carcinogenesis, and that genetic transpositions, including relatively large regions of the genome, may be more relevant.

The DNA adducts, deoxyadenosine and deoxyguanosine, which are induced by malondialdehyde, the end-product of lipid peroxidation, accumulate in human breast tissues. These adducts are present at relatively higher concentrations in breast cancer cells compared to normal breast cells. In a recent study, serum antioxidative vitamin levels and lipid peroxidation were compared in gastric cancer patients. The level of serum ascorbic acid, α-tocopherol, β-carotene, and retinol were assessed. The levels of ascorbic acid in patients with gastric carcinoma were less than one-fifth of that in the control group, and the production of β-carotene and *c*-tocopherol were decreased, as well.

Neuronal Disease

Lipid peroxidation of biological membranes gives rise to degeneration of synapses and neurons, and may be observed in stroke, or neuronal disorders such as Alzheimer's, Parkinson's, and Huntington's diseases. Oxidative stress and damage are accepted features of neural degeneration. The pathological presentation of Alzheimer's disease, the leading cause of senile dementia, involves regionalized neuronal death and accumulation of intraneuronal and extracellular lesions. 4-Hydroxynonenal mediates oxidation-induced impairment of glutamate transport and mitochondrial function in synapses. Amyloid β-protein may be involved in modulation of membrane lipid peroxidation. Amyloid β-protein fragments 25–35 [A-beta (25–35)] inhibit lipid peroxidation at low concentrations as a result of physicochemical interactions with the membrane lipid layer. Further, there is close association between increased levels of the antioxidant enzymes superoxide dismutase and heme oxygenase-1 and cytoskeleton abnormalities found in Alzheimer's disease.

Detection and Characterization of Free Radicals

ROS have been involved in the pathogenesis of a variety of human diseases. Their injury potential and pathologic role demand quantitative methods that are diagnostic of the process and that meet basic analytical criteria regarding accuracy, reliability, sensitivity and specificity. In addition, the determination and quantification of antioxidant activity is necessary for the discovery and evaluation of drug candidates. However, because of their reactive nature and short half-lives, it is difficult to quantify ROS. Alternatively, analyses involving secondary or end products produced by the attack of ROS on lipids, enzymes, or other cellular components are generally preferred. In spite of recent advances in technology, however, these indirect methods often give misleading results due to their poor specificity and sensitivity.

Chemiluminescence Measurements

Chemiluminescence is the production of light generated from chemical sources. The quantum yield of photons for intrinsic (non-stimulated) or native reactions are low but organic substances are able to undergo an oxidative reaction that can be sufficiently exothermic to produce an emitting state. Generally, the light produced is in the visible range (400–600 nm), but UV or infrared emission is possible.

Due to potential variability and low intensity of native chemiluminescence, enhancer compounds have been introduced. These compounds were selected primarily as a result of their high quantum efficiency and photon yield after oxidation. Luminol and lucigenin are enhancers for oxygenation when added to an in vitro biological system and form high levels of excited-state products and chemiluminescence. These compounds react with all species of oxidants to form 3-aminophthalate and N-methylacridone, respectively. The excited electrons in these compounds revert to their ground state with the emission of energy as light, which can be detected by photomultipliers. The sensitivities of luminol and lucigenin vary. Luminol detects H_2O_2, $HO^•$, hypochloride, peroxynitrile and lipid peroxy radicals, whereas lucigenin is particularly sensitive to the superoxide radicals. Chemiluminescence may be utilized as a direct non-invasive method for measuring ROS, and for detection of lipid hydroperoxide, phospholipid and cholesterol hydroperoxide if cytochrome c–heme is added prior to luminol.

Thiobarbituric Acid (TBA) Assays

The TBA test is perhaps the most widely used method for determining lipid peroxidation. The representative adduct of lipid peroxidation, malondialdehyde, forms a 1:2 adduct with TBA that can be measured by spectroscopy or fluorometry. The general procedure, of which there are numerous variations, simply involves heating a small quantity of the test substance for a defined period of time in an aqueous acidic solution of TBA, and then measuring the absorbance (535 nm) of the red color which is produced in the TBA reaction. It should be considered as an index of oxidative stress that represents primarily lipid peroxidation.

Chemical Measurement of Superoxide Radical

The reduction of yellow nitroblue tetrazolium (NBT) to blue formazan is applied as a probe of O_2^{-} generation in biological systems. This reaction is utilized in demonstrating the role of phagocytes (neutrophils and monocytes/macrophages) in the host response to infection and inflammation. Oxygen is rapidly reduced via a complex NADPH-oxidase system composed of a flavoprotein and a cytochrome. The cytochrome has a sufficiently low midpoint potential to allow the direct catalytic transfer of electrons from NADPH to oxygen resulting in the production of superoxide.

The respiratory burst of phagocytic cells can be assessed by incubating a suspension of cells in an isotonic solution of the yellow oxidized nitroblue tetrazolium dye. During this process, the soluble dye interacts with the cytoplasmic components associating with the oxidant species generated. NBT reduction by activation cells in the presence of superoxide dismutase has been shown to be markedly reduced, which suggests the major oxidant species responsible for the reduction of dye to a black-blue deposit called formazan is superoxide. The overall degree of NBT reduction in a given cell population can be quantified by measuring the concentration of reduced NBT or formazan spectrophotometrically.

Cytochrome c Reduction Assay Using a HL-60 Cell Culture System

HL-60 is an acute human premyelocytic leukemia cell-line derived by Collins, Gallo, and Gallagher, of which about 10% spontaneously differentiate. Various differentiation inducers, such as DMSO, TPA (12-*O*-tetradecanoylphorbol 13-acetate), or retinoic acid, lead to the differentiation of HL-60 cells through the monocyte or granulocyte pathways. HL-60 cells treated with DMSO appear as granulocytes with morphological and functional changes including production of superoxide anion and phagocytosis. Respiratory burst due to phagocytosis produce ROS such superoxide anion in the non-mitochondria oxidase system. In a simple assay procedure, HL-60 cells differentiated by treatment with 1.3% DMSO are stimulated to produce superoxide anion by addition of TPA, and cytochrome c oxidized by superoxide anion is measured by absorbance at 550 nm.

Xanthine/Xanthine Oxidase Assay

Xanthine oxidase is an obvious candidate for the production of oxygen free radicals. This enzyme is localized in the liver, small intestinal mucosa, and vascular endothelial cells, and catalyzes the hydroxylation of many purine substrates. It converts hypoxanthine to xanthine and then to uric acid in the presence of molecular oxygen to yield superoxide anion. During ischemia, xanthine dehydrogenase is converted to the oxidase form. At the same time, ATP is degraded to hypoxanthine that accumulates in ischemic tissue. On reperfusion, with the readmission of large quantities of molecular oxygen in the presence of high concentrations of hypoxanthine that is the other substrate for xanthine oxidase, there may be aburst of superoxide anion production. With in vitro systems, antioxidant activity can be measured by the absorbance of uric acid (292 nm) which is produced by xanthine oxidase. If a test sample inhibits the enzyme, xanthine oxidase cannot produce uric acid from xanthine.

DPPH Assay

DPPH (1,1-diphenyl-2-picryhydrazyl) is a purple-colored stable free radical that is reduced to the yellow-colored diphenylpicrylhydrazine by free radicals. The DPPH assay measures one electron, such as hydrogen atom donating activity and hence provides a measure of free radical scavenging activity. This assay is suitable for the initial screening of multiple samples, such as plant extracts. Reaction mixtures containing test samples dissolved in DMSO and DPPH in absolute ethanol are incubated at 37°C for 30 min in a 96-well plate and absorbance measured at 515 nm.

As summarized in this article, ROS are involved in reactions of importance in human disease states. A mechanistic understanding of these pathological processes is beginning to emerge. As a result, intervention strategies can be devised and antioxidants are receiving a great attention as potential drugs. While it is clear that prevention of oxidative damage should have a beneficial effect on human health in general, the possibility of prooxidant activity leading to adverse health effects must be strongly borne in mind. A number of assay systems are currently available for thorough characterization of the large number of potential antioxidants which are known, or for the discovery of new chemical entities. With these tools and prudent preclinical and clinical studies, it should be possible to devise dietary strategies or pharmaceutical preparations that will reduce morbidity and mortality.

10

Biosynthesis of Drug

Metabolism is the series of pathways operating when biological systems synthesize their constituents. Biosynthesis is the experimentally established pathway of formation of secondary metabolites; where experimental proof is absent, the term biogenesis is used.

Secondary Metabolites

Reaction products that are necessary for the generative functions (respiration and catabolism) of an organism are termed primary metabolites; those resulting in products used for other functions are known as *secondary metabolites*. Such compounds typically characterize the individuality of an organism or a group of organisms; this study is termed chemotaxonomy. Consequently, the biosynthetic pathways of secondary metabolism are not random but are highly conserved. Thus, a given plant family may produce substantial numbers of a certain type of metabolite (e.g., quassinoids in the Simaroubaceae), whereas another family produces quite different metabolites (e.g., monoterpene indole alkaloids in the Apocynaceae).

Precursors

A select group of primary metabolites, predominantly acetate, shikimic acid, isopentenyl pyrophosphate, and a few amino acids, is responsible for the diversity of the 135,000 plant-derived secondary metabolites in 12 major classes. Only those classes with some social or economic significance as bioactive agents are discussed here.

Significance of Biosynthesis

Biosynthetic knowledge is an integral and essential aspect of natural products chemistry and has recently assumed high-profile academic and commercial significance for biotechnological reasons. It is the foundation permitting a systematic and rational framework for organizing the bewildering structural diversity of mammalian, arthropod, insect, plant, microbial, and marine secondary metabolites. It provides structural clues for new metabolites through biogenetic possibilities based on established biosynthetic schemes. It permits the bioengineering of metabolic pathways for enhanced yields or the altering of desired product profiles for greater economic gain. Manipulations at the genetic level may afford a substantially new array of metabolites for future drug discovery. Finally, it is of fundamental human curiosity to discern how secondary metabolites are produced in living systems. The modification of such processes at the enzyme or gene level may be of critical importance in the treatment of mammalian processes involved in disease states; cholesterol synthesis-inhibiting drugs, such as mevinolin, are an example.

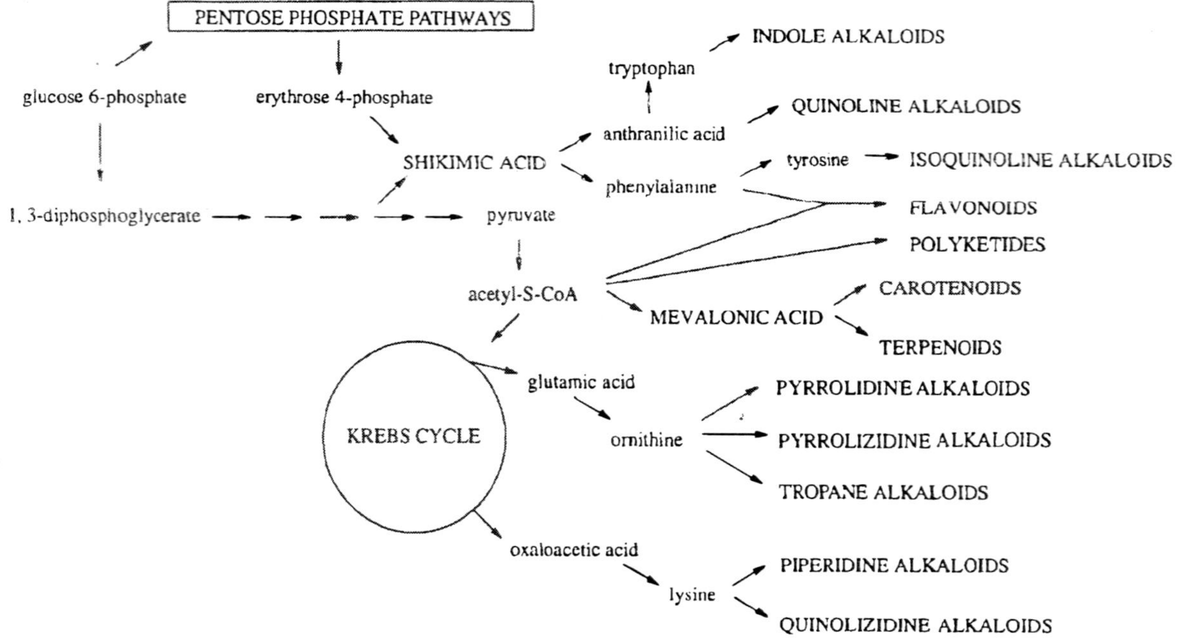

Fig. 10.1. The biosynthetic origin of secondary metabolites.

Methods in Biosynthesis

Biogenetic theories arose as the need to classify diverse secondary metabolites became apparent. Biosynthetic experimentation tested hypotheses when the precursors became available in radio-, and subsequently stable, isotope labeled forms. It focuses on the study of precursor relationships (including the stereochemistry of specific processes) and of the enzymes involved in the succinct steps in the pathway. A typical experiment involves the administration of a potential precursor in labeled form to the organism, at a time when it is known that the organism is actively producing the metabolite of interest. After an appropriate period of time, the organism is processed for the metabolite of interest and the isotope content located and measured. Most of the fundamental pathways of natural product biosynthesis were established using the radioactive isotopes of hydrogen and carbon, ^{3}H and ^{14}C. Extensive use is now made of the stable isotopes of the key atoms present in natural products, ^{13}C, ^{18}O, ^{15}N, and ^{2}H.

Evaluation of the structural complexity of natural products, coupled with prior biosynthetic knowledge, frequently offers a rational overview of the necessary chemical transformations. This may lead to isolation of the enzymes and perhaps the involvement of unanticipated intermediates. Although frequently these pathways are conserved, given the diversity of metabolic systems, it should not be assumed that the same compound will be produced by the same biosynthetic pathway in a different organism, i.e., in one plant family compared with another.

For biosynthetic experiments to be meaningful, the precursor must reach the site of synthesis at a time when the enzyme systems mediating metabolite formation are both present and active. Secondary metabolism occurs at a discontinuous rate in a given organism and at different points in the growth cycle in different organisms. Consequently, establishing a time for precursor administration to the organism is critical, if substantial degradation is to be avoided. Transportation and permeability factors may result in very low incorporations, even if the organism is known to be producing secondary metabolites at the time of the feeding and a known precursor is being used. Translocation of the precursor to the site of synthesis may be important in studies with whole plants or callus tissue. For microorganisms, metabolic degradation may occur because the growth of cell mass frequently precedes the initiation of secondary metabolite production.

Use of Radioisotopes

Although a single radiolabel may be adequate to demonstrate a preliminary precursor relationship through incorporation, it is preferable to use a precursor containing two, different, strategically placed labels. There are two types of these experiments, one in which two labeled precursors are physically mixed and the ratio of labels monitored. An example is a feeding experiment with [2-^{14}C, 4-$^{3}H_2$]-mevalonic acid. A second experiment involves using a precursor in which the two labels are in the same molecule; the use of [1,2-$^{13}C_2$]-acetate is an example. Double- or multiple- labeled substrates are used to examine bond-forming and bond-breaking reactions and to examine the stereospecificity of enzymatic processes if the precursor is labeled stereotopically (e.g., [4R-^{3}H]- mevalonic acid) and is selectively retained in the product or if the label in the product can be assigned stereotopically. Techniques are available for distinguishing between the prochiral hydrogens on a methylene or a methyl group.

Use and Detection of Stable Isotopes

The common stable isotopes used in biosynthetic studies are ^{13}C, ^{2}H, ^{15}N, and ^{18}O . Stable isotope-labeled precursors have replaced radiolabeled precursors in many biosynthetic studies for the following reasons: (1) no appropriate radiolabeled isotope is available (e.g., N and O); (2) the detection methods frequently permit location of the label in the product directly; and (3) radio-contamination and safety issues are reduced. The negative aspects of stable isotope studies are: (i) detection methods are relatively insensitive (higher incorporation levels needed); (ii) high levels of enrichment of the label in the precursor are required; and (iii) reasonable quantities of the precursor are necessary, which can be expensive.

Mass spectrometry and NMR spectroscopy are the dominant techniques for detecting stable isotopes. MS offers the advantage that less sample is needed to establish incorporation, whereas NMR typically permits direct determination of the labeled site.

Administration of Precursors

When the system under examination is microbial, i.e., a plant in tissue culture or a cell-free system, administration of the precursor is straightforward. For meaningful conclusions, a profile of formation of the compound of interest over time is necessary so that feeding is conducted when there is active product formation. When intact plants are used, precursor feeding is more difficult; options are wick feeding through the stem, root feeding, isolated leaf feeding, or even direct injection into the stem.

Examining Intermediates

Conclusively establishing the role of potential intermediates in a biosynthetic pathway is a difficult aspect of biosynthesis. Typically, intermediates accumulate because subsequent enzymatic reactions are slow. Organisms also produce shunt metabolites that are off the main pathway and may not be further metabolized; these will also accumulate. Isolation of an "*intermediate*" does not, therefore, establish intermediacy. Trapping experiments are sometimes used to overcome these problems. In the pathway A $\rightarrow$ B $\rightarrow$ C, where A is a known precursor of C, labeled A and non-labeled B are fed at the same time. The latter is metabolized to C and labeled B is produced from A; B is then temporarily available for isolation. An alternative approach for microbial metabolites is to mutate the organism or add specific enzyme inhibitors. This may allow intermediates to accumulate. Incorporation of a labeled, potential intermediate into a product does not prove that the intermediate lies on the main biosynthetic pathway. It may simply serve as a substrate for the enzymes involved. Only when each of the enzymes in a pathway has been isolated and characterized, and the substrate specificity determined, can the intermediates in a biosynthetic route be characterized.

Enzymes and Genes

Biosynthetic pathways are characteristically under enzymatic control and proceed with a very high degree of stereospecificity. Compared with the number of steps in the pathways of significant natural products, very few enzymes have been isolated and characterized and even fewer cloned and expressed. In the future, it will be very important to be able to express these enzymes heterologously in more productive systems so that these biocatalysts can be used for both known metabolite production and new metabolite generation. One dream of the biosynthetic chemist is to develop a system of stabilized enzymes on solid supports, permitting a continuous flow process from precursors to products. With no variability due to climate or soil conditions, yields would be totally controllable and reproducible, and product clean-up would be greatly simplified, or ideally, unnecessary. With the isolation, characterization, cloning, and expression of more enzymes in biosynthetic pathways, the reality of the dream moves inexorably closer. Already the use of enzyme systems for directing stereospecific reactions in organic synthesis has risen dramatically, with a corresponding increase in efficiency and enantio selectivity.

Combinatorial Biosynthesis

Another biosynthetic dream is the ability to modulate predictably the product profile of an organism. In the microbial and plant tissue culture areas, this can be achieved randomly by modifying the growth medium or by challenging the organism with a chemical or other external agent (such as a fungus), producing metabolic stress metabolites (allelochemicals). A more controllable route to altering a metabolic profile in the polyketide area can be achieved through selectively modifying the gene sequence of the biosynthetic pathway. Known collectively as combinatorial biosynthesis, this way allows new products to be formed for chemical analysis and biological evaluation.

Compounds Derived from Acetate

Acetyl coenzyme A is the biosynthetically active form of the two-carbon building block, acetate. It is of central importance in mammalian, plant, and microbial biochemistry, giving rise to the fatty acids, the polyketides, and through mevalonic acid, the terpenes.

Fatty Acid Biosynthesis

The common fatty acids, such as palmitic (C_{16}), stearic (C_{18}), and arachidonic (C_{20}), have an even number of carbons. Their chain building process initially involves a reaction of acetyl CoA with carbon dioxide to afford the more chemically reactive malonyl CoA, which condenses with a second acetate unit. The carbon dioxide subsequently lost is the same carbon that was added. It is this specificity that allows correlative experiments with [1,2-$^{13}C_2$]-acetate. Reduction of the beta carbonyl group is followed by dehydration and reduction of the cis-olefin to the saturated fatty acid. Repetition causes chain extension by two-carbon fragments. Unsaturated fatty acids can also result from dehydrogenation, as shown in the conversion of oleic acid to arachidonic acid. The latter compound is the precursor of the prostaglandins. Branching in fatty acids may occur either through the initiating acid, through acylation with a preformed fatty acid, or through reaction of an intermediate olefin with methionine.

Polyketide Pathway

Aromatic compounds are predominantly formed through either the shikimate (vide infra) or the polyketide pathway. Collie first suggested the polyketide pathway in 1893, and this was extended theoretically (acetate hypothesis) and experimentally by Birch. Factors involved in the diversity of products include the chain-initiating unit, the number of units in the cyclizing chain, condensation reactions occurring between separately formed polyketide chains, and secondary processes, such as alkylation or halogenation. The 1,3-diketone nature of the intermediate chain leads to a characteristic *meta*-relationship between ether or phenolic groups; in shikimate-derived metabolites these groups are typically *ortho*-related.

Penicillic acid provides an example of a simple tetraketide whose aromatic ring is cleaved and cyclized, as shown by experiments with [1,2-$^{13}C_2$]-acetate. On the other hand, the pentaketide citrinin is the result of the cyclization of a linear polyketide chain wherein three methyl groups are introduced from methionine. Hexaketide derivatives are rare. The naphthoquinone plumbagin is an example where cyclization followed by decarboxylation occurs. Griseofulvin is a heptaketide and was one of Birch's very early demonstrations of the accuracy of the acetate hypothesis. Anthraquinones, such as islandicin, are octaketide derivatives; the two alternative modes of cyclization of the polyketide chain can be distinguished through the use of [1,2-$^{13}C_2$]-acetate. Xanthones can be produced through oxidative cleavage of the quinone ring, cyclization and decarboxylation.

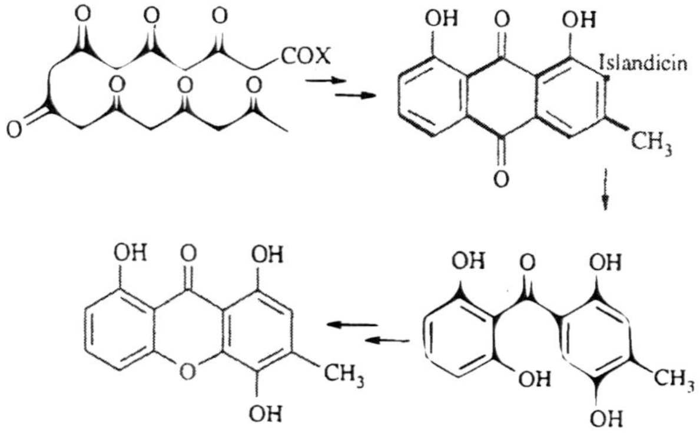

Fig. 10.2. The biosynthesis of anthraquinones and xanthones.

The most clinically significant polyketides are the anthracyclinone and tetracyclinone antibiotics produced in *Streptomyces* cultures. The tetracyclines demonstrate that chain initiation can occur with a malonamide unit and that a wide range of reactions can occur after the initial aromatic cyclization. Mixed biosynthesis is very evident in the macrolide antibiotics, where various combinations of acetate and propionate form the chain (e.g., tylosin and nystatin) or only propionate (e.g., erythromycin) and cyclize to a ring of varying size. Several plant-derived anthraquinones are of clinical significance, including the sennosides of senna (*Cassia angustifolia*), the aloins of aloe (*Aloe vera* and related species), the cascarosides of cascara sagrada (*Rhamnus purshiana*), and hypericin of Saint John's Wort (*Hypericum perforatum*).

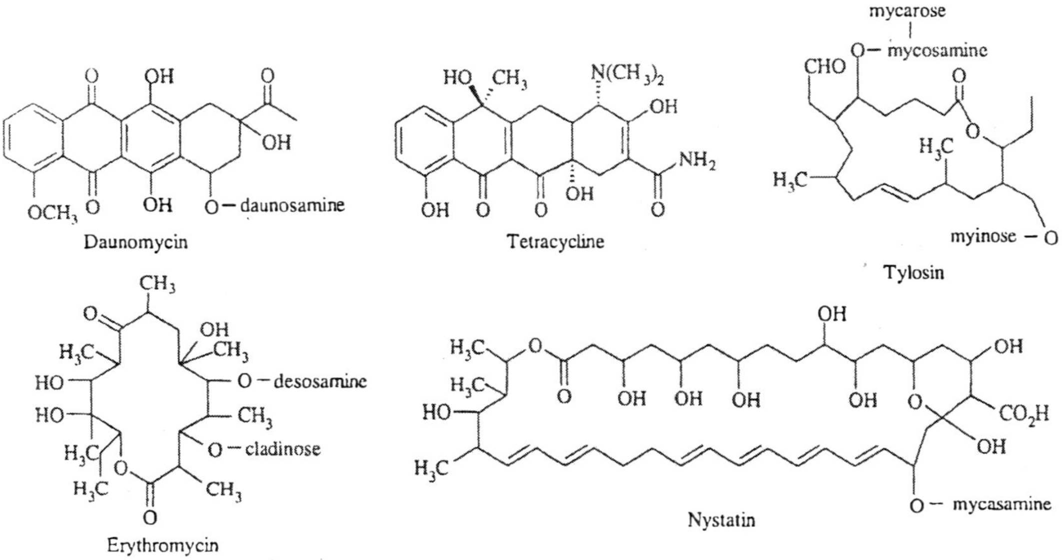

Fig. 10.3. Representative polyketide antibiotics.

Shikimate Pathway

The majority of aromatic compounds, including most alkaloids, are derived through the shikimate pathway. At the branching point of chorismic acid, either anthranilic acid, the precursor of tryptophan,

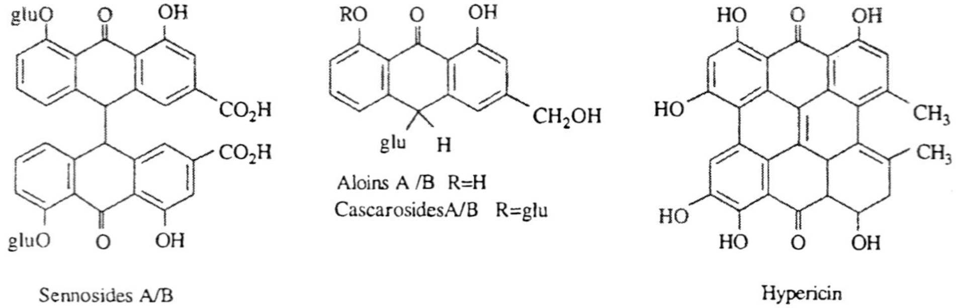

Sennosides A/B

Aloins A/B R=H
Cascarosides A/B R=glu

Hypericin

Fig. 10.4. Representative plant-derived anthraquinones.

or prephenic acid, the precursor of phenylalanine, itself the precursor of tyrosine and dopa (3,4-dihydroxyphenylalanine), is formed. Phosphorylation at the 3-position, condensation with phosphoenol-pyruvate, and elimination of phosphoric acid yields chorismate from shikimate. Chorismate is also the precursor of a number of simple, and very important, aromatic compounds, including salicylic acid, 4-amino-benzoic acid (PABA), a constituent of folic acid, and 2,3-dihydroxybenzoic acid, a key acylating group of enterobactin.

Amination at the 2-position and loss of pyruvate yields anthranilic acid, the precursor of the quinoline alkaloids, distributed widely in the Rutaceae, and tryptophan, the precursor of the indole alkaloids. Internal Claisen rearrangement on chorismic acid yields prephenic acid en route to phenylalanine. During the course of the hydroxylation of phenylalanine to tyrosine, there is a characteristic NIH shift of the

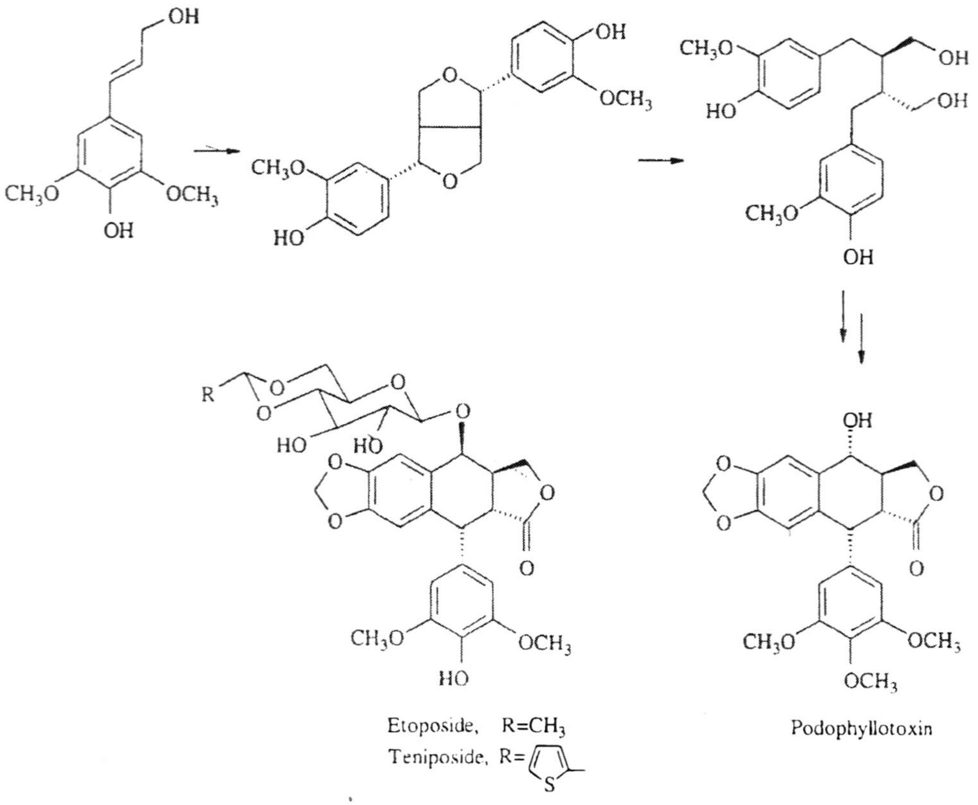

Etoposide, $R=CH_3$
Teniposide, R= (2-thienyl)

Podophyllotoxin

Fig. 10.5. The biosynthesis of lignans.

proton at C-4´. Further hydroxylation yields dopa, used in the treatment of Parkinson's disease. Dopa can oxidize and polymerize to yield the melanin group of hair, skin, and eye pigments. 4´-amination of chorsimic acid, a Claisen rearrangement, and amination yields 4´-aminophenylalanine, whose importance is as a precursor of chloramphenicol. Oxidative deamination of phenylalanine by phenylalanine ammonia lyase (PAL) and 4-hydroxylation affords *p*-coumaric acid, whose derivatives are the fundamental building blocks of lignin, as well as the lignans, such as the potent anticancer agent podophyllotoxin. The latter is the template for the drugs, teniposide and etoposide.

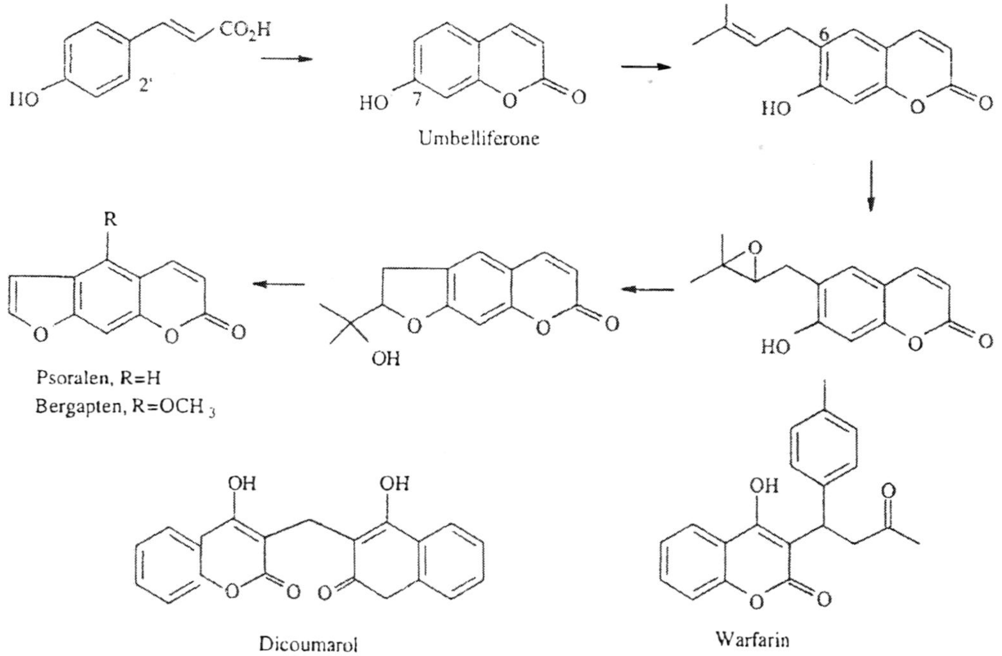

Fig. 10.6. The biosynthesis of furanocoumarins.

2´-Hydroxylation of p-coumaric acid, followed by photocatalyzed isomerization of the double bond and lactonization, affords 7-hydroxy coumarin (umbelliferone). Prenylation at the 6-position, epoxidation, cyclization, and a retro-aldol reaction afford the furanocoumarins; some (psoralen, bergapten) are known as photosensitizers and find use in the treatment of vitiligo and psoriasis. Coumarin stimulates the reticulo-endothelial system and served as a model for anticoagulant drugs, such as dicoumarol and warfarin.

Flavonoids are essentially universal plant pigments and exist in at least nine different structure classes, frequently with attached sugar units. They are derived from a mixed acetate-shikimate biosynthesis. 4-Coumaroyl CoA reacts with a triketide unit to afford 4,2´,4´,6´-tetrahydroxychalcone, which cyclizes to naringenin under the influence of chalcone isomerase. 3-Hydroxylation and dehydrogenation leads to the flavanol, kaempferol, which, along with quercetin (3´-hydroxykaempferol), is widely distributed. There is very substantial interest in the flavonoids present in the diet for their wide range of in vitro activities. Silybum marianum (milk thistle) is used in Europe as an antihepatotoxic agent for mushroom poisoning, where the active ingredient is silymarin (a mixture of flavonolignans).

Isoflavonoids are of limited distribution (Fabaceae, bean family) and are probably formed through the epoxidation and rearrangement of the enol form of a flavone (e.g., the conversion of naringenin to genistein). Several isoflavonoids are associated with strong estrogenic activity, and there is interest in their potential in the prevention of hormone-dependent breast cancer. Rotenoids (e.g., rotenone) from *Derris* and *Tephrosia* species are noted for their insecticidal and cytotoxic activity.

Compounds Derived from Isopentenyl Pyrophosphate

Numerous natural products contain units derived from a terpene precursor. Built up of five carbon "*isoprene*" units, they are successively known as hemiterpenes (C_5), monoterpenes (C_{10}), sesquiterpenes (C_{15}), diterpenes (C_{20}), sesterterpenes (C_{25}), triterpenes (C_{30}), and tetraterpenes (C_{40}). Successive units may join through head-to-tail (e.g., farnesol) or tail-to-tail linkages (e.g., squalene). Isopentenyl

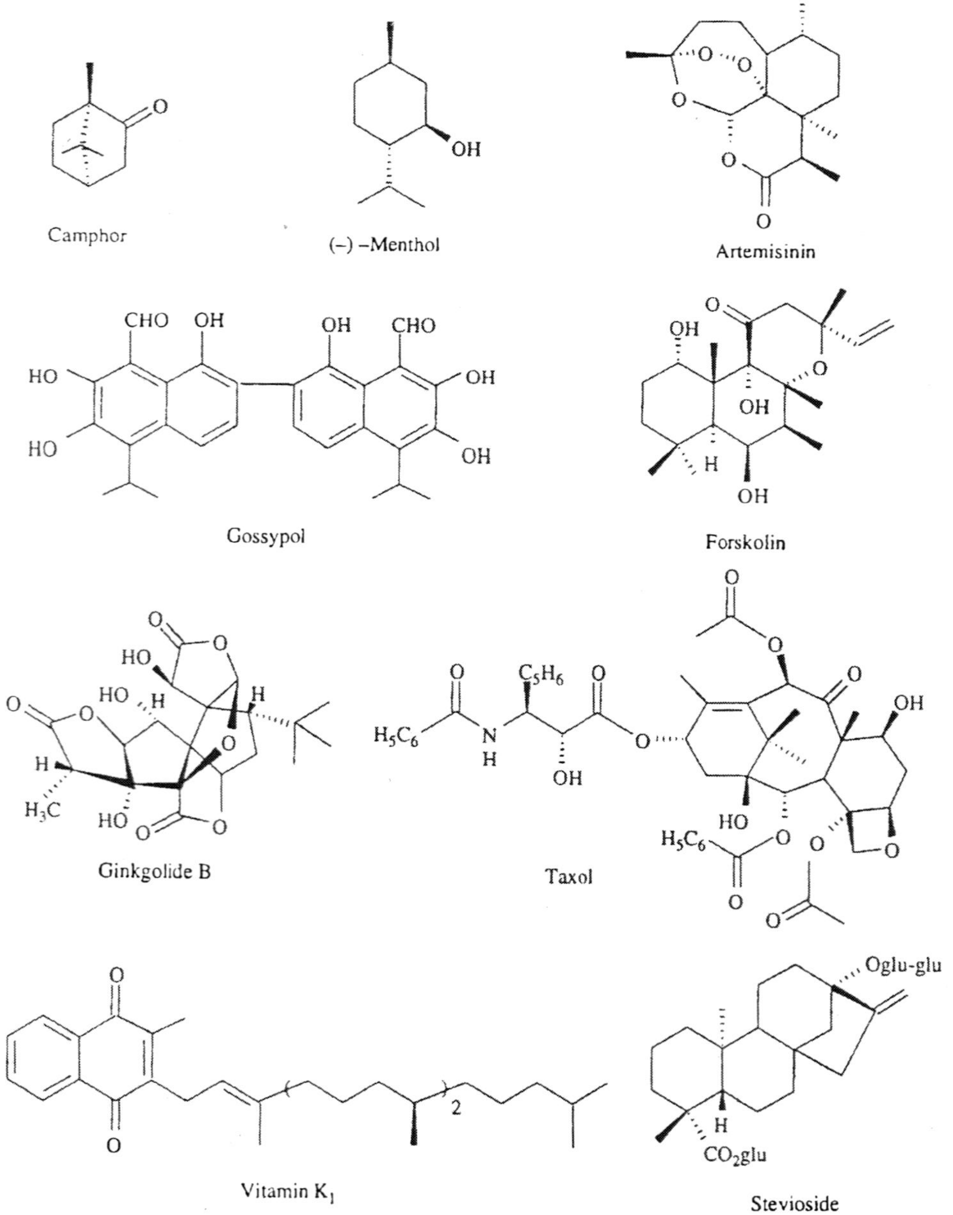

Camphor

(–) –Menthol

Artemisinin

Gossypol

Forskolin

Ginkgolide B

Taxol

Vitamin K_1

Stevioside

Fig. 10.7. Representative mono-, sesqui- and diterpene derivatives.

pyrophosphate (IPP), derived from either mevalonic acid or 1-Deoxyxylulose, is the moiety isomerizing to dimethylallyl pyrophosphate (DMAPP) and is also the chain extending unit. The formation and occurrence of these metabolites is widespread, and many derivatives are essential for mammalian functions (e.g., cholesterol, steroid hormones, bile acids, vitamin D, and retinols).

Geraniol is the primordial monoterpene, and its simple derivatives and cyclization products occur in the oils of many plants, used as flavoring and aromatic agents (e.g., caraway, coriander, dill, eucalyptus, lavender, orange, peppermint, rose, and sandalwood), as well as drugs (e.g., camphor, menthol), and insecticides (e.g., pyrethrins). Chain extension leads to farnesol, which can dimerize to squalene or undergo its own molecular modifications to yield the diverse sesquiterpenes. One of these, artemisinin from *Artemisia annua*, is of significance as an antimalarial agent, and another, (–)-gossypol, is a male contraceptive agent.

Several diterpene derivatives are commercially significant drugs. Forskolin, from the Indian medicinal plant *Coleus forskohlii*, is a potent inhibitor of adenylate cyclase and shows promise for congestive heart failure and bronchial asthma. The gingkolides, from the leaves of *Gingko biloba*, are potent inhibitors of platelet activating factor, and in a specified mixture with associated flavonoids, they improve peripheral and cerebrovascular function, hence, their wide use for senile dementia and memory loss. Taxol, originally isolated from the yew *Taxus brevifolia*, is a potent agent against many forms of cancer, including ovarian and breast cancer. It acts by promoting the assembly of microtubules (compare podophyllotoxin, colchicine, and vincristine). Geranylgeranyl units are also found in the side chains of chlorophyll a and vitamin K1. Many *Euphorbia* species have a latex containing tigliane esters noted for their powerful skin irritant and cocarcinogenic activity. Derivatives of an entkaurene alcohol (stevioside, rebaudioside) are non-cariogenic sweetening agents.

Through a series of cyclizations, squalene oxide (C_{30}) affords lanosterol in animals and fungi and cycloartenol in plants. In both instances, the intermediate is a protosteryl cation that can also undergo a series of Wagner-Meerwein rearrangements to afford the cytotoxic cucurbitacins of melons and cucumbers. Squalene oxide in a chair-chair-chair-boat conformation yields the dammarenyl cation, a parent of numerous triterpene skeleta (e.g., lupane, oleanane, ursane, and taraxerane) contained in the saponins found in many foodstuffs, in soaps, and in several drugs from complementary systems of medicine (e.g., ginseng, liquorice, Bupleurum, and horsechestnut).

Steroids are degraded triterpene derivatives, and the different nuclei are classified based on carbon number. The most significant, from a drug perspective, are the cholane, pregnane, androstane, and estrane systems. When a carbon, such as a methyl group, is lost from the nucleus, the term nor is used. In animals, lanosterol undergoes a series of degradative steps, whose sequence depends on the organism to afford cholesterol. In photosynthetic organisms, this role is played by cycloartenol where the cyclopropane ring is opened. Cholesterol is in almost every animal tissue, and is derived from cattle brains and spinal chords, as well as lanolin from sheep wool. High levels of blood cholesterol are correlated with a high risk of heart disease and atherosclerosis (through deposition of cholesterol and its esters in the artery wall). Thus, an agent that can selectively inhibit an early stage (HMG-CoA reductase) in cholesterol biosynthesis in humans, such as mevinolin (lovastatin), has the effect of reducing serum cholesterol levels.

The steroidal saponins, typically based on a C_{27} sterol nucleus, are distributed in the Dioscoreaceae, the Agavaceae, and the Liliaceae, and have a spiroketal at C-22 (e.g., diosgenin). They are also characterized by numerous sugar units attached at C-3 and sometimes elsewhere. Although not employed as drugs, steroidal saponins are critical for the semisynthesis of important hormones (estrogens, androgens, and progestins) and selected anti-inflammatory agents. An example is the conversion of diosgenin to a dehydropregnenolone acetate for elaboration to the hormones (progesterone, testosterone,

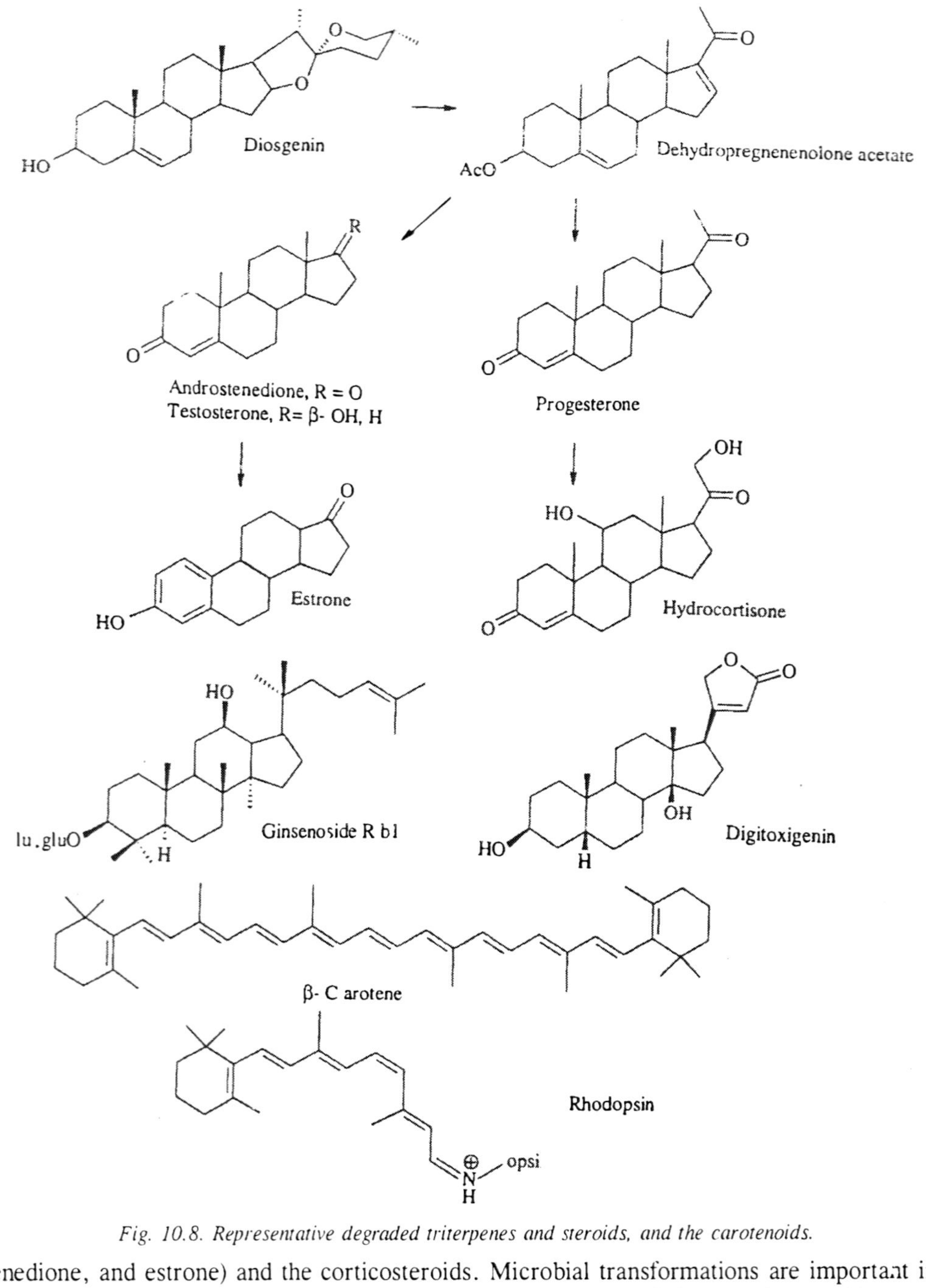

Diosgenin

Dehydropregnenenolone acetate

Androstenedione, R = O
Testosterone, R= β- OH, H

Progesterone

Estrone

Hydrocortisone

Ginsenoside R b1

Digitoxigenin

β- Carotene

Rhodopsin

Fig. 10.8. Representative degraded triterpenes and steroids, and the carotenoids.

androstenedione, and estrone) and the corticosteroids. Microbial transformations are important in several of the reaction sequences. Ginsenosides, the adaptogenic principles of Korean ginseng (*Panax ginseng*), are polysaccharide derivatives of a trihydroxylated (3β, 12β, and 20S) dammarane nucleus, and sugar variation occurs at C-3 and C-20.

Cardiac glycosides, such as those of *Digitalis lanata*, are composed of a polysaccharide unit of three or four sugars, including some 2,6-dideoxyhexoses, linked at C-3 to a modified polyhydroxy (C-

3β, C-12β, and C-14β in the case of digitoxigenin) steroid nucleus. The modification takes place on a 20- keto-pregnane through hydroxylation, the addition of acetate, and cyclization to yield an α,β-unsaturated butyrolactone. Cucurbitacins, withanolides, ecdysones, guggulsterone, limonoids, and quassinoids are also modified triterpene derivatives with potent biological effects, including high cytotoxicity. The carotenoids are tetraterpenes and are formed through the tail-to-tail coupling of geranyl pyrophosphate, followed by cyclizations at each terminal (e.g., β-Carotene in carrots). They are widely used as coloring agents for foods, confectionery, and drugs. β-Carotene is under investigation as an antioxidant for the prevention of cancer. Cleavage of β-carotene yields retinol (vitamin A1). The retinoids are important signalling agents and regulate many aspects of cell differentiation, embryonic development, growth, and vision (rhodopsin is a derivative of 11-cis-retinal with the protein opsin).

Alkaloids

Alkaloids are nitrogenous secondary metabolites primarily derived from amino acids for both their nitrogen content and a portion of their carbon framework. However, the approximately 27,000 known alkaloids defy a simple definition. Many alkaloids and their derivatives display profound biological effects and are of enormous commercial, pharmaceutical, and social significance. Ornithine, lysine, phenylalanine, and tryptophan are the principal amino acid precursors.

Alkaloids Derived from Ornithine and Lysine

There are three principal groups of alkaloids derived from ornithine: nicotine, the pyrrolizidines, and the tropanes, all having significant biological effects. From lysine are derived the piperidine alkaloids (e.g., lobeline, an antismoking agent) and the quinolizidine alkaloids, such as sparteine (an oxytocic agent) and cytisine (a teratogenic agent). Only the alkaloids derived from ornithine will be discussed here. Two very different taxa, the Asterales (Solanaceae) and Geraniales (Erythroxylaceae), formulate the tropane nucleus through similar, but distinct, pathways. Using[2-^{14}C]-ornithine in solanaceous plants, the bridgehead carbon C-1 was labeled, precluding an unbound symmetrical intermediate. In *Atropa belladonna*, ornithine is N-methylated prior to decarboxylation to N-methylputrescine. By contrast, in *Erythroxylum coca*, the bridgehead carbons C-1 and C-5 were equally labeled, suggesting that an unbound putrescine is methylated. Oxidative deamination affords an aldehyde that undergoes Mannich closure to yield N-methyl-pyrrolinium; condensation with acetoacetate affords hygrine-1′-carboxylic acid.

Decarboxylation is followed by oxidative cyclization to tropinone, followed by stereospecific reduction to the α-Hydroxy group, which is esterified to hyoscyamine. The esterifying ester, tropic acid, is an intramolecularly rearranged phenyllactic acid (derived from phenylalanine). Further elaboration of hyoscyamine yields scopolamine. The enzymes for this transformation are known.

In the biosynthesis of cocaine, the carboxylic acid is retained as the methyl ester, and after stereo-specific reduction to afford the β-alcohol, benzoylation affords cocaine. Although cocaine is widely recognized as a drug of abuse, for many populations in South America, the chewing of coca leaves is a routine aspect of the working day and has been for thousands of years.

There are no drugs based on the pyrrolizidine alkaloids of the Asteraceae (e.g., *Senecio* and *Symphytum*) and Boraginaceae (*Crotolaria*). However, these alkaloids pose a great threat to human and animal health because of their potential for inadvertent consumption. In the case of 1,2-dehydro derivatives, such as senecionine, ingestion leads to non-reversible hepatotoxicity.

Alkaloids Derived from Phenylalanine and Tyrosine

The isoquinoline alkaloids are the second largest group of alkaloids, numbering about 6000, and can be viewed as five subgroups—the simple tetrahydroisoquinolines, the benzylisoquinolines, the phenethylisoquinolines, the Amaryllidaceae alkaloids, and the monoterpene isoquinolines. In addition, there are a number of simple phenethylamine derivatives, including ephedrine (originally from *Ephedra* species, but now synthesized) and pseudoephedrine, used for asthma and nasal decongestion, respectively. Khat (*Catha edulis*) is widely used as a stimulant in the southeastern Arabian peninsula and contains cathinone. Tyrosine is the precursor of the neurotransmitter noradrenaline and the hormone adrenaline. The hallucinogen mescaline, from the mushroom *Lophophora williamsii*, is also a member of this series. An aldehyde, 4-hydroxy-phenylacetaldehyde, operating under the influence of the enzyme norcoclaurine synthase, condenses with dopamine to afford (*S*)-norcoclaurine, the progenitor of all benzylisoquinoline alkaloids. Robinson, in 1917, was the first to suggest the biogenetic derivation of the pavines, aporphines, morphinans, and protoberberines from a benzylisoquinoline precursor. These ideas led to a correct proposal for the structure of morphine and were expanded to embrace numerous alkaloid classes.

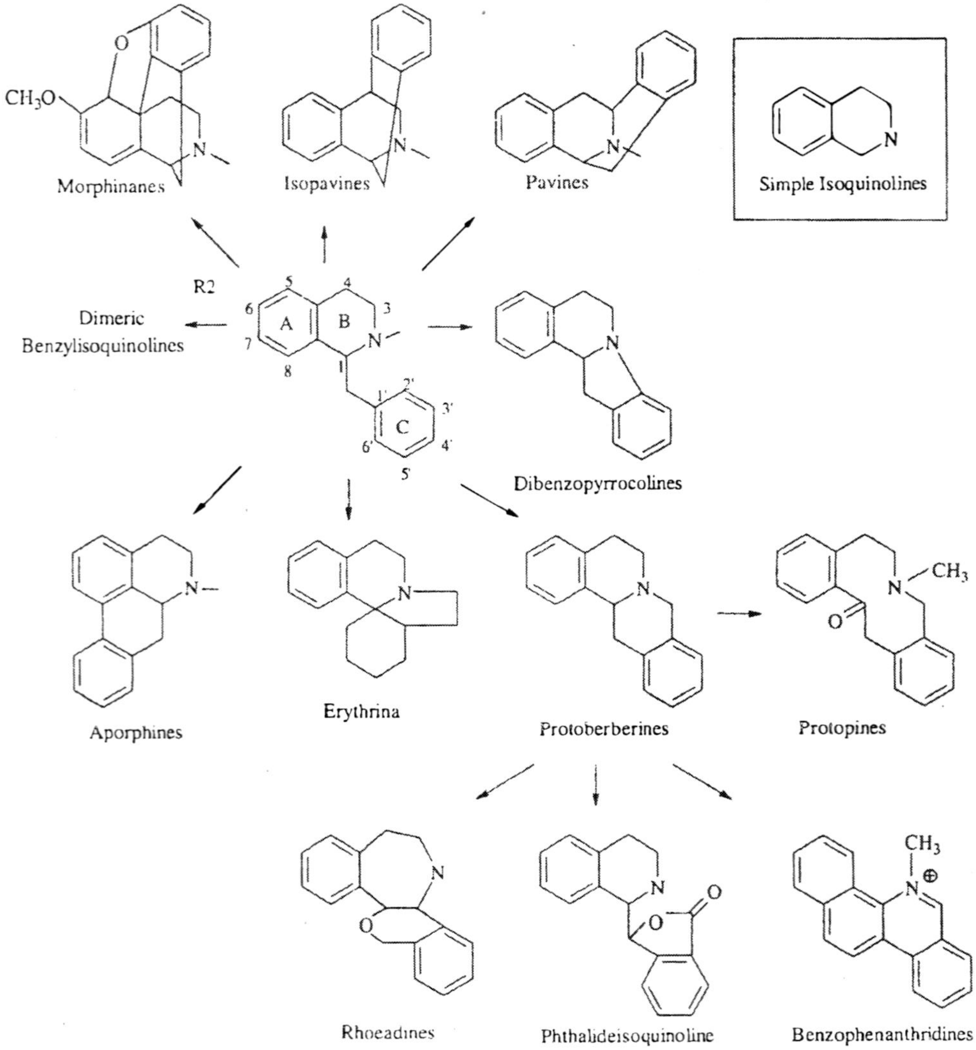

Fig. 10.9. Biosynthetic interrelationships of the major classes of benzylisoquinoline alkaloids.

Papaverine is one of the few commercial alkaloids synthesized, rather than isolated. It is used either alone for various vascular disorders or in combination as an antispasmodic. The several classes of bisbenzylisoquinoline alkaloid are based on the number of bridges between the units and their orientation. The alkaloids are common in the Menispermaceae and the Ranunculaceae. One member of the series, tubocurarine, is the prototype for several neuromuscular blocking agents; an activity based on the ethnobotanical use of the tube curares (*Chondrodendron* species) is its use as arrow poisons in the upper Amazon.

Phenol oxidative coupling was proposed by Barton and Cohen in 1957 to enumerate the relationships between many of the benzylisoquinoline alkaloid groups and accounts for the importance of reticuline as a precursor. In the case of berberine, phenolic oxidative coupling occurs between the *ortho* benzylic position and the N-methyl carbon (berberine bridge) to afford scoulerine. Many of the enzymes in this pathway have been elucidated by Zenk and coworkers. The protoberberines themselves are the precursors of several groups of alkaloids, including the protopines, the benzophenanthridines (e.g., sanguinarine, used as an antiplaque agent) and the phthalideisoquinolines (e.g., β-Hydrastine, a constituent of *Hydrastis canadensis*). Berberine is a widely used antimicrobial agent, being active against *Staphylococcus*, *Streptococcus*, *Proteus*, *Vibrio*, etc.

Morphine and related alkaloids are specific to the genus *Papaver* (Berberidaceae), although the antipodal series of alkaloids is distributed in the Menispermaceae. Early in the biosynthesis of morphine, an inversion at C-1 of (S)-reticuline occurs, followed by *ortho–para´* benzylic coupling to afford salutaridine. Stereospecific reduction and cyclization-elimination affords the 4,5-Ether bridge and thebaine. The dominant pathway from this point involves neopinone, codeinone, codeine, and morphine. Again, most of the enzymes in this sequence were isolated and characterized by Zenk's group.

Morphine binds with very high affinity to several receptors in the CNS and is a potent analgesic and central depressant. It is also the prototype for many semisynthetic derivatives (e.g., naloxone, oxycodone, ethorphine, nalbuphine, and buprenophine) with various degrees of analgesic and narcotic properties. Heroin is diacetyl morphine.

Colchicine is a phenethylisoquinoline alkaloid from the autumn crocus, *Colchicum autumnale* (Liliaceae), a plant used since at least the fifth century to treat gout. *Gloriosa superba* (Liliaceae) is an alternative source. Colchicine inhibits microtubule formation at a specific site, and at a dose of 10 mg, it causes fatal respiratory arrest and renal insufficiency. It is used for the prevention and treatment of gout. The biosynthesis remains unclear; autumnaline has been proposed as an intermediate which undergoes *para–para´* coupling to afford O-methyl androcymbine. Hydroxylation, cyclopropane ring formation, and ring expansion affords colchicine.

The Amaryllidaceae alkaloids (e.g., lycorine) are derived from the phenol oxidative coupling of a $C_6C_2NC_6C_1$ unit. One unit (C_6C_2N) is derived from tyrosine, whereas the other (C_6C_1) is projected to be derived from phenylalanine, followed by oxidative deamination, hydroxylation, and cleavage of a two-carbon unit to afford a dihydroxylated benzaldehyde. *Para–ortho´* coupling leads to lycorine, whereas *para–para´* coupling affords galanthamine, of interest as a cholinesterase inhibitor.

The monoterpene isoquinoline alkaloids are constituents of the genus *Cephaelis* and selected other Rubiaceae species. *C. ipecacuanha* (ipecac) is a powerful emetic whose active principle is emetine, derived through the condensation of dopamine and secologanin. Emetine is also a powerful amebicide, antiviral, and inhibitor of protein synthesis. It is now largely replaced by synthetic dehydroemetine.

ALKALOIDS DERIVED FROM TRYPTOPHAN

Numerous clinically important alkaloids are also derived from-tryptophan and are frequently referred to as *"indole alkaloids."* They range in molecular complexity from the mammalian hormone serotonin to the complex bisindolic anticancer alkaloid vincristine. In addition, a number of indole alkaloids, particularly those in the carbazole series, are found in peppers (*Murraya* sp.), and simple derivatives of tryptamine (e.g., N,N-dimethyl-5-methoxy-tryptamine and psilocybin) are found in several sources (e.g., snuffs, mushrooms, and toad skins) with attributed hallucinogenic properties.

Physostigmine, under investigation for potential use in Alzheimer's disease, is possibly formed from N_b-methyltryptamine through a radical mechanism involving C-3 methylation and concomitant C-2 cyclization, followed by N_b-methylation.

The powerful biological effects of ergot have been known for over 1000 years. Ergot is a fungus (*Claviceps purpurea* and species) that grows parasitically on rye and some other grains, and it produces three types of ergot alkaloids—the clavines, the simple lysergic acid-derived, and the peptide lysergic acid-derived alkaloids. The alkaloids find therapeutic use as agents for postpartum hemorrhage (methylergonovine) and as vasoconstrictors and vasoregulators (ergotamine and 9,10-dihydroergotamine) for migraine headaches. More elaborate synthetic derivatives are also available, including lisuride (for Parkinsonism) and 2-bromo-*a*-ergocryptine (for prolactin-secreting adenomas and Parkinsonism).

The biosynthetic pathway to the ergoline nucleus proceeds through 4-dimethylallyl tryptophan (4-DMAT), chanoclavine-I, agroclavine, and lysergic acid. Two *cis, trans* isomerizations occur: one before chanoclavine-I and the other before agroclavine, as shown by experiments with [2-^{14}C]-mevalonic acid and [Z-CH_3]-4-DMAT. The peptide unit is derived from a combination of three amino acids, one of which is always proline. Several genera in the plant family Convolvulaceae (*Rivea*, *Ipomoea*, etc.) also produce ergot alkaloids. The largest group of alkaloids is the monoterpene indole alkaloids, distributed in the Apocynaceae (mutual exclusion with cardenolides) and in the Rubiaceae and Loganiaceae. The molecular acrobatics of the various systems derived from deglucosylation of the primordial alkaloid strictosidine accounts for this stunning structural diversity.

Strictosidine is produced, stereospecifically, from tryptamine and secologanin by strictosidine synthase, isolated from several species producing monoterpene indole alkaloids. The enzyme was cloned and can be expressed in large quantity. After deglucosylation, the pathway proceeds through a 4,21-Dehydrogeissoschizine derivative to ajmalicine (an α-Blocking spasmolytic agent, used for tinnitus and cranial trauma with an ergot derivative). If cyclization occurs between C-17 and C-18, the yohimbine nucleus is produced, whose derivatives include the *Rauvolfia* alkaloids reserpine and rescinnamine (antihypertensive activity). Ajmaline, formerly used as an antiarrythmic, also occurs in *Rauvolfia* species, and several of the enzymes in the pathway have been isolated. Recent considerations suggest that the C-16–C-5 bond may be formed before the N-4–C-21 bond.

The subsequent steps from geissoschizine to form the *Strychnos* alkaloids, the secodines, the *Aspidosperma* alkaloids and the iboga alkaloids remain speculative, based on low levels of incorporation of early precursors or alkaloid time course studies. Joining C-2 and C-16 while moving C-3 to C-7, yields the strychnan skeleton of strychnine (lethal dose 0.2 mg/kg), still used as a rodenticide in some countries.

If the C-1 5, C- 16 bond is oxidatively cleaved, the secodine skeleton results (the proposed progenitor of the *Aspidosperma* and the iboga systems) through alternative Diels–Alder type cyclizations to afford tabersonine and catharanthine. The bisindole alkaloids of *Catharanthus roseus* reflect the union of vindoline and catharanthine to afford anhydrovinblastine; modification affords the clinically significant alkaloids, vinblastine (VLB) and vincristine (VCR). The alkaloids, particularly VCR, are important as anticancer agents and have led to the development of the semisynthetic derivatives vindesine and vinorelbine. Synthetic approaches are available to join the monomeric precursors. The enzymatically controlled sequence of reactions from tabersonine to vindoline has been elucidated.

Through a biomimetic approach, tabersonine is also the semisynthetic precursor of vincamine, a Eburna alkaloid isolated from *Vinca minor*, and is used for cerebral insufficiency in Europe. *Tabernanthe iboga* has a long history of use as a stimulant in tropical Africa; its main active principle is ibogaine,

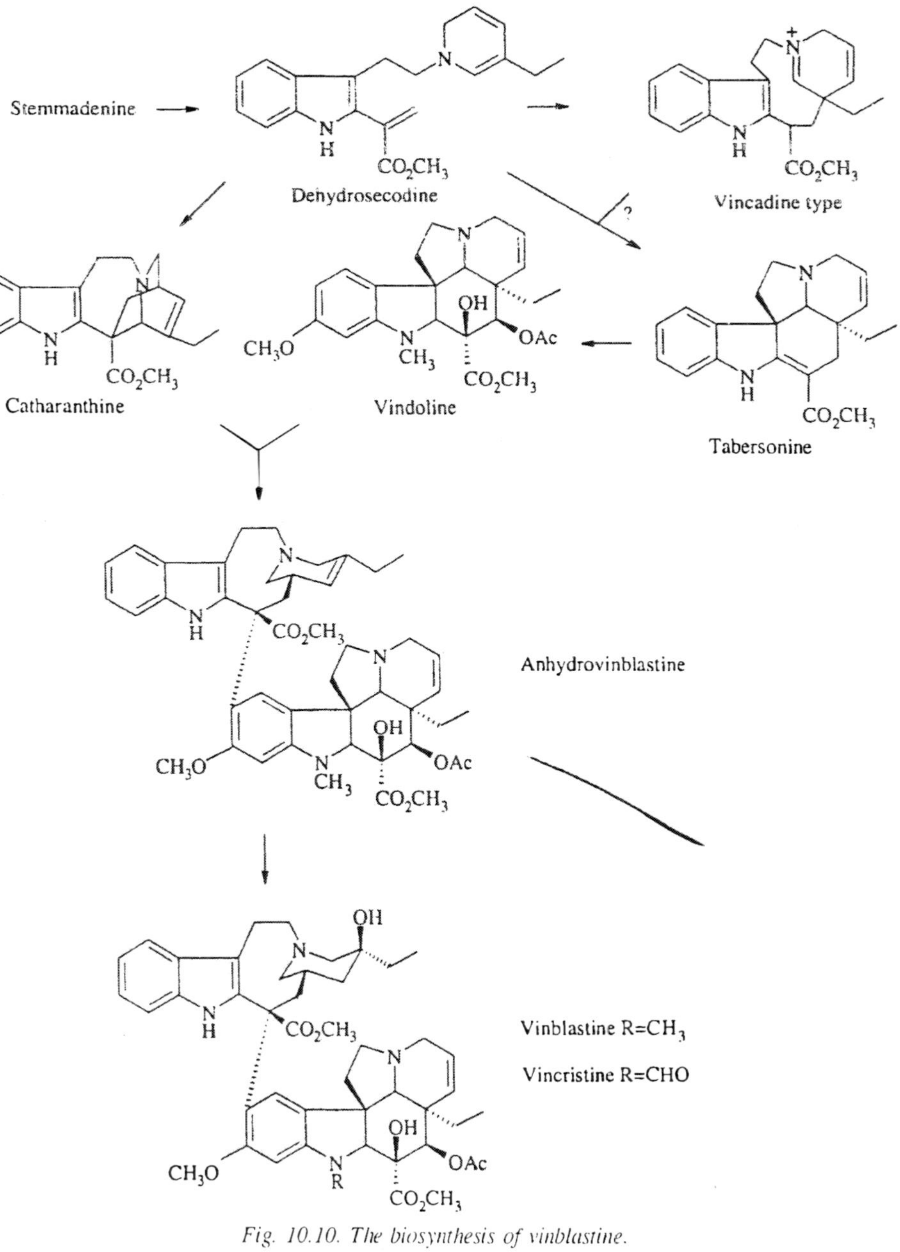

Fig. 10.10. The biosynthesis of vinblastine.

a controlled substance in many countries. It is being actively investigated in the United States for its potential to induce opium addiction withdrawal.

Camptothecin, a quinoline alkaloid from *Camptotheca acuminata* (Nyssaceae), is derived from strictosidine through strictosamide. Originally isolated in 1966, it biologically inhibits topoisomerase I, and in 1996, two derivatives, topotecan and irinotecan, were approved for the treatment of ovarian cancer and colon cancer, respectively. Other derivatives are in clinical trial.

Cinchona species (Rubiaceae) are sources of quinine and quinidine, containing a quinoline nucleus and derived through the extensive elaboration of strictosidine. The intriguing history of the antimalarial quinine and its role in world politics over the past 350 years are legendary. It is frequently the only antimalarial drug to which patients are not resistant. Its widest use, however, is in the beverage industry in tonic water. Quinidine, an isomer of quinine, is used to treat cardiac arrythmias.

Alkaloids Based on a Terpene Skeleton

Although a variety of monoterpene alkaloids and some sesquiterpene alkaloids are known, they are of little biological interest. By contrast, the diterpene alkaloids of the Ranuculaceae, for example from *Aconitum* and *Delphinium* species, have profound biological effects. The principal alkaloids of interest are those related to aconitine, acting by exciting and paralyzing peripheral nerve endings. The plants are some of the most toxic known, with merely 10 g of aconite root being lethal. Detoxified root preparations are used as drugs in several major systems of traditional medicine. Formation of the acontine nucleus is thought to occur through a rearrangement of the kaurane skeleton.

The steroidal alkaloids have a nucleus based on 21, 24, or 27 carbon atoms. The C_{21} alkaloids are pregnane-derived with nitrogen inserted at C-3, at C-20, or at both positions. They are characteristic of the Apocynaceae (*Funtumia* and *Holarrhena* species) and the Buxaceae (*Buxus* species). The Buxaceae also produces C_{24} alkaloids based on the cycloartane skeleton. The most interesting alkaloids are those in the Solanaceae and the Liliaceae. These are C_{27} alkaloids, and examples include solasodine and solanidine; many derivatives are glycosylated. The alkaloids from the Liliaceae, such as veratramine of the white hellebore (*Veratrum album*), were formerly used for cardiac insufficiency. Other alkaloids, for example cyclopamine, are potent teratogens. Biogenetically, they are derived through nitrogen insertion at C-22, followed by a rearrangement generating a C-nor-D-homo steroid nucleus. They are not used therapeutically, but the glycoalkaloids of *Solanum tuberosum* (potato) are very toxic and are not destroyed in cooking.

Alkaloids Derived from a Nucleotide Precursor

Caffeine is one of most widely consumed alkaloids on a daily basis. As well as being a significant constituent of coffee (*Caffea arabica*) and tea (*Camellia sinensis*), caffeine is also present in kola (*Kola* species), guarana (*Paullinia cupana*), and mate (*Ilex paraguariensis*). All of these species are used in various parts of the world to produce beverages that reduce fatigue.

Although some steps remain to be fully elucidated, caffeine is probably derived though a pathway beginning with inosine 5′-monophosphate and proceeds through xanthosine, 7-methylxanthosine, 7-methylxanthine, 3,7-dimethylxanthine (theobromine) to caffeine. The final methyltransferase has been characterized in coffee and tea, whereas the methylation of xanthosine has only been studied in tea.

Caffeine is noted for its ability to stimulate the CNS and also has positive inotropic and mild diuretic activity. Theophylline (1,7-Dimethylxanthine) is noted for its smooth muscle relaxant activity and its use for chronic asthma.

Alkaloids Derived from Other Precursors

Acetate is also a precursor of several groups of alkaloids in the form of a polyketide chain that interacts with an unknown nitrogen source (as in the terpene alkaloids). Examples of acetate-derived alkaloids are coniine—the toxic principle of *Conium maculatum*, pinidine—from several *Pinus* species, and the naphthylisoquinoline alkaloids (e.g., ancistrocladine)—showing antimalarial and anti-HIV activity. The latter alkaloids are apparently derived from the oxidative coupling of two pentaketide units. Huperzine A, currently in clinical trials for the treatment of Alzheimer's disease and isolated from the club moss (*Serrata huperzia*), is derived from a polyacetate precursor.

Histidine is a precursor of a very limited number of alkaloids. The most well-known is pilocarpine from *Pilocarpus jaborandi*. The plant was formerly used as a truth serum (diaphoretic activity), and the alkaloid is used to counter the mydriatic effects of atropine.

The penicillins, from the fungus *Penicillium chrysogenum*, are the oldest and most widely used antibiotics. They are formed through stepwise build-up from a tripeptide (ACV) derived from α-Amino adipic acid, cysteine, and valine. Successive oxidation steps form the β-lactam and close the thiazolidine ring to form isopenicillin N. Action of an acyltransferase then yields penicillin G. Alternatively, hydrolysis of isopenicillin N (or penicillin G) yields 6-aminopenicillanic acid, a key precursor for the wide range of semisynthetic pencillins used therapeutically.

Cephalosporins are modified penicillin derivatives produced by *Cephalosporium acremonium*, wherein isomerization occurs to afford penicillin N followed by a ring expansion involving one of the methyl groups and hydroxylation to produce descetylcephalosporin C. Once again, removal of the acylating side chain to afford 7-Aminocephalosporanic acid was the key to generating the diversity of available cephalosporin derivatives. The monobactams, such as SQ26,180 from *Chromobacterium violaceum*, contain a 3-Methoxy group and an N-Sulphonate moiety. The carbon framework is derived from serine. More complex derivatives, such as nocardicin-A, are formed through a tripeptide pathway similarly to the penicillins.

11

Drug Delivery

A drug can be administered via many different routes to produce a systemic pharmacologic effect. The most common method of drug administration is via the peroral route, in which the drug is swallowed and enters the systemic circulation primarily through the membranes of the small intestine. Although this type of drug administration is commonly termed oral, per-oral is a better term because oral administration more accurately describes drug absorption from the mouth itself. The mouth is lined with a mucous membrane and among the least known of its functions is its capability of serving as a site for the absorption of drugs. In general, drugs penetrate the mucous membrane by simple diffusion and are carried in the blood, which richly supplies the salivary glands and their ducts, into the systemic circulation via the jugular vein. Active transport, pinocytosis, and passage through aqueous pores usually play only insignificant roles in moving drugs across the oral mucosa.

Buccal Route

The administration of drugs by the buccal route has several main advantages over peroral administration, including the following:

1. The drug is not subjected to the destructive acidic environment of the stomach.
2. Therapeutic serum concentrations of the drug can be achieved more rapidly.
3. The drug enters the general circulation without first passing through the liver.

This last phenomenon is important for drugs that are highly metabolized during their first passage through the liver. This metabolism (governed by the hepatic extraction ratio) can lead to a dramatic reduction in the amount of drug available systemically from a given peroral dose but is avoided by buccal absorption.

Two sites within the buccal cavity have been used for drug administration. Using the sublingual route, as for glyceryl trinitrate (GTN), the medicament is placed under the tongue, usually in the form of a rapidly dissolving tablet. The second anatomic site for drug administration is between the cheek and gingiva. Although this second application site is itself known as *buccal absorption*, the absorption from all areas within the buccal or oral cavity are considered in this article.

Of the range of pharmaceutic preparations available for administration into the oral cavity, the most popular form is that of a rapidly dissolving tablet that releases its drug contents for absorption across the oral mucosa. Alternatively, a tablet or capsule can be chewed to release its contents. This latter method is less successful because mastication tends to produce a large volume of saliva that increases the probability of premature swallowing. The same problem occurs in the administration of drug in the form of a chewing gum.

The aim of the present article is to review the published literature on the absorption of drugs through the oral mucosa. Special attention is given to the prevention of presystemic metabolism via drug administration by the buccal and sublingual routes. Consideration is also given to the types of pharmaceutical preparations that are commercially available for drug administration into the mouth. Before progressing to drug absorption, however, the structure and blood supply of the oral mucosa are discussed because of the important role they play in the transfer of drugs from the mouth into the systemic circulation.

Structure and Secretions of the Oral Mucosa

Epithelial lining

The major function of the oral epithelium is to provide a protective surface layer between the oral environment and the deeper tissues. The oral epithelium has a squamous epithelium of tightly packed cells that form distinct layers by a process of maturation from the deeper layers to the surface. The pattern of maturation differs in different regions of the oral mucosa due to the variation in the specific function of the tissues. The surface layer of the hard palate and tongue forms keratin to yield a tough, non-flexible epithelial surface resistant to abrasion, but the epithelium of the cheek, floor of the mouth, and soft palate is non-keratinized and facilitates distensibility. The major features of the keratinized and non-keratinized oral epithelium have been extensively investigated by Squier and Rooney. Together with the presence or absence of keratin, the second main feature likely to influence regional differences in drug absorption is the epithelial thickness. This varies in different regions of the mouth: the hard palate, buccal mucosa, lip mucosa, and floor of the mouth have been found to have thicknesses of 100–120 μm, 500–600 μm, 500–600 μm, and 100–200 μm, respectively.

Secretion of saliva

In addition to the protective function afforded by the oral mucosa, it also has the ability to maintain a moist surface, which enhances permeability of the membrane to drugs. Although the mucous membrane lining in the mouth contains many minute glands called *buccal glands*, which pour their secretions into the mouth, the chief secretion is supplied by three pairs of glands, namely, the *parotid* (under and in front of the ear), the *submaxillary* (below the jaw), and the *sublingual* (under the tongue) glands. Blood is richly supplied to the salivary glands and their ducts by branches of the external carotid artery and afterwards, travelling through the many branch arteries and capillaries, returns to the systemic circulation via the jugular veins. The presence of saliva in the mouth is important to drug absorption for two main reasons:

1. Drug permeation across moist (mucous) membranes occurs much more readily than across nonmucous membranes.
2. Drugs are commonly administered to the mouth in the clinical setting in a solid form. The drug must, therefore, first dissolve in saliva before it can be absorbed across the oral mucosa; that is, the drug cannot be absorbed directly from a tablet.

Vascular System of the Oral Mucosa

The vascular system and blood supply to the oral mucosa have been clearly described by Stablein and Meyer. Netter's excellent drawings of the blood supply to the mouth and pharynx, venous drainage of the mouth and pharynx, and lymphatic drainage of the mouth and pharynx have been published by Ciba. This latter publication also includes definitive documentation of the blood supply and drainage from the mouth.

The blood supply to the mouth is delivered principally via the external carotid artery. The maxillary artery is the major branch, and the two minor branches are the lingual and facial arteries. The lingual artery and its branch, the sublingual artery, supply the tongue, the floor of the mouth, and the gingiva, and the facial artery supplies blood to the lips and soft palate. The maxillary artery supplies the main cheek, hard palate, and the maxillary and mandibular gingiva. The internal jugular vein eventually receives almost all of the blood derived from the mouth and pharynx. Drugs diffusing across the membranes have easy access to the systemic circulation via the internal jugular vein.

Factors Influencing Drug Absorption from the Oral Cavity

Because the oral mucosa is a highly vascular tissue, the two main factors that influence drug absorption from the mouth are the permeability of the oral mucosa to the drug and the physicochemical characteristics of the drug that is presented at the site of absorption.

Permeability of the oral mucosa to drugs

The lipid membranes of the oral mucosa are resistant to the passage of large macromolecules; however, small un-ionized molecules tend to cross the membrane with relative ease. This passage is in either direction, and indeed passage of drugs from the circulation into the mouth can be used in therapeutic drug monitoring by measuring drug concentrations in saliva. The permeability of the oral mucosa has been comprehensively reviewed by Siegel.

Mechanisms involved in drug absorption across the oral mucosa

The mechanisms by which drugs cross biologic lipid membranes are passive diffusion, facilitated diffusion, active transport, and pinocytosis. Small, water-soluble molecules may pass through small, water-filled pores. The main mechanism involved in drug transfer across the oral mucosa, common with all regions of the gastrointestinal tract, is passive diffusion, although facilitated diffusion has also been shown to take place, primarily with nutrients. *Passive diffusion* involves the movement of a solute from a region of high concentration in the mouth to a region of low concentration within the buccal tissues. Further diffusion then takes place into the venous capillary system, with the drug eventually reaching the systemic circulation via the jugular vein. The physicochemical characteristics of a drug are very important for this diffusion process. Although passive diffusion is undoubtedly the major transport mechanism for drugs, the absorption of nutrients from the mouth has been shown to involve carrier systems (*facilitated diffusion*), which lead to a more rapid absorption than the concentration gradient would promote. Such a carrier system, unlike passive diffusion, exhibits stereospecificity, and indeed the absorption of D-glucose and L-arabinose across the buccal mucosa has been shown to be stereospecific. The same authors also showed that the absorption of D-glucose, galactose, and 3-0-methyl-D-glucose was at least partially dependent on the presence of sodium ions in the luminal fluids. Furthermore, the transport of D-glucose was inhibited by galactose and 3-0- methyl- D-glucose, suggesting at least one common carrier system. Similarly, Kurosaki et al. demonstrated that the absorption of cefadroxil (a cephalosporin antibiotic) from the human oral cavity occurs through a carrier-mediated mechanism; this absorption was inhibited by the presence of cephalexin, which shares a common carrier-mediated process with cefadroxil in the small intestine of rat.

Membrane storage during buccal absorption of drugs

The absorption of a drug from the mouth is not synonymous with drug entry into the systemic circulation. Instead, the drug appears to be stored in the buccal membranes, sometimes known as the membrane reservoir effect. Due to this phenomenon, buccal partitioning has been suggested as a more accurate term to describe the diffusion of drugs across the oral mucosa. Although several authors have devised schematic representations of the kinetics of oral drug absorption the mucosal constituents responsible for drug binding have not been identified.

Regional differences in mucosal permeability

The epithelial lining of the mouth differs in both composition (keratinized and non-keratinized) and thickness in different regions of the mouth. Therefore, drug absorption may vary from different oral sites. This site-dependent absorption has been shown to take place by Pimlott and Addy, who measured the absorption of isosorbide dinitrate into the systemic circulation after applying tablets to the buccal, palatal, or sublingual mucosa in six healthy volunteer subjects. Serum levels of drug were detected from the buccal and sublingual sites after 1 min. The drug concentration progressively increased, peaking at 5 min, and then decreased during the 30 min sampling period. At most of the time periods, serum concentrations were higher from sublingual sites than from buccal sites. The drug was not detected in the serum of any subject after application to the palatal mucosa. These authors concluded that the keratinized layer of the oral mucosa may be an important barrier to drug absorption because the palatal epithelium is keratinized, but the buccal and sublingual mucosa are not. Absorption across the sublingual epithelium is likely to be greater than across the buccal epithelium because the former is thinner and is immersed in a larger volume of saliva.

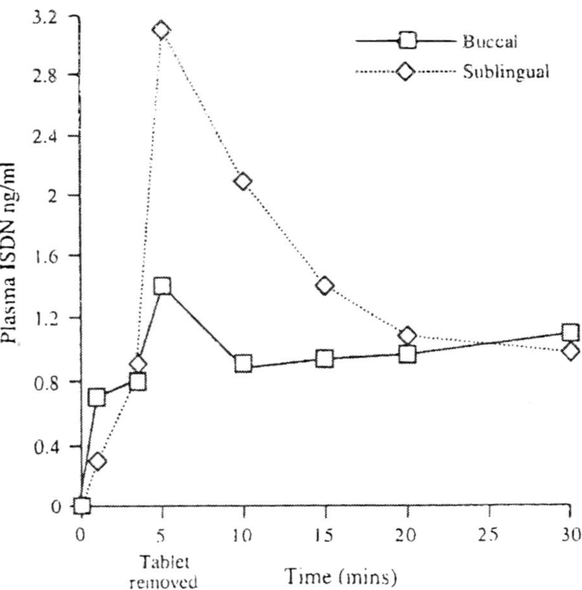

Fig. 11.1. Mean plasma isosorbide dinitrate concentrations after application of isosorbide dinitrate (5 mg) to the buccal and sublingual mucosa in six healthy male volunteer subjects.

Rapid absorption from the sublingual mucosa was also demonstrated through work by Al-Furaih et al., who reported that sublingual administration of captopril led to a more rapid attainment of plasma captopril concentrations and had a more rapid pharmacological effect (i.e., lower systolic blood pressure) compared to peroral administration of the drug.

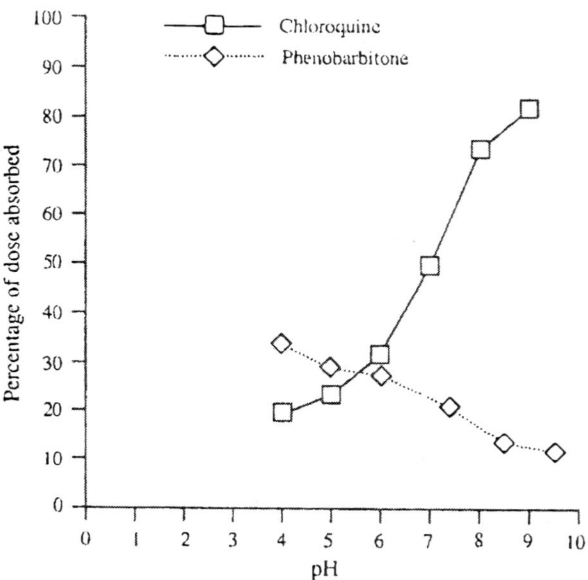

Fig. 11.2. The influence of pH on the absorption of the weak acid phenobarbitone and the weak base chloroquine from the buccal cavity in three healthy volunteer subjects.

Physicochemical characteristics of the drug

Various experimental techniques have demonstrated that cell membranes have a large lipid component, and most drugs cross such membranes by simple passive diffusion. In order to cross these lipid membranes, a drug should be in the lipid-soluble or un-ionized form and also be in solution. The various physicochemical characteristics of the drug are, therefore, of paramount importance as far as drug penetration across the oral mucosa is concerned.

Molecular weight

In general, molecules penetrate the oral mucosa more rapidly than ions, and smaller molecules penetrate more rapidly than larger molecules. However, this rule is not absolute because dextrans with a molecular weight of up to 70,000 cross keratinized rabbit oral mucosa, but horseradish peroxidase (molecular weight 40,000) does not. High-molecular-weight mucopolysaccarides such as heparin are not well absorbed, although inclusion of penentration enhancers in some insulin formulations have improved bioavailability.

Degree of ionization

The average pH of saliva is 6.4. Because the un-ionized form of a drug is the lipid-soluble-diffusible form, the pK_a of the drug plays an important role in its absorption across the lipid membranes of the oral mucosa. The degree of ionization of a drug at a specified pH can be calculated using the Henderson–Hasselbalch equation as follows:

For an acid:

$$pH = pK_a + \log_{10} \frac{[\text{un - ionized species}]}{[\text{ionized species}]}$$

For a base:

$$pH = pK_a + \log$$

The importance of pH on drug absorption from the mouth has been extensively studied using the buccal absorption model, in which loss of drug from buffered drug solutions placed in the mouth is monitored.

However, pH does not always influence the rate or extent of absorption. For example, McElnay et al. found that captopril pharmacodynamic parameters (blood pressure, heart rate, and plasma renin activity) did not differ significantly between buffered and unbuffered sublingual administration, suggesting that manipulation of pH had little effect. It was, therefore, proposed that a mechanism other than passive diffusion was involved in the buccal absorption of this drug.

Although many studies illustrate the importance of ionization on drug absorption, the pH of saliva is relatively constant, and in the absence of a buffer, the pK_a of the drug plays the deciding role as to the state of drug ionization. Also, due to the relatively large surface area available for absorption and to the maintenance of an equilibrium between ionized and un-ionized drug, only a small percentage of drug has to be present in the un-ionized form before significant absorption can take place.

Lipid solubility

Although the undissociated (un-ionized) form of a drug has the higher lipid solubility, the un-ionized moieties themselves have differing lipid solubilities. A common way of assessing the lipid solubility of a drug is to measure its oil–water partition coefficient. As with pH, buccal absorption has been shown to be positively correlated with a drug's oil–water partition coefficient. Beckett and Moffat, for example, found a correlation of partition coefficients in n-heptane/aqueous systems with buccal absorption data for a series of amines and acids when the degree of ionization was held constant.

In conclusion, to penetrate the oral mucosa to a significant degree, a drug should have a relatively low molecular weight and exhibit biphasic solubility patterns, that is, be soluble in both the aqueous salivary fluid and the lipid membrane barrier to penetration. A significant amount of the drug should be un-ionized at salivary pH, and the drug should also not bind strongly to the oral mucosa.

Buccal Administration as a Method of Preventing Presystemic Metabolism

The systemic availability of a drug is a measure of the fraction of the administered amount of drug that is absorbed into the general circulation in an unchanged form from its site of administration. Disregarding pharmaceutical reasons (e.g., poor tablet disintegration) and inappropriate physicochemical properties of the drug, the two main reasons for poor bioavailability after peroral administration are drug destruction by stomach acid and drug modification by metabolic enzyme systems prior to its entry into the systemic circulation. The principal organs involved in presystemic elimination are the gut wall, the liver, and the lung. Drug metabolism of this type is known as first-pass metabolism. A number of drugs have high affinities for the enzyme systems in these organs and are, therefore, highly extracted during their flow through the organs. These drugs, which are said to have a *high extraction ratio*, include propranolol, terbutaline, levodopa, imipramine, aspirin, morphine, pentazocine, nitroglycerin, lignocaine, hydralazine, verapamil, and methyldopa. The main metabolizing organ in the body is the liver. Because blood draining from the gut via the portal vein must pass through the liver prior to entry into the general circulation, the total drug absorbed from the gut must pass through the liver before it can reach its site of action. Once the drug has entered the systemic circulation, it is distributed to other areas of the body (depending on its volume distribution); although the extraction ratio remains constant, the proportion of the total drug in the body that is metabolized on subsequent passes through the liver is reduced due to a lowered drug concentration in the plasma after distribution has taken place. The liver receives only 20% of the cardiac output (as compared with 100% from the portal vein), which also protects the drug that has already been absorbed from the metabolic systems of this organ. Presystemic elimination can, therefore, be avoided by choosing a site of administration from which the drug enters the systemic circulation directly, without first passing through the liver, lung, or gut wall. Because blood draining from the oral cavity enters the general circulation via the internal jugular vein, oral administration by the buccal or sublingual routes provides a useful strategy for improving bioavailability of drugs that are susceptible to exténsive first-pass metabolism. A high first-pass effect does not, however, mean that drugs with a high extraction ratio cannot be given perorally. If a sufficient dose of the drug is given, an adequate amount of drug (to produce the required therapeutic effect) often remains intact during its first passage through the liver. Also, a high peroral dose of drug or, indeed, serum levels of the drug from previous doses may saturate the high-affinity metabolizing systems in the liver and, thereby, decrease the first-pass effect and increase bioavailability. With some drugs, moreover, the metabolites themselves may have good pharmacologic activity.

Drugs and Pharmaceutical Formulations for Administration by the Buccal and Sublingual Routes

Although the data produced using the buccal partitioning model of drug absorption have shown that numerous drugs are absorbed efficiently from the oral cavity, few drugs have been assessed clinically after administration by this route, and not all drugs that have given encouraging clinical data have specific formulations available for intraoral administration. Drugs within the cardiovascular and strong analgesic pharmacologic classes have received the most attention.

Cardiovascular drugs

Glyceryl trinitrate (GTN)

This vasodilator has been used for over 100 years in the treatment of angina pectoris, and today, many clinicians consider it the most effective drug despite exhaustive efforts to find alternatives. It is also used in the treatment of congestive heart failure. This drug is rapidly absorbed from the mouth, with much of the drug bypassing the liver. The liver has a high metabolic capacity for organic nitrates by virtue of the enzyme glutathione reductase. Sublingual administration of GTN is the most appropriate action to alleviate the pain of an acute angina attack because of its rapid action, its long-established efficacy, and its low cost. The traditional pharmaceutical formulation of the drug is a rapidly dissolving tablet for administration under the tongue. This approach, however, has two main disadvantages:

1. The time taken for the tablet to disintegrate and dissolve may vary from person to person. A delayed and varied onset of action may result.
2. The tablets of GTN lose significant potency after only 8 weeks of the initial opening of the manufacturer's bottle and should be discarded after that period because exposure to moisture and to the atmosphere accelerates nitrate breakdown. Heat also accelerates drug deterioration.

In an attempt to overcome the previously noted problems with the sublingual tablet formulations, GTN is now widely available in metered-dose aerosol preparations. The sprays usually contain 0.4mg GTN per unit dose. The manufacturers suggest that 1 or 2 metered doses be sprayed on the oral mucosa (preferably under the tongue) and then the mouth should be closed.

A slightly different approach has been taken by Pharmax, the manufacturer of Suscard Buccal tablets. Instead of the traditional 300-, 500-, and 600-μg sublingual tablets, the Pharmax tablets contain 1, 2, 3, or 5mg of GTN and are placed between the upper lip and the gum on either side of the front teeth. During the dissolution phase, the tablet softens and adheres to the gum, after which dissolution continues in a uniform and gradual manner. Because this is a prolonged- release dosage form, the patient should not increase the tablet's dissolution rate by moving it around the mouth. The tablet should be replaced if accidentally swallowed, and the placement of successive tablets should be alternated on either side of the mouth. As well as an effective prophylactic in angina, this formulation has been shown to be effective in congestive heart failure.

Isosorbide dinitrate

This nitrate is also active sublingually and is a more chemically stable drug for those who require nitrates only infrequently. It is a longer-acting drug than GTN. The activity of isosorbide dinitrate may depend on the production of active metabolites, the most important of which is isosorbide 5-mononitriate. Isosorbide mononitrate is also available for angina prophylaxis, though the advantages over isosorbide dinitrate have not yet been firmly established. The general consensus is that the activity of the dinitrate is also longer than that of GTN Kattus et al., for example, found that sublingual isosorbide dinitrate offered protection against angina for 2.5–3 h compared to 1 h relief with GTN The finding of equal bioavailability of chewable (buccal absorption) and slow-release capsules (intestinal absorption) "infers that buccal or sublingual absorption does not circumvent the first pass effect, that presystemic metabolism occurs in the buccal mucosa, that buccal absorption is not as effective as believed or that isosorbide dinitrate is swallowed and not absorbed by the buccal mucosa. The identical pattern of metabolites after buccal and intestinal administration favours the theory that buccal absorption is slow and that isosorbide dinitrate is swallowed with the saliva in which it is dissolved." Current knowledge concerning the buccal absorption route supports this theory. The main advantage of sublingual and buccal dosing may be the rapid disintegration and dissolution of the tablet in saliva. Present knowledge suggests using the drug buccally for the treatment of acute attacks of angina and using a sustained-release formulation for prophylactic purposes. Iga and Ogawa demonstrated that a sustained release buccal formulation of both GTN and isosorbide dinitrate increased the bioavailability of both drugs when administered to dogs, compared to oral administration. A number of isosorbide dinitrate preparations are available for administration by the buccal or sublingual routes, the usual strengths being 5 or 10mg. Although chewable preparations are available, the more traditional quick-disintegrating tablets predominate. Because mastication tends to increase saliva production, in order to prevent premature swallowing of the drug, the traditional tablet type may also be preferable. Sublingual rather than buccal administration may also be preferable because higher plasma concentrations have been found in healthy volunteers when the former route was used.

Nifedipine

In the past, the difficulties presented in the administration of drugs in the treatment of hypertensive emergencies were largely overcome with the use of nifedipine administered sublingually. The onset of action was rapid, and the drug was also used sublingually for the treatment of acute attacks of angina pectoris. Presently, two types of formulation of nifedipine are available, both intended primarily for peroral administration. The sustained-release formulation is solely used perorally; however, the rapid-release capsule, which contains nifedipine in solution form, was formerly administered to the buccal cavity. However, the manufacturers now state in their literature that "nifedipine should not be used for the treatment of acute attacks of angina" as it has been associated with large variations in blood pressure and reflex tachycardia.

Captopril

Two studies have indicated the usefulness of sublingual captopril in the treatment of severe hypertension. The hypertensive patients thus treated showed a marked decrease in systolic and diastolic blood pressure, with the onset of action being 2–5 min and the peak effect at 10 min. Perorally administered captopril takes 1–2h to achieve a maximal therapeutic effect and, therefore, is unsuitable for the treatment of hypertensive crisis. Al-Furaih et al. reported that sublingual administration of captopril (followed by plasma monitoring of drug levels) led to a more rapid attainment of plasma captopril concentrations and had a more rapid pharmacological effect (i.e., lower systolic blood pressure) compared to peroral administration of the drug.

Iscan et al. compared a number of parameters of a specially formulated buccal bioadhesive captopril tablet with that of a conventional tablet. The buccal formulation provided controlled release of captopril with a smooth plasma level profile and a long duration of action; however, its bioavailability was 40% via the buccal route as compared to 65% following an oral dose. This was attributed to the intestinal mucosa being more permeable than the buccal mucosa, and it was concluded that further work was required to improve its bioavailability.

Analgesics

Buprenorphine

In common with other phenolic opiate analgesics, buprenorphine shows low peroral potency, suggesting a high first-pass metabolism effect; indeed, work in rats has shown this to be the case. Intravenous studies have estimated that the extraction ratio of buprenorphine is 85% and that peroral systemic availability is consequently expected to be 15% or less. Although absorption from the mouth is slow and, therefore, not as useful as parenteral administration in the treatment of acute pain, it offers a major bioavailability advantage over the peroral route for this drug. If required, the patient can be given a parenteral dose of buprenorphine to achieve rapid pain relief and thereafter be maintained on sublingual drug. The drug is available as a sublingual tablet containing 200 or 400 μg of buprenorphine hydrocholoride for the treatment of moderate to severe pain.

Morphine

Although not routinely given by the buccal or sublingual routes, several research studies have shown that absorption of morphine from the mouth gives rise to effective analgesia and that these routes may provide suitable alternatives to parenteral administration. Clinical studies have suggested that the bioavailability of morphine is 40–50% greater after buccal than intramuscular administration; as plasma morphine concentrations decline more slowly after buccal administration, buccal morphine may be associated with enhanced analgesia. Anlar et al. administered buccoadhesive morphine sulphate tablets to six healthy volunteers, resulting in up to 30% of active drug being absorbed; this is in contrast to absolute bioavailability of a morphine sulphate solution of 23%. Christrup et al. found that buccal delivery of morphine sulphate could be enhanced further by using ester prodrugs with higher lipophilicity than the parent drug itself.

Ketobemidone

Ketobemidone is a narcotic analgesic that has been used clinically in Scandinavia and other European countries. The mean bioavailability in humans has been reported to be approximately 35% following oral administration, but this can be substantially improved when administered by the sublingual or buccal route. To date, in vitro work has focussed on the use of the ketobemidone prodrugs (largely esters), and published results suggest that, as with morphine sulfate, buccal mucosa permeation is greatly improved.

Flurbiprofen

Studies have suggested that this nonsteroidal anti- inflammatory drug may be useful in the treatment of peridontal disease. Manipulation of pH was shown to influence the amount of drug absorbed; an increase in pH resulted in a reduction of drug absorbed, thus resulting in a poor local effect. Gonzalez-Younes et al. reported that the drug was tightly bound to the membrane of the tissues in the mouth.

Peptide drugs

The oral mucosa has been cited as a route of administration for peptide drugs as a way of avoiding parenteral delivery, although permeability is low, which reduces its value as a viable option. However, modifications to drug formulation may offer greater success. The addition of penetration enhancers to dosage forms appears to improve bioavailability to the greatest extent, by improving the permeability of the epithelium and/or affecting the nature of the drug. To date, much of the experimental work has been conducted in animals.

Insulin

To achieve hypoglycemia with insulin, the traditional route of administration has been via subcutaneous injection. Peroral preparations are not feasible due to the degradation of insulin by gastric acid and enzymes. However, studies carried out in animals utilising buccal formulations have been more successful. Ritschel et al. administered insulin to beagle dogs using solutions of different pHs. Bioavailability (22.3%) was maximized at pH 7.5, and the addition of penetration enhancers (bile salts) did not increase this further. Experimental work in rabbits found that in the absence of penetration enhancers, insulin solutions over a range of pHs did not show any significant hypoglycaemic response, indicating that insulin was not absorbed to a significant degree through the buccal mucosa.

Buserelin

This luteinizing hormone-releasing hormone has been used in the treatment of endometriosis and hormone- dependent tumors. Modes of administration have included injections, nasal sprays and subcutaneous implantations. One study, conducted in pigs, demonstrated the value of glycodeoxycholate (a penetration enhancer) in improving the bioavailability of buserelin by up to five-fold after buccal delivery.

α-Interferon

α-Interferon has broad antiviral and antiproliferative activity and has been used in HIV and certain forms of hepatitis. As with other peptide drugs, ways have been sought to improve the buccal delivery of α-interferon to avoid gastro-intestinal degradation and first-pass metabolism. Using a range of penetration enhancers, Stewart, Bayley, and Howes noted improved bioavailability, particularly with sodium taurocholate, in rats. As with all of the studies reviewed under the category of peptide drugs, extrapolation to the human situation should be done with caution.

Miscellaneous drugs

Nicotine

The absorption of nicotine from chewing tobacco has been widely used for many years. Buccal absorption of nicotine is also the route of absorption for pipe and cigar smokers if the smoke is not inhaled. Nicotine replacement therapy has been used in smoking cessation strategies. Nicotine in the form of chewing gum carries no cancer risk and is a useful part of a smoking cessation strategy. A recent innovation has been the development of a sublingual tablet (available in 2 mg); a clinical trial has shown that this formulation is a safe form of administration, and patients may use one tablet every 1–2h.

Zinc

Zinc gluconate in the form of a lozenge has been marketed for the treatment of the common cold; there has been no definitive conclusion as to whether it is effective in treating cold symptoms, although differences in study methodology may partially explain the conflicting results that have been reported.

Midazolam

Midazolam administered bucally in solution has been shown to be rapidly absorbed and produces changes in EEG readings. The authors suggested that this may offer an alternative to rectal administration of diazepam in the emergency treatment of seizures.

The buccal cavity provides a highly vascular mucous membrane site for the administration of drugs. The epithelial lining of the oral cavity differs both in type (keratinized and nonkeratinized) and in thickness in different areas, and the differences give rise to regional variations in permeability to drugs. Although some macromolecules have been shown to cross the absorption barrier (lipid membrane), the absorption of smaller drug molecules occurs more reproducibly and rapidly. The main absorption mechanism is passive diffusion of the un-ionized (lipid-soluble) form of the drug. Facilitated diffusion has also been shown to take place with nutrients. Drugs are often stored or bound to the buccal mucosa prior to entry into the bloodstream. The blood drainage from the mouth enters the general circulation directly without first passing through the liver. This feature enhances the bioavailability of certain drugs as compared with peroral administration because first-pass metabolism is avoided. To ensure adequate absorption from the mouth, a drug administered as a solid dosage form must exhibit *biphasic solubility*, that is, be soluble in saliva and in the lipid membranes of the buccal cavity. The major drugs currently available for buccal administration fall within the vasodilator and strong analgesic pharmacologic classes. Although the main type of formulation available for buccal absorption is rapidly disintegrating tablets, new approaches include mucoadhesive tablets and spray formulations. Much of the current knowledge on the mechanism and characteristics of drug absorption from the buccal cavity has been gained from volunteer studies in which buffered drug solutions are placed in the mouth (buccal absorption model) rather than from clinical pharmacologic studies in patients. This former method provides useful information on the bioavailability of new and existing drugs. The main advantages of the buccal route of administration over the traditional peroral route are that drug degradation in the stomach is avoided, first-pass metabolism is avoided, and therapeutic blood levels of drug can be achieved rapidly. Clearly these advantages are presently clinically relevant for only a limited number of drugs. However, with the recent developments of formulation types, such as mucoadhesive preparations and the use of peptides as drugs, this number may increase in the future. The main disadvantage of the buccal route is that the drug may have an unwanted local effect in the mouth, such as bad taste, or may be absorbed slowly and, therefore, be swallowed prior to sufficient absorption taking place. The buccal route, like the rectal and intranasal routes, has been largely neglected by clinicians and manufacturing companies in the past and clearly merits further intensive research.

Monoclonal Antibodies

The selective delivery of drugs to their site of action should increase their therapeutic effectiveness while minimizing unwanted side-effects. In the early 1900s, Paul Ehrlich proposed the potential use of antibodies as carriers of biological agents to the target sites, thus inventing the "*magic bullet*" concept. With the development of hybridoma technology, it is now possible to produce virtually unlimited quantities of homogenous antibodies having a defined specificity, that is, monoclonal antibodies (MoAbs), which have potential to fulfill Ehrlich's vision. While MoAbs have found use in sensitive diagnostic tests, the therapeutic use of MoAbs and their conjugates are only beginning to realize the promise that was predicted with the advent of the core technology.

Basic Terminology

In simplistic terms, an antibody is an immunoglobulin synthesized by the body's immune system in response to a foreign molecule (an antigen, i.e., an antibody generator), and is capable of binding the antigen with high specificity. In general, an antigen must have a relatively large molecular weight (> 1000) to elicit an immune response; smaller molecules can be made to be antigenic by coupling it to a suitable macromolecule, e.g., albumin.

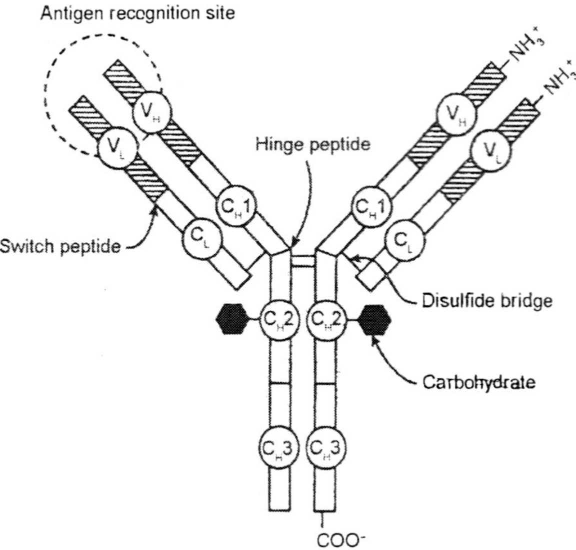

Fig. 11.3. Diagram of an monoclonal antibody molecule.

An antibody is a Y-shaped molecule, and contains two light chains and two heavy chains joined together by disulfide bonds. Each of the heavy chains also contains a carbohydrate residue. The bottom "trunk" portion of the antibody molecule is known as the constant (Fc) region because its amino acid sequence is often similar within a given animal species. The upper "arms," the antigen binding regions (Fab), are known as the variable regions because its amino acid sequence is determined by the antigen responsible for its formation. The variable region, in turn, has several "hypervariable" regions, also known as the "*complementarity determining regions*" (CDR), which show greater variability than the rest of the variable region.

Antibodies can be classified in the following:

Polyclonal antibodies

After an antigen is injected into an animal by a regimen designed to induce an optimal immune response, serum can be collected from the animal and the immunoglobulin fraction isolated. This "*antisera*" is enriched with antibodies specific for the original antigen. Because a large number of lymphocytes are involved in the production of the anti- sera, antibodies produced by this classical method are called polyclonal.

Monoclonal antibodies

An antibody is called "*monoclonal*" when each immunoglobulin is produced by a single clone of cells and hence is identical to every other molecule in the preparation, in terms of heavy as well as light chain structure. Thus they are highly specific and offer more consistent efficacy and predictable toxicity in vivo than the polyclonal counterparts.

Antibody fragments

The earliest MoAbs examined in animal and clinical studies were murine antibodies. Because of their non-human origin, they are immunogenic in humans, i.e., they have a tendency to elicit a human antimouse antibody (HAMA) response. They also have been shown to have much shorter clearance rates than human MoAb's. One approach to overcome these problems has been to cleave the antibody (e.g., by papain digestion) into its respective Fc and Fab fragments. In general, the Fab fragments are less immunogenic than the corresponding intact antibodies, and their smaller molecular size may facilitate penetration into tumor tissue and result in a longer half-life. However, they can lose some of their antigen binding capacity, and in some cases the therapeutic effect may depend on the Fc portion of the antibody.

Chimeric antibodies

The obvious solution to the problems encountered with murine antibodies would be to clone a fully human antibody. However, human hybridomas required for human MoAb production have been notoriously difficult to culture, and it may be impossible to obtain many of the appropriate antibodies. A strategy that has been devised to overcome the HAMA problem of murine MoAbs is by constructing a chimeric antibody, which contains the Fc region of human IgG, but the Fab regions are murine in origin. These can be made chemically by joining murine Fab fragments to the Human Fc fragment, but the preferred method is to use recombinant DNA technology, as detailed in a later section.

Humanized antibodies

Although human studies have suggested that chimeric antibodies elicit less HAMA response than murine antibodies, they are still immunogenic due to their murine regions (generally about 30% of the total molecule). A major advance was achieved when it was recognized that only a small portion of an antibody molecule was actually responsible for antigen binding, in fact only the CDR regions. One can envision construction of a "humanized" antibody in which the majority of the antibody framework is human in origin, but the CDR's are murine. Synthesis of such humanized antibodies have been successfully achieved by recombinant DNA technology, and can have up to 95% homology with human antibodies. (Some confusion in the literature exists regarding the terminology for humanized and chimeric antibodies, in that some authors use the terms interchangeably.)

Bispecific antibodies

Antibodies can be constructed using recombinant DNA technology in which each of the two arms are specific for two different antigens. For example, bispecific MoAbs reactive with CD 15 antigen, and composed of Fab fragments of anti-CD64 MoAb 32 and a whole IgM antimyeloid cell MoAb, PM-81, have been investigated for the therapy of patients with CD15 positive tumors, e.g., acute myelogenous leukemia, small cell carcinoma of the lung, colorectal cancer, and breast carcinoma.

Immunoconjugate

For MoAb targeted drug delivery, a drug is bound covalently to an antibody that is chosen to target it to the desired site of action. The resulting immunoconjugate may contain a spacer between the drug and antibody, or a polymer to increase the number of drug molecules that can be bound to each antibody. Another possibility is a radio-immunoconjugate, which is designed to be concentrated at the target site by the targeting antibody, allowing the radiation from the bound radioisotope to exert its cytotoxic affect. Alternatively, the drug can be incorporated non-covalently into a liposome or microsphere to which the targeting antibody is bound to the surface, yielding an immunoliposome or immunomicrosphere, respectively.

Preparation and Manufacture of Antibodies and Antibody-based Delivery Systems

Manufacture

Every B-lymphocyte in an animal expresses an antibody of only one specificity. After it is triggered to differentiate, the B-cell turns into a plasma cell with the cytoplasmic machinery to synthesize and secrete large quantities of its own unique immunoglobulin. To prepare MoAbs, usually a mouse is immunized with the antigen of interest, e.g., human tumor cells. When an immune response ensues, B-lymphocytes from the spleen or lymph nodes of the animal are harvested in a single cell suspension. These cells are then fused with myeloma cells from the same species, using a fusogenic substance (e.g., polyethylene glycol) or electric current. Mutant myeloma cells are used which are deficient in an enzyme, hypoxanthine guanine phosphoribosyl transferase (HGPRT), which is needed for their survival in the presence of the folic acid antagonist, aminopterine. The resulting fused cells have the cytoplasmic machinery to promote cell division and produce large amounts of immunoglobulin. The cell suspension is then transferred to the wells of a microtiter plate in a medium such as hypoxanthine/aminopterine/thymidine. Only the hybridomas that have acquired the HGPRT from lymphocytes via cell fusion usually survive. The hybrids are cloned by limited dilution to one cell per well so that it is easy to identify an antibody of the desired titer, specificity, and avidity for propagation in mass culture. The cell supernatant is then purified by column or affinity chromatography to harvest the pure antibody.

For chimeric and humanized MoAb the above procedures are modified somewhat. The preferred method for the latter is to use recombinant DNA technology and construct a gene that expresses the chimeric or humanized antibody, by splicing the appropriate DNA sequences together in the plasmid of the hybridoma. Synthesis of such humanized antibodies have also been successfully achieved by recombinant DNA technology; the portions of gene encoding the murine CDR regions are spliced into the gene encoding the human antibody by transfection. Although these constructs proved to be much less immunogenic than murine or chimeric antibodies, early work indicated that they had lower antigen binding capacity than the original murine MoAb. This was apparently because of the absence of certain residues in the human framework that while not directly involved in antigen binding, are required to retain the CDR regions in the correct conformation. Choice of human framework IgG, which is as homologous as possible with the murine antibody, will aid in this regard. In addition, sophisticated molecular modeling techniques based on X-ray crystallography and computer modeling has been used to identify these required residues, which has allowed introduction of the residues into the framework region by recombinant technology.

Due to the increased application of MoAbs in diagnostics and therapeutics, considerable effort has been made to develop technology for the large-scale production of MoAbs. Examples of the currently employed culture systems are hollow-fiber systems, suspensions, solid-phase cell immobilization, perfusion reactor, and encapsulation in semipermeable vesicles. The system of choice is dependent on the cell line and on the desired characteristics and quantity of the final product. To increase the mixing efficiency of cell-culture equipments and to provide aeration, several different devices have been designed, e.g., vibromixer, marine propeller, turbine propeller, spinning magnetic bar, magnetic spinner, and airlift.

Perfusion systems have also been used for successful scale-up of MoAb production. During the culture period, cell growth occurs exponentially until the cell density reaches a maximum. At that point, the medium needs a continuous supplementation of fresh nutrients and elimination of waste. In perfusion systems, fresh nutrients are supplied and wastes are removed continuously so that the medium meets the physiological needs of the cells. At steady state, the cell concentration is determined by space and other limitations. High cell densities have been achieved by immobilizing the cells in porous ceramic matrices or hollow fiber devices. Intermediate cell densities have been achieved by perfusion reactors with a spin filter, or in a fluidized bed reactor in which the cells are embedded in sponge-like microcarriers.

Coupling methods for antibody drug conjugates

An important part of the design of an antibody-directed drug delivery system is the type of linkage and coupling method between antibody and drug. The drug can be covalently bound to the MoAb directly or through a short spacer, or the two can be conjugated through a linker such as a water-soluble polymer. Alternatively, a carrier such as a liposome or a polymeric microsphere can be used, wherein the drug is entrapped in or bound to the carrier, and the MoAb is bound to the surface of the carrier. Characteristics that would comprise an ideal antibody directed delivery system could include, preparation by a method that has high efficiency and yield, and is capable of scaleup; high stability of the conjugate, both under shelf storage conditions and in the circulation after injection; and retention of antigen-binding ability of the antibody while it is carrying the drug to the target tissue. Finally, upon reaching the target, either the immunoconjugate itself should have the desired pharmacological effect equivalent to the free drug, or must release free drug or a derivative that is fully efficacious. Although such a system is probably impossible to achieve for most therapeutic applications, a variety of coupling reagents are fortunately available that aid in optimizing the properties of an immunoconjugate.

Amino, sulfhydryl, and carboxyl groups are the most common functional groups on the antibody, carrier, and drug molecules used for coupling. If the drug lacks the desired group, it may be possible to introduce it. For example, succinic anhydride can convert an alcohol or amino group to a carboxyl group; 2-iminothiolane (Traut's reagent) can convert an amino group to a sulfhydryl.

For linkage of drug to antibody, "classical" protein cross-linking reagents have been used to prepare immunoconjugates. For example, carbodiimide reagents link amino groups with carboxyls via amide bonds. In an "*active ester*" method, carboxyl groups of the drug are linked to *N*-hydroxy succimide (NHS) in the presence of a carbodiimide to form an active ester derivative of the drug, which then reacts with the amino group of the antibody. Linkers such as dextran, allow conjugation of a much larger number of drug molecules with each antibody molecule. Thus, dextran and similar carbohydrate linkers are oxidized with periodic acid to form aldehyde groups, which are then linked to amino groups of drug and antibody with formation of an imine. This product can be stabilized by reduction with sodium cyanoborohydride.

These simple reactions are often not specific enough for efficient immunoconjugate formation. More recently, a number of bifunctional reagents have been developed that are more specific in forming linkages of antibody to drug. Heterobifunctional reagents, which have two different reactive groups at the two ends of the molecule, have become the method of choice for preparation of immunoconjugates. Among the most widely used is *N*-succimidyl 3-(pyridyldithio) propionate (SPDP). Generally, the reagent is used to derivatize the drug with a pyridyl disulfide group; reaction of this species with the antibody containing free sulfhydryl groups yields the immunoconjugate. *N*-[-6 maleimidocaproyl)oxy]succinimide (EMCS) is a reagent that reacts with amino groups at the succimide end and sulfhydryl groups at the maleimide end. A similar reagent, *N*-[-4 maleimidoethoxy succinyloxy]succinimide (MESS), has a metabolizable ester linker between the two active functionalities, thus providing a method to control release of free drug. Combinations of classical coupling methods with bifunctional reagents have also been used to advantage for preparation of immunoconjugates. For example, a 6 carbon spacer ending in a carboxyl group was introduced into dextran (MW 70,000), and then mitomycin C (MMC) was coupled to the spacer with a carbodiimide. The remaining carboxyl groups of the spacers were modified to amino groups, which were then coupled to MoAb A7 by means of SPDP, with a final MMC/MoAb ratio of 40. The antibody activity of the resulting conjugate was almost equivalent to native MoAb A7, and released free MMC by chemical hydrolysis to maintain cytoxicity. Similarly, Zara et al. modified an IgM against human carcinoma by oxidation of its carbohydrate residues, which were then coupled to a bifunctional reagent, S-(2-thiopyridyl)-L-cysteine hydrazide (TPCH) via the hydrazide. After Ricin A was coupled to the other end of the reagent by a disulfide bond, the immunoconjugate retained full toxin and antibody activity with up to 16 TPCH molecules incorporated per antibody, suggesting that carbohydrate residues of the antibody were not involved in the antigen-binding process.

Plasma or intracellular enzymes such as esterases or proteases can potentially degrade immunoconjugate linkages. Glutathione reductase and related enzymes are instrumental in cleavage of disulfide bonds of immunoconjugates. The local pH of the target tissue or of its intracellular environment (e.g., lysosomes) may also increase the rate of release of drug from the immunoconjugate. Thus it is important to consider the possible physiological destinations after injection of the immunoconjugate, and to monitor its degradation under conditions mimicing the biological milieu, which it may encounter. Ideally, an immunoconjugate should be sufficiently stable in the circulation to allow targeting to take place; once the antibody binds to its antigen on the target cell surface, the entire immunoconjugate should be internalized into the cell and be degraded to release free drug or an active derivative. However, for many cell types internalization of the immunoconjugate does not always occur in response to antibody binding. In that case, degradation of the immunoconjugate linkage should be sufficiently rapid to provide high local concentrations of free drug or active derivative for the desired pharmacological response. An advantage of bifunctional reagents is that they allow incorporation of a metabolizable linker into the immunoconjugate, thereby releasing free drug or an active derivative at a predictable rate.

A number of studies have explored coupling methods that allow control of the in vivo rate of release of active drug. Kaneko et al. designed hydrazone linkers to release drug at lower pH: free doxorubucin was released from conjugated antibody within 6 h at 37°C at pH 4.5, conditions which mimic the environment of the lysosomes; the particular antibody used was known to be internalized. Similarly, Lavie et al. constructed daunomycin conjugates linked to MoAb L6 via a polylysine and aconitate linkage, such that the conjugate releases free drug at pH 6. Although this antibody is not internalized, the lower pH of tumor tissue was suggested to lead to increased concentrations of free drug in tumors. New heterobifunctional reagents have been reported with greater versatility in release rate. The disulfide bond of SPDP conjugates has been shown to be labile in the circulation and release drug prematurely; an analog, NHS-ATMBA, is up to two orders of magnitude more stable than SPDP conjugates because of steric hindrance around the disulfide bond, and thus leads to more efficient targeting. Several new substituted 2-iminothiolane reagents, which exhibit increased stability of the disulfide bond of the resulting immunoconjugate, have also been synthesized.

Appropriate choice of spacer can also significantly improve the success of an immunoconjugate. For example, O'Neill and co-workers conjugated *N,N*-bis-(2-chloroethyl)-*p*-phenylenediamine (PDM) to the globulin fraction of rabbit anti-EL4 serum, which reduced the toxicity by as much as 20-fold relative to free drug. However, the conjugate was found to aggregate, making it difficult for clinical applications. Hence poly-L-glutamic acid (PGA) was tried as a spacer and it allowed preparation of a water-soluble PDM-PGA-Ig conjugate in molar ratio of 90:2: 1 retaining 66% of the original antibody activity.

In the case of immunotoxins and other protein– antibody conjugates, a unique choice exists for their construction, viz. the conjugate can be made entirely by recombinant DNA techniques. This would require splicing the two genes together and expression of the chimeric gene in a monoclonal system. For example, the gene for angiogenin (a human toxin-like molecule) was fused to the gene for an antitransferrin receptor, and the chimeric gene was introduced into a transfectoma to clone cell lines that secrete the hybrid antibody-angiogenin protein. The conjugate was active as a cytotoxic agent, and the activity was mediated by the transferrin receptors. Similar techniques were used to construct a conjugate of urokinase-type plasminogen activator and a humanized antifibrin antibody, resulting in a 12-fold enhancement of fibrinolytic activity of the conjugate relative to the parent (unconjugated) urokinase. Construction of an immunoconjugate by this approach has the advantage that once the clones are expressed, the immunoconjugate can be made in one step without chemical modification. Also, a single species is generally produced by this method. It has the disadvantage that generally only a 1:1 or perhaps 2:1 ratio of drug to antibody can be accommodated by the immunoconjugate.

Immunotherapy with Unconjugated Monoclonal Antibodies and Radioimmunoconjugates

Results from the clinical trials of these and other MoAbs in development have shown that unconjugated MoAbs are able to kill cancer and other cells. When the circulating MoAb binds to its target antigen, several mechanisms may be initiated that are responsible for the therapeutic effect. One is antibody-dependent cellular toxicity (ADCC), wherein neutrophils, mononuclear phagocytes, eosinophils, natural killer, and T-cells, which have receptors for IgG (Fc), are triggered to mediate cell destruction. Also important is complement dependent cytotoxicity (CDC) wherein complement binds to the Fc portion of the MoAb after antigen binding and initiates the complement cascade ending in cell death. MoAb binding to the target antigens on cell surfaces can also act as "blocking" antibodies, interfering with the binding of certain peptides or growth factors needed for cell growth, or elicit a regulatory effect on the metabolism of the cell, especially for B-cell lymphocytes and B-cell lymphomas. The interaction of MoAbs with growth factor receptors (such as transferrin receptors) may also have an antitumor effect via a regulatory mechanism because transferrin is essential for the growth of cells and its receptors are predominantly present on proliferating cells.

Among the most successful has been Rituximab (Rituxan). This MoAb binds to the CD20 antigen of B-lymphocytes, which is expressed on >90% of non-Hodgkin's lymphoma B-cells. Upon binding, the Fc region of the MoAb recruits immune effector functions to mediate B-cell lysis, possibly by both CDC and ADCC mechanisms. In a multicenter clinical trial with 166 non-Hodgkin's lymphoma patients, who received 375 mg/m^2 over 4 doses, the overall response rate was 48% (6% complete, 42% partial). A second study with 37 patients gave similar response rates, and single doses of up to 500 mg/m^2 were well-tolerated.

Tratsuzumab (Herceptin) binds to the extracellular domain of a transmembrane protein, human epidermal growth factor receptor 2 (HER2), which is over-expressed in 20–30% of primary breast cancer cells. It is thought to act primarily by ADCC. In a phase III trial, 222 breast cancer patients, who exhibited over-expressed HER2, were dosed weekly with 2mg/kg tratsuzumab after a 4mg/kg loading dose. There was a 14% overall response (2% complete response and 12% partial response), which appeared to be correlated to the degree of HER2 overexpression. Overall response was much better when tratsuzumab was combined with standard chemotherapy (viz., paclitaxel, doxorubicin + cyclophosphamide, or epiubicin + cyclophosphamide): sphamide): 45% compared to chemotherapy alone. Similarly, tratsuzumab combined with cisplatin, either in pegylated liposomes or in saline/mannitol solution, was significantly better than either treatment alone in retarding tumor growth in a mouse xenograft tumor model.

Some workers have proposed use of anti-idiotypic antibodies as type of "*tumor vaccine.*" In this approach, a MoAb is prepared against a given tumor antigen. Rather than using it for immunotherapy directly, it is used to inoculate mice, which produces a second antibody against the idiotypic site of the original antibody (hence, the anti-idiotype). After cloning and administration to patients, this anti-idiotypic MoAb would mobilize the patient's own immune system to produce a third antibody (i.e., an anti-anti-idiotype), that would have the same idiotype of the first antibody and thus bind to the original antigen and lead to cytotoxicity. The perceived advantage of the approach is the multiplicative effect of the "vaccine," and it is believed to be more specific and safer than using the antigen itself as a vaccine. When 15 melanoma patients were treated with a mouse anti-idiotypic antibody homologous to a melanoma antigen, 7 patients developed the desired immune response, and there were 3 partial responses. Thus, although the approach may be promising, it has to be more fully evaluated to determine its utility.

Although MoAbs have many potential uses for tumor therapy, there are inherent problems associated with this approach: (i) Cancer cells are heterogeneous, so those cells that are not recognized by the MoAb can escape and proliferate; (ii) Some tumors contain semidead cores with poor circulation and thus cannot be reached by monoclonals; (iii) MoAbs can interact with circulating target antigens before reaching their target; and (iv) Patients can experience possible immunogenic reactions. For these reasons, it has frequently proven more effective to combine MoAb treatment with standard chemotherapeutic agents.

Radioimmuno-conjugates are MoAbs to which radio-nuclides have been conjugated, to provide cytotoxic radiation after the MoAb binds to its target antigen. The isotopes most commonly used are Iodine-131 and Yttrium-90, both of which are β^- emitters having half-lives of 8 and 2.5 days, respectively. The former is covalently bound to tyrosine residues of the MoAb by standard chemical techniques, whereas the latter is chelated to a ligand that has been conjugated to the MoAb by techniques described in the previous section (e.g., diethylenetriaminepentaacetic acid ligand coupled with a mixed anhydride method). Radionuclide emissions from both ^{131}I and ^{90}Y can extend to 1–5 mm of their final location, corresponding to several cell diameters. Thus, their chief advantage resides in their ability to kill tumor cells that are poorly accessible and/ or antigen-negative. Unlike conventional radiation therapy, radioimmunoconjugates provide continuous radiation from the decay of the radionuclide, which allows less opportunity for the tumor cells to repair sublethal damage. Depending on the type of MoAb, the antibody itself may trigger CDC and ADCC mechanisms that supplement the effect of the radionuclide.

Although no radioimmunoconjugates have progressed to the market, a number have been examined in clinical trials. Bexxar (^{131}I-tositumomab) is an anti-CD20 MoAb examined in Phase III trials for non-Hodgkin's lymphoma. In an early trial of this radioimmunoconjugate, 19 patients with non-Hodgkin's lymphoma, who had been prescreened for favorable biodistribution of the MoAb, received 234–777 mCi of the ^{31}I-anti-CD20 MoAb. Because this was considered a myeloablative dose, the patients received autologous marrow reinfusion following the therapy. Although adverse effects were substantial due to the high dose of radiation, the regimen resulted in a complete response in 16 patients and a partial response in 2 patients; the MTD in terms of tissue exposure was determined to be $\leq$ 2700 cGy. A Phase II trial with a similar regimen in 21 patients achieved 17 complete responses, with an 81% progression-free survival at 12 months.

Applications of Monoclonal Antibodies in Drug Delivery

Principle of targeting

Several classes of drugs lack specificity for diseased cells; for example, the cytotoxic action of chemotherapeutic agents is directed against any rapidly proliferating cell population. Due to this non-specificity, many drugs have low therapeutic indices and often cause serious side effects. One way of circumventing this problem is to deliver the drug in a manner such that it is preferentially localized at the desired site of action, or it predominantly attacks the diseased cells. This process is called targeting. Targeted drug delivery systems can be classified into three categories, viz. passive, physical, or active targeting. Passive targeting refers to the natural in vivo distribution pattern of the drug delivery system, which is determined by the inherent properties of the carrier (e.g., hydrophobic and hydrophilic surface characteristics, particle size and shape, surface charge, and particle number). For example, modulation of particle size makes it possible to passively target the lungs or reticuloendothelial system (RES) using particles >7 μm or 0.2–7 μm, respectively.

In physical targeting, some characteristics of the environment are utilized to guide the carrier to a specific site or to trigger selective release of its content at the site. Usually, it is accomplished via an external mechanism, such as induced local hyperthermia (e.g., using thermally sensitive liposomes) or a localized magnetic field (e.g., using magnetically responsive albumin microspheres). In active targeting, the natural disposition pattern of a carrier is modified to target it to specific organs, tissues, or cells. Athough cell-specific ligands have been used to target carriers to specific cell types, this approach is probably limited to a small number of tumor types. MoAbs would thus appear to be the more generally applicable mode of active targeting. While the field is less advanced than unconjugated MoAb and radioimmunoconjugates, there has been some success in targeting toxins (i.e., immunotoxins) and drugs (i.e., drug immunoconjugates) using MoAbs as targeting agents.

Toxin conjugates

Over the last two decades, several toxin proteins like diphtheria toxin and ricin have been conjugated to tumor specific antibodies, with moderate to high degree of success in tumor drug delivery. There are several toxins produced by plants (e.g., ricin, abrin, saporin, and gelonin) or bacteria (e.g., diphtheria toxin and pseudomonas exotoxin) used to construct immunotoxins. These toxins are highly potent, and generally a single toxin molecule is sufficient to lead to cell death. Most of the native toxins consist of two chains (e.g., Ricin A and B chains) one of which bind non-specifically to cell surfaces and the other is responsible for the cytotoxicity. To construct an immunotoxin, the non-specific binding chain (viz. Ricin B) must be removed or masked, and the cytotoxic chain (viz. Ricin A) conjugated to a MoAb chemically or by recombinant methods. Most toxins of plant origin exert their cytotoxicity by deactivating the ribosomal protein synthesis, and thus require internalization. A few others do not require internalization and are membrane-acting by a cytolytic mechanism; these include bacterial α-hemolysin, streptolysin, and the equinatoxin of sea anemone. In one of the first Phase I trials of an immunotoxin, an antiCD22 MoAb Fab′ fragment was conjugated to Ricin A and administered to 15 patients. The MTD was 75 mg/m^2 and there was a 38% partial response. Of the total of 200 patients in 9 clinical trials, which examined a variety of ricin-based immunotoxins, there was only a 3% complete response and a 12% partial response. This mediocre success may be due in part to the high inherent immunogenicity of immunotoxins. For ricin-based conjugates, the dose limiting toxicity arises from the vascular leak syndrome, a condition characterized by extravasation of fluid into interstitial space. Clinical trials have also indicated that poorly vascularized tumors are not suitable for immunotoxin therapy, perhaps because of their high molecular weight. To be more penetrating and to be less immunogenic, immunotoxins and similar targeting molecules need to be made smaller.

Drug immunoconjugates

Over the last several decades, a number of antitumor agents, including chlorambucil, methotrexate, daunomycin, and doxorubicin conjugated to tumor specific antibodies, have been investigated, with varying degrees of success in tumor drug delivery. The most extensively studied has been a doxorubicin-BR96 immunoconjugate (BMS-182248-1). BR96 is a chimeric MoAb specific for a Lewis antigen found on the surface of tumor cells. The immunoconjugate is formed using an acid- labile hydrazone linkage attached through the thiol groups of the MoAb, with 8 moles of doxorubicin/ mole of MoAb. After rapid internalization into antigen-bearing cells, the conjugate is designed to release free doxorubicin from the MoAb hydrazone linkage in the acidic environment of the lysosome. When tested in mice with xenografted human lung, breast, and colon carcinomas, there was an 89% and 72% cure rate (tumor reduction to non-detectable levels) in the lung and colon models, respectively. In breast carcinoma xenograft, results were less spectacular, with 10% complete response and 60% partial response. Doxorubicin or MoAb alone gave <1% cures in any of the models. In a rat lung carcinoma xenograft model, there was a 94% cure rate, even though, unlike mice, the Lewis antigen is expressed in normal tissue of rats.

Because of the encouraging in vivo results, clinical development of this immunoconjugate was initiated. The pH-rate profile was determined using a stability- indicating size-exclusion HPLC assay, and exhibited a maximum stability at pH 7.5. The predominant route of degradation was hydrolysis at the hydrazone linkage to release free doxorubicin, with aggregation being a secondary pathway. This was supported by ELISA assay that demonstrated no loss of conjugate after 1 week of storage at 2–8° C. However, because the stability even at this temperature was insufficient for clinical development, a lyophilized formulation was developed. Formulations that remained amorphous due to the use of sucrose or lactose as lyoprotectant showed the greatest stability, with a shelf life of the lyophilized product of more than 12 months at 2–8°C. In a Phase II study, the BR96 Doxorubicin conjugate (BMS182248-1) was administered to 14 metastatic breast cancer patients. However, there was only 1 partial response (7%), in contrast to doxorubicin alone, which gave 44% response. The toxicity profile of the two regimens was markedly different, with the doxorubicin showing the usual cardiotoxicity and hematologic toxicity, whereas the immunoconjugate showed GI associated toxicity, similar to the Phase I studies. It was proposed that the lack of correlation of the Phase II trial with the preclinical in vivo data could be because of the presence of the Lewis antigen at sites in the GI tract. This may act as an "*antigen sink*," preventing targeting to the tumor tissues and instead exacerbate the GI toxicity. Colon and lung cancer models showed better clinical responses than the breast cancer models, suggesting that clinical trials in these cancers may be more promising than breast cancer.

Another promising immunoconjugate is CMA-676, which is a conjugate of an anti-CD33 MoAb and calicheamicin, an anticancer drug shown to be 1000-fold more potent than doxorubicin in animal models. A Phase II trial of 39 acute myeloid leukemia patients resulted in 2 patients with complete remission and 7 patients who showed temporary removal of leukemia cells from the blood. CMA-676 is now in pivotol clinical studies in a number of centers in North America and Europe.

Preliminary clinical studies with chlorambucil-antimelanoma globulin conjugates in patients with disseminated diseases have also indicated improvement in patient survival. The evaluation of vindesine-anti-CEA antibody conjugates in patients with advanced metastatic cancer (and probably expressing CEA) has demonstrated positive localization of the conjugate. In this study, 8 patients received escalating doses of antibody (1–42 mg) conjugated to 24–1800 μg vindesine, and no toxicity or hypersensitivity was noticed in any patient. However in most instances, the tumor versus normal tissue distribution ratio of antibodies approximated 2:1, and it rarely demonstrated specificity leading to a more desirable ratio like 10:1.

Some studies have demonstrated synergism in antitumor response with drug–antibody conjugate. For example, a clinical trial with bronchial carcinoma patients compared chemotherapy with immunochemotherapy. The latter group received chemotherapy immediately prior to the administration of antibodies against a resected portion of the primary tumor. The group receiving chemotherapy alone demonstrated a 60% recurrence rate along with a 41% death rate; however, the immunochemotherapy group demonstrated only a 25% recurrence rate along with a 16% death rate.

Bispecific MoAbs composed of anti-CD3 or anti-CD2 MoAb, chemically conjugated to antitumor antibody and coated on lymphokine-activated killer (LAK) cells, have been clinically investigated for the treatment of malignant glioma, lymphoma, and ovarian cancer with encouraging results. In a trial involving malignant glioma therapy, bispecific MoAb-coated LAK cells were injected intracranially following surgical removal of tumor and whole brain irradiation and/or chemotherapy. This resulted in 76% of the patients being tumor-free after 2 years, as opposed to 33% of the patients tumor-free with LAK cell treatment alone.

Because of the ability to achieve higher drug–antibody ratios, various water-soluble polymeric carriers have been examined as linking agents in immunoconjugates. For example, encouraging results have been demonstrated with daunomycin conjugated to MoAbs via dextran bridge in rats bearing AH66 hepatoma cells. Similarly, MMC was conjugated to an anti-α-fetoprotein MoAb via a human serum albumin carrier in a molar ratio of 30: 1:1. Full antibody activity was retained, and the conjugate was 20-fold more cytotoxic than free MMC in vitro and was also more effective than free MMC in tumor-bearing mice. Poly(lysine) has also been successfully used as a carrier, e.g., for targeting methotrexate. and muramyl dipeptide. N-(2-hydroxypropyl)-methacrylamide copolymers have been extensively examined as carriers for tumor targeted drug delivery. Enzymatically cleavable spacers (e.g., oligopeptides) have been incorporated into these conjugates to allow release of active chemotherapeutic agent.

Immunoliposomes

Generally, the antigens expressed by tumor cells are not specific but are merely present in higher ratio than on the normal cells. Hence, systems such as immunoliposomes have been developed to exploit these opportunities, as they are expected to bind to a greater extent to high antigen density tumor cells than to low antigen density normal cells. In immunoliposomes, the number of antibody molecules per liposome can be varied by as much as two orders of magnitude. Using egg phosphatidylcholine, cholesterol, phosphatidylserine, and N-4-nitrobenzo-2-oxa-1-1,3-diazole phosphatidylethanolamine in molar ratio of 56:33:10:1, unilamellar liposomes with 12–55 antibody molecules per vesicle have been investigated for binding with RDM-4 lymphoma cells with varying antigen density. The increase in the valency of liposomes (i.e., number of antibody molecules per liposome) increased their binding with low as well as high antigen density cells, and thus the low valency immunoliposomes were found to allow better discrimination between target and normal cells. An additional advantage of immunoliposomes is that a relatively high drug loading can potentially be accommodated, with the result that a small number of antibody molecules conjugated to the surface of an immunoliposome can deliver many more drug molecules to the target than is otherwise possible. Once the drug is released into the target cell, no further transformation is needed, because the entrapment process does not involve any chemical modification of the drug.

Heath et al. have proposed the use of immunoliposomes for the intracellular delivery of compounds that intrinsically do not enter diseased cells. These compounds are cytotoxic if they are transported intracellularly. Methotrexate-γ-aspartate, a good example of this type of compound, has been encapsulated in liposomes composed of phosphatidylcholine, cholesterol, and 4-(p-maleimidophenyl)-butyryl-phosphatidylethanolamine in a molar ratio of 10:10:1. The liposomes were conjugated to either specific (anti-K2Kk IgG2A) or non-specific MoAbs (antisheep erythrocyte IgG2A). The binding of targeted liposomes was found to be six fold higher to L929 fibroblasts (which express H2Kk protein) than non-targeted liposomes, whereas their binding was comparable in a non-specific BALB/c 3T6 cell lines. The growth inhibition studies using L929 fibroblasts demonstrated the IC50 of free drug, targeted immunoliposomes, and non-targeted immunoliposomes to be 0.68, 0.066, and 1.2 μM, respectively. Hence, the targeted immunoliposomes appeared to be 10 times more effective than free drug and 18 times more effective than non-targeted immunoliposomes, whereas targeted liposomes actually had the least efficacy in the non-specific BALB/c 3T6 fibroblasts.

Extensive work is being pursued to assess the potential of immunoliposomes for the targeted drug delivery to CD4 positive cells in patients with HIV infection. The HIV infected cells possess CD4, which can be targeted by conjugating anti-Leu3A (CD4) MoAbs onto the surface of drug-loaded liposomes. Preliminary studies showed that immunoliposomes possessing surface-bound anti-Leu3A may be used to target antiviral agents to cells at risk from HIV infection. Cell adhesion molecules are glycoproteins expressed on cell surfaces during pathological inflammatory states such as rheumatoid arthritis, atopic dermatitis, and asthma; thus they also provide an opportunity for targeting. An F10.2 antibody against the cell adhesion molecule ICAM-1 was conjugated to liposomes; the immunoliposomes bound to human bronchial epithelial cells in a specific, dose-and time-dependent manner, correlating to the degree of ICAM-1 expression. Immunoliposomes of this type therefore have potential for targeted drug delivery in inflammatory disease states.

Heat-sensitive immunoliposomes have also been evaluated for the feasibility of drug delivery. These liposomes release the entrapped drug at temperatures above the phase transition temperature of the lipid(s). In vitro cell culture studies based on dipalmitoyl phosphatidylcholine liposomes with entrapped

^{3}H-uridine have demonstrated enhanced intracellular delivery of drug as compared to that observed with free drug and liposomes without MoAbs. Similarly, selection of appropriate lipids can also allow synthesis of pH-sensitive liposomes. Inclusion of target-cell specific immunogenic moieties in these colloidal particles leads to preparation of pH-sensitive immunoliposomes. Huang and co-workers have used 8:2 molar ratios of dioleoylphosphatidyl ethanolamine and oleic acid to develop pH-sensitive liposomes. Arabinofuranosylcytosine (ara-C) and methotrexate were encapsulated in the liposomes that were rendered immunospecific against L-929 cells by homing specific MoAbs. Compared to free drug, drug encapsulated in antibody-free liposomes and pH- insensitive immunoliposomes, the drug-encapsulated pH-sensitive immunoliposomes were found to significantly enhance the cytotoxic activity. Pretreatment of target cells with excess free MoAbs or placebo immunoliposomes was found to block the cytotoxic effect of the drug-loaded pH-sensitive immunoliposomes. In addition, it was shown that the drug release from these specific carrier particles occurs in cell endosomes.

Because of the complexities involved with distribution, uptake, and pharmacological effects of targeted drug delivery systems, in vitro results do not always adequately predict the efficacy of a proposed MoAb-targeted system such as an immunoliposome. In fact, there are only a few in vivo studies of immunoliposomes that clearly demonstrate the promise shown by in vitro studies. One encouraging example is a study by Onuma et al. that compared the in vivo efficacy of doxorubicin loaded immunoliposomes against free drug in cows. MoAb c143 against the antigen expressed by bovine leukemia cells was conjugated to liposomes containing doxorubicin. Two groups of antigen- positive cows received four i.v. injections of either 0.4 mg/kg free drug or an equivalent dose of drug via immunoliposomes at an interval of 4 days. Whereas the two animals receiving free drug demonstrated only a slight decrease in their antigen positive cells, the three animals receiving drug-immunoliposomes gradually became free of antigen-positive cells, and 2 of these animals became antigen-negative in 6- and 14-week periods after treatment, respectively. In another study, MoAbs against tumor-associated antigens expressed on bovine leukemia cells were conjugated with liposomes containing doxorubicin, and the formulation was administered intravenously to BALB/c nude mice inoculated with BLSC-KU cells on day 0, 3, and 7 after the initiation of treatment. The results were compared with untreated animals and the animals receiving doxorubicin liposomes conjugated to normal mouse IgG. The doxorubicin liposomes bearing target antigen specific antibodies significantly suppressed the tumor growth. The increase in tumor volume with this treatment, over 10 days after the initiation of therapy, was only 27% as opposed to 166% and 750% in the animals receiving non-specific therapy and no therapy, respectively. Histological screening of the tumors from animals receiving drug-loaded liposomes with specific antibody demonstrated scattered focal necrosis and marked proliferation of macrophages; however, in the untreated animals, active proliferation of tumor cells was observed with little involvement of macrophages. A great deal of attention has been paid in recent years to long-circulating (also called sterically stabilized or "stealth") liposomes, in which polyethylene glycol (PEG) molecules have been grafted to the surface of the liposomes by covalent attachment of PEG to liposomal phospholipids

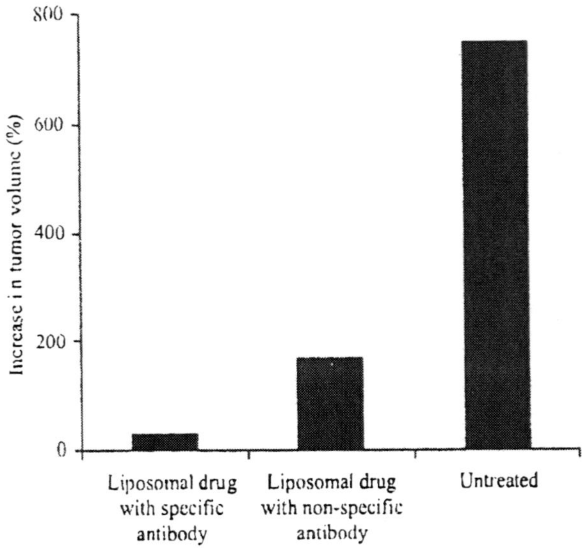

Fig. 11.4. Effect of treatment type on the increase in tumor volume in mice inoculated with BLSC-KU cells.

(specifically phosphatidylethanolamine). These long-circulating liposomes have been shown to avoid the rapid uptake by the reticuloendothelial system (RES), which normally plagues conventional liposomes without PEG; the circulating half-life can be increased by an order of magnitude. In fact, the presence of a MoAb on the surface of a conventional immunoliposome may actually increase the uptake by the RES system, suggesting that modification to insure long-circulation may be especially important for immunoliposomes. When designing PEG-modified immunoliposomes, the composition must be optimized for both antigen binding and extended circulating lifetimes. Antigen recognition by the liposomal antibody can be sterically hindered by the presence of the PEG. This can be overcome by either reducing the polymer size to 2000, or by moving the antibody out to the terminus of the PEG rather than the liposome surface.

Despite the extensive in vitro and in vivo research on immunoliposomes, these MoAb targeted systems have apparently not yet reached clinical trials. This may be because of a variety of factors, including the difficulty of clearly demonstrating efficacy in suitable animal models, and the obstacles associated with scaleup and manufacture of system as complex as a sterically stabilized MoAb-targeted liposome. Other potential problems of immunoliposomes are that they may not adequately penetrate the vasculature of solid tumors; they may not adequately release the loaded drug into the target cells; and they may demonstrate immunogenicity. Use of humanized antibodies may alleviate the latter effect to some extent. Recently, sterically stabilized liposomes conjugated to Fab′ fragments of a humanized anti-HER2 MoAb (similar to Herceptin) were studied in vitro using confocal microscopy techniques. The immunoliposomes bound selectively and were internalized by HER2-over-expressing breast cancer cells, reaching 8000–23,000 vesicles/cell at saturating liposome concentrations, which was at least two orders of magnitude greater than cells with low HER2 expression. These immunoliposomes, containing doxorubicin and optimized with respect to Fab′/lipid/PEG composition for intracellular tumor delivery, were subsequently examined in an in vivo human xenograft breast cancer model; they demonstrated significantly increased antitumor efficacy compared to free doxorubicin or non-targeted doxorubicin liposomes, and less systemic toxicity than free doxorubicin. The studies demonstrate the importance of optimizing a delivery system with respect to binding to the target epitope as well as uptake and/or release of available drug at the target site. Such considerations are necessary before successful demonstration of efficacy of immunoliposomes in the clinic. An ideal immunoliposome system should allow efficient encapsulation of intended compound so as to protect its degradation prior to and during endothelial transfer, and hence minimize inherent toxicity; it should also allow controlled release of drug in the extravascular compartment of target tissue. In this regard, it should be noted that the delivery systems based on particulate carriers may allow reversal of tumor cell drug resistance. Nevertheless, immunoliposomes fall short of meeting the above ideal criteria and much work remains to be done before they are clinically useful.

A related approach for lipophilic drugs is MoAb targeted emulsions. For example, a lung-targeted MoAb 34A was conjugated to the surface of a long-circulating emulsion composed of castor oil, phosphatidylcholine, and pegylated phosphatidylethanolamine. Upon intravenous injection into mice, 30% of the injected emulsion dose became preferentially associated with lung tissue within 30 min. A similar long-circulating emulsion conjugated to an anti-B-cell lymphoma MoAb LL2 was found to bind in vitro to three different Burkitt's lymphoma cell lines, and thus shows potential for delivery of anticancer drugs to B-cell malignancies.

Immunomicrospheres

In view of the availability of a wide variety of biocompatible and biodegradable polymers, and the ease of preparation of stable microparticles with predictable physicochemical characteristics, antibodies have been conjugated to polymeric microparticles for controlling their in vivo deposition.

Although a few in vitro studies have demonstrated promising results with immunomicrospheres, limited information has been published on the in vivo efficacy of immunomicrospheres for drug delivery. In one case, following promising in vitro results, an in vivo study was conducted in mice bearing human tumor xenografts, using ^{14}C-polyhexylcyanoacrylate nanoparticles with adsorbed anti-osteogenic sarcoma MoAbs 971T/36. However, the particles were found to deposit predominantly in liver and spleen, and hence the study failed to demonstrate any appreciable improvements in drug delivery due to the immunocarrier. Lack of optimal particle size and/or tumor tissue permeability, lack of expression of sufficient Fab portions on the surface of particles, particle opsonization leading to a secondary non-interactive coating, distribution of specific antigens in the liver, and competitive displacement of the adsorbed MoAbs by serum components were suggested as possible reasons for this undesirable in vivo distribution of the immunoparticles. Another study has evaluated the in vivo drug delivery potential of albumin immunomicrospheres in mice. The microspheres bearing Lewis lung carcinoma MoAbs demonstrated slightly higher localization in lung carcinoma at 24 h after its administration.

Regulatory Concerns

While a regulatory agency's prime concern remains the safety and efficacy of a new product in its proposed use, the technological issues concerning the manufacture of monoclonal-based therapeutics are not ignored. Indeed, because antibody-based systems involve specific immune reactions for their response, and they are comprised of components derived from biological origin, it is obvious that the proposed regulatory guidelines for the clinical use of these products are likely to be extremely strict. The technology for the development of antibodies and antibody-based delivery systems is relatively new and has been continuously expanding over the last several years. More and more practical changes in manufacturing process of these systems can therefore be expected over the next several years. Although most products are expected to be handled on a case-by-case basis, the following general guidelines should apply to all antibody-based systems: exhaustive characterization of the origin of cell lines, characterization of production procedures, product purification and characterization, quality control, and validation of processes involved during production and testings. For example, successful approval and use of a MoAb product will mandate declaration of the source, name and characteristics of the parent myeloma cell lines, and all pertinent details regarding the animal species used for hybridization. The rationale for selecting a particular cell line along with criterion for its acceptance, the genotype and husbandry of animals used for in vivo production, and steps taken to control contamination is expected to play a critical role. Once the product is made, extensive purification to reduce the level of contamination (using techniques like affinity, size exclusion or ion-exchange chromatography and/or ultracentrifugation) is likely to increase the probability of its approval. Measures would need to be undertaken to insure that the product does not contain any biological contaminant transferred from the original malignant hybridoma cell lines.

Once a bulk lot is in hand, its characterization for immunoglobulin and subimmunoglobulin class, and testings for potential aggregation, denaturation, fragmentation of immunoglobulin and immunologic specificity would be required. If a MoAb fragment is used, its degree of homogeneity would need to be confirmed. Finally, information on the sterility and polynucleotide contamination of the lot is likely to be required. It would be expected that the process validation allows rejection of lots with viral or nucleic acid contaminants. Additional tests may include determination of the product stability with respect to fragmentation, aggregation, and loss of potency. The preclinical toxicity testing with the final product would be required in at least one species bearing relevant antigen. Following the identification of an appropriate animal model, GLP-compliant pharmacokinetic evaluations involving in vivo distribution, metabolism and excretion, would be desired. As mentioned earlier, in most instances the antigens are preferentially associated with the target site rather than specifically present there, i.e., small amounts of the same antigens are present in one or more non-target organs. Because the probability of unacceptable levels of this cross-reactivity is reasonably high, regulatory guidelines recommend screening for cross-reactivity. For in vitro screening, blood cells, cell culture lines, fluorescent antibody tests, radioaudiography, and/or similar other techniques would be useful. If possible, tissues from unrelated human donors could be used to screen phenotypic expressions of potentially cross-reactive tissue antigens. If these tests demonstrate positive cross-reactivity, extensive in vivo testing in animals sharing similar phenomenon would be required to determine its frequency as well as intensity. Alternatively, an isolated perfused human organ system could be used. If these choices are not available, limited clinical testings may be advisable with particular emphasis on the quantitation of the product's biodistribution over a period of time.

It should be realized that the above guidelines, generally meant to assess and regulate the antibody or antibody-component of an overall product, would need to be expanded and/or modified according to the characteristics of the final product. For example, in antibody-based drug delivery systems, the effect of drug and antibody on the potency and biological activity of the final system would need to be assessed.

Future Prospective

Problems and possible solutions

Despite the promise of MoAb-directed drug delivery, there are still a multitude of problems that need to be worked out before the technology makes a large impact on therapy. A MoAb is often not as specific in vivo as would be predicted from in vitro studies; i.e., tumor antibodies may bind to normal cells as well as target cells. Despite the fact that antigens associated with tumor tissue have been identified, antigens are rarely specific enough to allow quantitative drug targeting. For example, CA 19-9, BW 494, and DU-PAN-2 have been identified as pancreatic tumor associated antigens. However, MoAb based therapy of pancreatic tumors has not been encouraging. In some cases, peak drug concentrations with MoAbs, in tumor tissue, have been found to be only 2–3 times higher than the surrounding normal tissues. Current literature suggests that the availability of high affinity MoAbs, which recognize specific antigens without cross-interaction with normal cells, is still scarce. The only exception to this observation is the surface immunoglobin idiotype expressed by certain B-cell lymphomas.

The lack of genetic stability of antigens on tumor cell surfaces is another cause of low density of target antigen on the tumor cell. Antigenic modulation may result in non-tumor specific antigen–antibody reaction, thus reversing the efficacy anticipated from the delivery system. Situations of low antigen density may readily saturate the MoAb-antigen binding. Quantitative evaluation of the localization of MoAbs in tumor tissue, at doses < 100 μg, have demonstrated a direct correlation between tumor mass and quantity of antibody localized, and at 2–3 days after administration only 8% of the dose could be detected in the tumor. However, the administration of larger doses of MoAbs have been shown to reduce the fraction localized in the tumor, with 1–2 mg doses almost saturating the tumor. The presence of circulating tumor-associated antigens is another factor that may decrease the overall efficacy of MoAb-directed delivery systems and complicate their evaluation. For example, the presence of circulating carcinoembryonic antigen has been shown to complicate the application of MoAbs against this antigen. In view of these problems, MoAb-directed delivery systems may ultimately be restricted to those few cases in which there are relatively high densities of known antigens in all cells of the target site.

The heterogeneity of tumor cells is another problem in targeting; i.e., a specific antigen may not be present in sufficient quantities in all cells of the target tissue to allow selection of suitable antibody. For example, it is now appreciated that multiple metastatic proliferation in a given host, and perhaps even in the same organ, can give rise to malignant tumors that contain heterogeneous subpopulation of cells with diverse biological characteristics, such as growth rate, antigenicity or immunogenicity, cell-surface receptors, response to individual and combined chemotherapeutic and immunological agents, invasiveness, and their overall metastatic potential. Trubetskoy et al. have proposed a method for MoAb-based drug delivery to target areas with heterogeneous antigens. The proposed method requires sequential administration of a mixture of modified antibodies against different antigens in the target area followed by administration of drug-carrier that recognizes and interacts with accumulated antibodies. The practical feasibility of this strategy was confirmed following administration of a mixture of biotinylated antibodies to target components followed by administration of biotinylated and avidin bearing liposomes. The binding of biotinylated liposomes via avidin was found to be higher than that achieved with liposomes bearing single antibody.

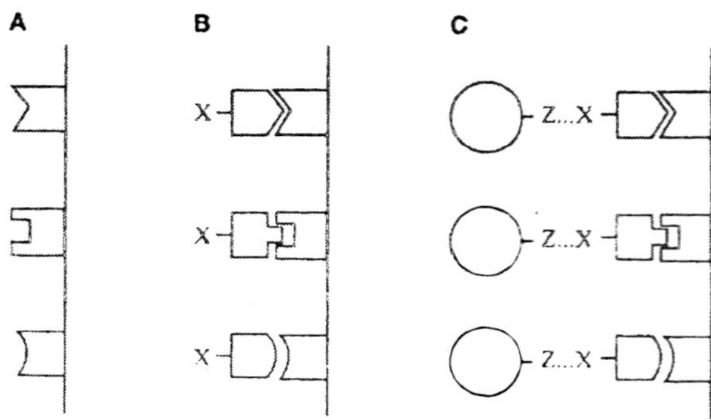

Fig. 11.5. A schematic representation of the unification of delivery systems to optimize therapeutic outcome with MoAbs: A–exposed target antigens; B–initial treatment with bridge molecules; and C–specific binding of unified carrier systems.

Solid tumors present special problems due to their frequent lack of vasculature; there is generally poor penetration of MoAbs, their fragments, and drug- or toxin-conjugates into solid tumor tissue. Because of the relatively intact microvascular barrier, and hence difficulties in carrier extravasation, the accumulation and uptake of immunoliposomes by solid tumor tissue is also generally low. On the other hand, the natural existence of increased transvascular permeability favors the use of MoAb-drug conjugates for the treatment of general lymphomas and leukemias.

The uptake of MoAb-based delivery systems by the reticulo-endothelial system (RES) is another drawback to these systems. It has been suggested that only 0.1–1% of the administered dose of antibody-based systems reaches non-RES sites, with ~8% dose reaching non RES sites under optimal situations. However, a study comparing the in vivo tumor localization of anti-CEA MoAbs, and their F(ab´)2 and Fab´ fragments, to human colon carcinoma grafts in nude mice has demonstrated greater tumor uptake of F(ab´)2 and Fab´ fragments than the intact MoAbs, due to the smaller molecular size of the former. Often multiple intravenous injections, over a course of weeks, have been found to be more effective than single injections, and continuous infusion is more efficient than bolus regimen.

As mentioned earlier, the immunogenicity of "foreign" MoAbs has always been a major factor in the lack of success of MoAb-based therapeutic systems. It has been suggested that use of (Fab´)2 fragments may improve drug delivery without sacrificing the specificity of antigen-MoAb binding because elimination of Fc portion would likely reduce immunogenicity and nonspecific binding to normal cells. Humanized antibodies probably hold the greatest promise in decreasing the immune response of MoAb-based therapies. While immunotherapy with these entities is promising and indicates greatly decreased immune responses, little work has been reported on humanized immunoconjugates. These entities may still be immunogenic due to the non-antibody portion of the conjugate. For example, rats injected with an unconjugated murine MoAb failed to elicit an antibody response, whereas rats injected with a MoAb-Vinca alkaloid conjugate mounted a strong antibody response directed against the linker portion of the conjugate.

New applications in the field of antibody-directed drug delivery may be developed by combining the technology with another form of targeting or other means of optimization. For example, in photodynamic therapy a photosensitizing drug (e.g., a porphyrin, chlorin, purpurin, or phthalocyanine) is localized in a tumor, which is then irradiated to effect cell-killing. Several reports have described the use of MoAbs to further increase the localization. For example, Sn (IV) chlorin e_6 was linked to the oligosaccharide moiety of an antimelanoma MoAb via a dextran carrier. In vitro studies indicated that phototoxicity was relatively specific for cells that exhibited the target antigen. Similarly, a chlorin derivative, meso chlorin e6 mono (*N*-2-aminoethylamide), was linked via a tetrapeptide linker to an antibody directed against ovarian cancer cells. Targeted conjugates were taken up rapidly by cells and detected within the lysosomes, and the conjugate had higher photodynamic effects on ovarian carcinoma cells than non-targeted conjugates (IC_{50} of 0.38, 290, and 0.34 μM for MoAb-HPMA-e_6, HPMA-e_6, and free e_6, respectively.

Another recent approach combines MoAb targeting with enzymatic prodrug activation. In this therapeutic method, called antibody-directed prodrug therapy (ADEPT), an enzyme–antibody conjugate is administered and allowed to accumulate in the target site (e.g., tumor). A latent, non-toxic prodrug is then injected, which on contact with the enzyme is converted into the active parent drug and subsequently kills the tumor cells. For example, a glutamic acid derivative of benzoic acid mustard was administered to choriocarcinoma-bearing mice, followed by a carboxypeptidase-antibody conjugate that cleaved glutamic acid from the active drug. Tumor contained the highest concentration of targeted enzyme conjugate, and was the only site in which all prodrug reaching the site was activated. The ADEPT technique has been tested clinically in colorectal cancer patients using para-*N*-(mono-2-chloroethyl monomesyl)-aminobenzoyl glutamic acid as the prodrug and an antibody conjugate of glutamate hydrolase as the activating enzyme, with temporary regression of disease in two out of five patients.

Despite the problems described in earlier sections, MoAbs should hold an important place in drug delivery and therapy in the future. Although the number of therapeutic applications that will eventually lend themselves to this technology may be small, the problems should not be insurmountable for these applications and may yield important advantages over other therapies. Proper attention to detail must be taken in the choice of antibody, coupling method, drug, route of administration, dose, and other factors in order to design an effective therapy for a particular disease; possible mechanisms of distribution, uptake, metabolism, and pharmacological effect must be properly understood to develop a rationale for a particular MoAb directed therapy. Humanized antibodies hold great promise to alleviate the immune response encountered in past clinical trials using murine derived antibodies. Many of the problems in the scaleup of MoAb manufacture have been solved, primarily because of the rapid growth of diagnostic applications of MoAbs and the coming to market of therapeutic MoAbs. Much work remains to be done, however, in the scaleup of immunoconjugates and complex systems such as immunoliposomes and immunomicrospheres. Nevertheless, it is likely that the next decade will see a number of MoAb-directed therapies reach extended clinical trials and perhaps come to the market.

Nanoparticles

Nanoparticles are small colloidal particles which are made of non-biodegradable and biodegradable polymers. Their diameter is generally around 200 nm. One can distinguish two types of nanoparticles: nanospheres, which are matrix systems; and nanocapsules, which are reservoir systems composed of a polymer membrane surrounding an oily or aqueous core. These systems were developed in the early 1970s. This approach was attractive because the methods of preparation of particles were simple and easy to scale-up. The particles formed were stable and easily freeze-dried. Due to these reasons, nanoparticles made of biodegradable polymers were developed for drug delivery. Indeed, nanoparticles were able to achieve with success tissue targeting of many drugs (antibiotics, cytostatics, peptides and proteins, nucleic acids, etc.). In addition, nanoparticles were able to protect drugs against chemical and enzymatic degradation and were also able to reduce side effects of some active drugs. This review focuses on the preparation and characterization methods of nanoparticles. The main applications of these systems are also described.

Preparation of Nanoparticles

Polymer nanoparticles including nanospheres and nanocapsules can be prepared according to numerous methods that have been developed over the last 30 years. The development of these methods occurred in several steps. Historically, the first nano-particles proposed as carriers for therapeutic applications were made of gelatin and cross-linked albumin. Then, to avoid the use of proteins that may stimulate the immune system and to limit the toxicity of the cross-linking agents, nanoparticles made from synthetic polymers were developed. At first, the nanoparticles were made by emulsion polymerization of acrylamide and by dispersion polymerization of methylmethacrylate. These nanoparticles were proposed as adjuvants for vaccines. However, since they were made of non-biodegradable polymers, these nanoparticles were rapidly substituted by particles made of biodegradable synthetic polymers. Couvreur et al. proposed to make nanoparticles by polymerization of monomers from the family of alkylcyanoacrylates already used in vivo as surgical glue. They succeeded in making nanoparticles by polymerization of the monomers in oil-in-water type emulsions prepared with an acidified aqueous phase. During the same period of time, Gurny et al. proposed a method based on the use of another biodegradable polymer consisting of poly(lactic acid) used as surgical sutures in humans. In this method, nanoparticles were formed directly from the polymer. Based on these initial investigations, several groups improved and modified the original processes mainly by reducing the amount of surfactant and organic solvents. At that time, the methods developed were only able to produce nanospheres. A breakthrough in the development of nanoparticles occurred in 1986 with the development of methods allowing the preparation of nanocapsules corresponding to particles displaying a core-shell structure with a liquid core surrounded by a polymer shell. From 1986, there was also an acceleration in the development of new methodologies for the preparation of all types of nanoparticles. The nanoprecipitation technique was proposed as well as the first method of interfacial polymerization in inverse microemulsion. In the following years, the methods based on salting-out, emulsion–diffusion, and double emulsion were described. Finally, during the last decade, new approaches were considered to develop nanoparticles made from polysaccharides based on the gelation properties of these natural macromolecules. These nanoparticles were developed for peptides and nucleic acid delivery. Another goal was the development of surface modified nanoparticles to produce long circulating particles able to avoid the capture by the macrophages of the mononuclear phagocyte system after intravenous administration.

All the methods can be classified into two groups depending on whether the nanoparticles are formed at the same time than the polymer itself requiring a polymerization reaction or are directly obtained from a polymer. There are numerous valuable reviews on the subject. The general principles of the methods leading to nanoparticle preparation are described and details of the most representative over are given.

Preparation of Nanoparticles by Polymerization

Nanospheres are mostly prepared by emulsion polymerization whereas nanocapsules are obtained by interfacial polymerization performed in emulsion or in microemulsion. In emulsion polymerization, the monomer itself, if liquid, is dispersed under agitation in a continuous phase in which it is non-miscible. The polymerization is usually initiated by the reaction of the initiators with the monomer molecules that are dissolved in the continuous phase of the emulsion. The polymerization continues by further addition of monomer molecules that diffuse toward the growing polymer chain through the continuous phase. The growing polymer chain remains soluble until it reaches a certain molecular weight for which it becomes insoluble. Therefore, phase separation occurs leading to the nucleation of the polymer particles and the formation of the tyndall scattering effect. Further growth of the nucleated particles occurs according to a mechanism that depends on the stability conditions of the whole system. This includes capture of new growing polymer chains, fusion or collision between nucleated particles. Throughout the polymerization, the monomer input in the continuous phase of the emulsion takes place by diffusion from the monomer droplets, which play the role of monomer reservoirs. When the reaction is completed, the particles formed contains a large number of polymer chains. Emulsion polymerization can be performed in emulsifier free systems and in both oil-in-water and water-in-oil emulsions.

The poly(alkylcyanoacrylate) nanospheres, widely used as drug carriers, are prepared by emulsion polymerization according to a method initially introduced by Couvreur et al. The monomers (isobutylcyanoacrylate, isohexylcyanoacrylate, *n*-butylcyanoacrylate) are dispersed in a continuous acidified aqueous phase under magnetic agitation. The anionic polymerization of the alkylcyanoacrylate is rapidly and spontaneously initiated by the remaining OH^- ions of the acidified water and is completed within 3–4 h depending on the monomer type. The preparation is performed at low pH (pH ~2.5) to slow down the anionic polymerization of the alkylcyanoacrylate, therefore allowing the polymer to arrange as colloidal particles. Dextran 70 or Pluronic F68 are usually dissolved in the aqueous phase to ensure the stability of the polymer particles. The size of the nanospheres can be controlled by the amount of Pluronic F68 from a diameter of 40–250 nm for concentrations ranging from 3 to 0%, respectively. Numerous drugs have been associated with these nanospheres including doxorubicin, an anticancer agent, a peptide growth hormone, and several antibiotics. Antisense oligonucleotides were adsorbed on the nanosphere surface via the formation of an ion-pair with a cationic surfactant, cethyltrimethylammonium bromide. Finally, it should be mentioned that some drugs can lose their biological activity during the preparation of poly(alkylcyanoacrylate) nanospheres. Generally, these molecules contain chemical functions that are able to initiate the polymerization of alkylcyanoacrylates and be covalently attached to the polymer constituting the nanospheres. The mode of such an interaction has been elucidated for two molecules including phenylbutazone (an anti-inflammatory drug) and vidarabine (an antiviral molecule). In contrast, the side reactions can be used to achieve the covalent linkage of defined compounds to give specific properties to the nanospheres. This has been used with poly(ethylene glycol) that initiated the polymerization of isobutylcyanoacrylate to give poly(ethylene glycol)-coated nanospheres, therefore presenting a more hydrophilic surface than those prepared according to the original method.

Methylidene malonates are other monomers that give biodegradable polymers and polymerize according to a similar mechanism than alkylcyanoacrylates. These monomers were also used to make nanospheres by emulsion polymerization for drug delivery.

Nanocapsules can be prepared by interfacial polymerization of alkylcyanoacrylates. The main advantage of using these monomers is their very fast polymerization rate when they come into contact with water. Oil containing nanocapsules were prepared by the rapid dispersion of an ethanol phase including ethanol, the oil, the monomer, and the molecule to be encapsulated in an aqueous solution of surfactant. When the ethanol diffuses in the aqueous phase, tiny individual oil droplets form, and because of the contact with water at the oil/water interface, the polymerization of the alkylcyanoacrylate takes place on the droplet surface. This method is mainly adapted for the encapsulation of oily soluble substances. However, surprisingly, highly water-soluble molecules such as insulin could be entrapped in these nanocapsules with high encapsulation yields (up to 97%).

Water containing nanocapsules were prepared by interfacial polymerization of the alkylcyanoacrylate in water-in-oil microemulsions. In these systems, water swollen micelles of surfactants of small and uniform sizes are dispersed in an organic phase. To prepare nanocapsules, the monomer is added to the oily phase of the already prepared microemulsion. The anionic polymerization of the alkylcyanoacrylate is initiated at the surface of the water swollen micelles and the polymer formed locally to make the shells of the nanocapsules. In the method first introduced by Gasco and Trotta, the microemulsions were prepared with hexane as the organic phase and Aerosol-OT as the surfactant. Both of these constituents are not compatible for the development of an acceptable drug carrier system. Thus, the method was recently adapted to microemulsions formulated with more biocompatible compounds, but still quite high concentrations of surfactant (up to 14wt%) are required for their preparation. The nanocapsules obtained by this method are dispersed in an organic medium and can mainly be used for oral administration. Indeed, for intravenous administrations, it is necessary to transfer the nanocapsules into an aqueous continuous phase. Such a transfer still remained a problem until recently, since the total elimination of the organic phase and the redispersion of the nano- capsules, in water is a difficult task to achieve avoiding the aggregation of the nanocapsules. Recently, Lambert et al. proposed to perform this operation by ultracentrifugation of the nanocapsule dispersion over a layer of pure water. Using this simple approach, the nanocapsules transferred from the organic phase to the aqueous phase without any aggregation problem during the centrifugation. In addition, this technique allows the elimination of the excess surfactant, which remains in the organic phase. This nanoencapsulation method has special interest for the encapsulation of water soluble molecules such as peptides and nucleic acids including antisense oligonucleotides.

Preparation of nanoparticles using a polymer

In this group of methods, the nanoparticles are obtained from a polymer, which was prepared according to a totally independent method. This approach presents the major advantage that the polymers entering the composition of the nanoparticles are well characterized and their intrinsic physicochemical characteristics will not depend on the conditions encountered during the preparation of the nanoparticles as it can be the case with the previously described methods. Most methods starting from polymers have taken advantages of the physicochemical properties of the polymer used in terms of its solubility or its faculty to form a gel under certain conditions. Basically, two approaches are followed. One is based on the spontaneous formation of colloidal particles of the polymer that are then stabilized in a second step of the procedure. The second approach is based on the adaptation of methods initially developed to make micro- particles. In this case, the goal is to reduce the size of the particles formed with these methods. A third approach leading to the formation of very specific particles named SupraMolecular BioVectors by their authors is described separately.

Methods based on the spontaneous formation of the nanoparticles

Spontaneous formation of nanoparticles can be achieved by taking advantage of the solubility and gelling properties of a dissolved polymer. Usually, the step allowing polymer colloidal particles to form is reversible, and it is necessary to complete the procedure by a second step required to stabilize the particles.

Based on the solubility properties of a polymer, the general principle is to prepare a solution of the polymer and to induce a phase separation by the addition of a non-solvent of the polymer or by a salting-out effect The occurrence of the phase separation can be followed by turbidimetric measurements or investigated using ternary phase diagrams. Phase separations leading to polymer colloid particles are usually obtained with diluted solutions of polymers. In a ternary phase diagram, it corresponds to a small domain. Using higher polymer concentrations in the solvent, the colloidal particles formed at the limit of the phase separation as followed by turbidimetric measurements in the case of proteins. To facilitate the formation of colloidal dispersion of polymer particles, it is better to induce the phase separation in totally miscible solvent–non-solvent systems. At that stage, the particles form spontaneously and quasi-instantaneously.

Once the proper conditions to obtain the polymer colloidal nanoparticles are identified, the particles must be stabilized. This is usually achieved either by the elimination of the polymer solvent by evaporation or by chemical cross-linking of the polymer as it is the case with proteins. This method, also known as the nanoprecipitation method, can be applied to numerous synthetic polymers. In general, the polymer is dissolved in acetone and the polymer solution is added into water. The acetone is then evaporated to complete the formation of the particles. Surface active agents are usually added to water to ensure the stability of the polymer particles. This easy technique of nanoparticle preparation was scaled up for large batch production. It leads to the formation of nanospheres. Nanocapsules can easily be prepared by the same method just by adding a small amount of an organic oil in the polymer solution. When the polymer solution is poured into the water phase, the oil is dispersed as tiny droplets in the solvent–non-solvent mixture and the polymer precipitates on the oil droplet surface. This method leads to the preparation of oil-containing nanocapsules and can be valuably used for the encapsulation of liposoluble drugs. Techniques based on the use of proteins are much more adapted to the encapsulation of hydrosoluble compounds and were recently developed to produce gelatin nanospheres as carrier systems for gene delivery.

Based on the gelation properties displayed by certain polymers, nanoparticles are formed spontaneously by controlling the gelation process. This approach has been developed with alginate and chitosan that form highly water-swollen gels. The gelling agents for these two natural polysaccharides are respectively calcium and tripolyphosphate. Nanoparticles are formed in a certain domain of concentrations of the polysaccharide and of the gelling agent. With the alginate, it has been shown that nanoparticles can be prepared when the respective concentrations of alginate and calcium are comprised in the domain of the pregel stage of the alginate gelling process (alginate 0.6 wt%, calcium chloride 0.9 mM). At this composition, tiny particles of gels form resulting from inter and intramolecular aggregations of alginate molecules caused by the interaction with calcium. These aggregates are stabilized by the formation of a polyelectrolyte complex with polylysine. Alginate and chitosan nanoparticles are interested for nucleic acid and protein delivery as recently reviewed by Vauthier and Couvreur.

Methods derived from microencapsulation techniques

Methods derived from microencapsulation techniques require the formation of an emulsion as a first step of the procedure. To produce nanometer-scale-sized particles, the size of the emulsion droplets must be small enough. This can be achieved by the use of special equipments such as high pressure homogenizers and microfluidizers. The energy input produced by these apparatus is important and is mainly due to high turbulence and cavitation forces. It allows an efficient dispersion of the polymer solution in the continuous phase. Once the desired emulsion is prepared, the formation of the nanoparticles can be induced according to two routes including the gelation of the polymer and the precipitation of the polymer either by solvent displacement or by solvent evaporation. Gelation can be induced by increasing the pH, adding calcium, or decreasing the temperature of emulsions containing respectively, chitosan, alginate, and agarose. In the solvent displacement technique, the emulsion is formed with a solvent of the polymer, which is partially soluble in water and with an aqueous phase saturated with the solvent. Once the emulsion is formed with ethylacetate as an example, it is diluted by the further addition of water to displace the solvent from the dispersed phase inducing the polymer precipitation. This principle was also developed on the base of an inverse salting- out method. In this procedure, a solution of polymer in acetone is dispersed in an aqueous phase containing a high concentration of salt to keep the acetone non-miscible with water. Just by diluting the emulsion with a large amount of pure water, the acetone is then extracted from the dispersed phase inducing the polymer precipitation. The total elimination of the acetone can be achieved by evaporation. Finally, precipitation of the polymer solubilized in the dispersed phase can also be induced by the removal of the solvent by evaporation. In this method named emulsification-solvent evaporation, the polymer solvent diffuses through the aqueous continuous phase and evaporates at the air/water interface. The emulsion should remain under agitation during the time required for the total evaporation of the solvent. These methods produce nanospheres. To make nanocapsules, small amounts of oil can be added in the dispersed phase of the emulsion that will form the nanocapsules by solvent displacement. Nanocapsules can also be prepared with the solvent evaporation technique from a double water-in-oil-in-water emulsion. The removal of the organic solvent of the intermediate phase of this double emulsion by evaporation causes the polymer to precipitate at the surface of the inner aqueous phase. Whereas nanocapsules made by the solvent displacement method is more adapted for the encapsulation of lipophilic compounds, this last method allows the encapsulation of hydrosoluble compounds.

Preparation of SupraMolecular biovector

SupraMolecular BioVector consists of polysaccharide nanospheres surrounded by a bilayer of phospholipids. At the origin, these systems were developed to mimic the low density lipoproteins that are natural colloidal structures encountered in the blood circulation and designed for the transport of cholesterol and cholesterol esters in vivo. SupraMolecular Bio-Vector are prepared in several steps including the functionnalization and chemical cross-linking of a polysaccharide (starch or dextran), the purification and the drying of the modified polysaccharide followed by the fragmentation of the resulted powder under high pressure to produce small polysaccharide nano-particles. Finally, a lipid bilayer is adsorbed on the surface of the nanoparticles. The chemical modification of the polysaccharide forming the core of the Supra Molecular BioVector lead to various possibilities in terms of the type of molecules that can be associated with such a carrier system. Indeed, the polysaccharide core can be either negatively or positively charged or even neutral opening large application potential.

Preparation of surface modified nanoparticles

Once intravenously administered, the body distribution of the nanoparticles is controlled by their surface properties. Indeed, despite their small size, nanoparticles display an enormous specific surface area that makes the interaction with the surrounding medium very important especially for their fate in vivo. Thus, the preparation of surface modified nanoparticles received much attention during the last decade to produce nanoparticles that are able to circulate for a long period of time in the blood stream at first and, more recently, to achieve an effective targeting of the device or to improve their bioadhesivity to mucosae.

Nanoparticles that are able to circulate for a long time in the blood stream should not be recognized by macrophages of the mononuclear phagocyte system. To achieve this goal, at least one of the two major known mechanisms involved in the recognition of foreign particles by macrophages should be avoided. These two mechanisms include the particle opsonization and the complement activation, which consists in protein adsorption and subsequent recognition by macrophages. A barrier to protein adsorption could be achieved by creating an efficient barrier of steric hindrance, therefore, by coating or adsorbing hydrophilic polymers to nanoparticle surface.

Nanospheres coated with poly(ethylene glycol) were first obtained by the simple adsorption of triblock copolymers of poly(ethylene glycol)–poly(propylene glycol)–poly(ethylene glycol) on the surface of already prepared nanospheres. To improve the stability of the poly(ethylene glycol) coating, nanospheres were prepared by nanoprecipitation or by emulsification- solvent evaporation using copolymers of poly(lactic acid)–co-poly (ethylene glycol) or of poly(alkylcyanoacrylate)–co-poly(ethylene glycol). Finally, poly (ethylene glycol) can initiate the polymerization of alkylcyanoacrylate to produce poly(ethylene glycol)-coated poly-(alkylcyanoacrylate) nanoparticles by emulsion polymerization.

To make nanoparticles able to escape complement activation, Passirani et al. proposed to coat nano- spheres with heparin. This compound, which is a polysaccharide, is a physiological inhibitor of complement activation in vivo. Heparin-coated poly(methylmethacrylate) nanoparticles were prepared by emulsion polymerization. In the method, the radical polymerization of methylmethacrylate was initiated by heparin according to an original method involving cerium ions and allowing heparin to covalently attach to poly(methylmethacrylate).

The next step now is the development of targeted nanoparticles toward a specific cell type. This has recently been investigated by Stella et al. who prepared poly(alkylcyanoacrylate) nanoparticles showing residues of folic acid on their surface. These nanoparticles will be used to target cancer cells overexpressing a membrane receptor for the folic acid. The targeting moiety, consisting on the folic acid, was grafted on the surface of poly(aminopoly(ethylene glycol) cyano-co-hexadecylcyanoacrylate) nanoparticles that were obtained by nanoprecipitation.

In another way, chitosan was used as a coating agent for nanoparticles to improve their bioadhesive properties after oral and nasal administration. Indeed, chitosan is known to have bioadhesive properties as well as an interesting absorption enhancing capacity.

Characterization of Nanoparticulate Drug Carriers

Nanoparticles can be characterized by all the different physico chemical techniques that apply for polymer colloids. Concerning the development procedure of nanoparticles as drug carriers, the main physico chemical parameters that are investigated are the shape, the size, the surface properties, the density, and the concentration of the particles. The size as well as the size distribution are important parameters to be determined to achieve safe intravenous administration. Surface properties are also important to consider as nanoparticles display considerable specific surface area responsible for the interactions with the surrounding medium. Finally, the density and the concentration are required to deduce the specific surface area of the particles together with the size.

Nanoparticles can be visualized using different microscopy techniques. Transmission electron microscopy is usually applied to nanoparticles after negative staining with phosphotungstate acid or with uranyl acetate after it has been checked that the staining agents do not modify the particles. Recent progress in transmission electron microscopy now allows direct observations of the nanoparticles without the use of any staining agent that may cause artefacts in some cases. In particular, direct observations of the nanoparticles after a sample of the nanoparticle dispersion has been freezing at very low temperature can be carried out by cryotransmission electron microscopy. Scanning electron microscopy is performed on samples coated with a thin layer of gold metal to produce the contrast. These techniques as well as those based on atomic force microscopy give useful images of the nanoparticles showing their shape. Measurements of the size and of the size distribution require determination of the diameters number of individual nanoparticles that may be assisted by the use of valuable image analysis softwares. The internal structure of the nanoparticles can be observed by freeze fracture and cryotransmission electron microscopy.

Generally, mean size and size distribution of nano- particles are evaluated by quasi-elastic light scattering also named photocorrelation spectroscopy. This method is based on the evaluation of the translation diffusion coefficient, D, characterizing the Brownian motion of the nanoparticles. The nanoparticle hydrodynamic diameter, d_H is then deduced from this parameter from the Stokes Einstein law.

Other techniques can be used to determine the size and the size distribution of the nanoparticles. The field flow fractionation method is based on the separation of particles according to their size in a thin glass channel in which the flow carrying on the nanoparticles is submitted to an external perpendicular force produced either by a crossed flow or a sedimentation. This technique, which can be applied for particles in a wide range of size (10 nm to several hundred μm), will gain more attention in the future for size determination and also for nanoparticle surface analysis. Size and size distribution of nanoparticles can also be determined by size exclusion chromatography performed on appropriate gels. This approach, requiring less equipment than the previous methods, presents the main limitation that only particles having a diameter lower than 120 nm can be characterized by this method.

As mentioned earlier, surface characteristics of the nanoparticles are of primary importance for the interaction of the nanoparticles with the surrounding medium. The main nanoparticle surface characteristics that are considered are the charge, the hydrophilicity, the chemical composition and the capacity to adsorb proteins and to induce complement activation. The charge of the nanoparticle surface is usually evaluated by the measurement of their zeta potential, which gives information about the overall surface charge of the particles and how it is affected by changes in the environment. Zeta potential is affected by the surface composition of the nanoparticles, the presence or the absence of adsorbed compounds, and the composition of the dispersing phase, mainly the ionic strength and the pH.

The hydrophilicity of the nanoparticle surface can be evaluated by hydrophobic interaction chromatography. This technique, based on affinity chromatography, allows a very rapid discrimination between hydrophilic and hydrophobic nanoparticles. The nano- particles are passed through a column containing a hydrophobic interaction chromatography gel. The nanoparticles that are retained by the gel and only eluted after the addition of a surfactant are considered as hydrophobic, whereas the nanoparticles that do not interact with the gel and that are directly eluted from the column are considered as hydrophilic. Apart from the hydrophobic interaction chromatography, the field flow fractionation techniques recently appeared to present interesting potential for the characterization of nanoparticles with different surface characteristics. X-ray photoelectron spectroscopy (ESCA) can be use to determine the chemical composition of the nanoparticle surface. This technique is a very useful tool for the development of surface modified nano- particles providing a direct evidence of the presence of the components that are believed to be on the nano- particle surface.

The capacity of the nanoparticles to adsorb proteins and to activate the complement in vivo after intravenous administration will influence the fate of the carrier and its body distribution. To approach this aspect, in vitro tests have been developed to investigate the profile of the type of serum proteins that adsorbed onto the nanoparticle surface after incubation in serum and to evaluate the capacity of the nanoparticles to induce complement activation. The analysis of the protein adsorbed onto the nanoparticle surface can be performed by 2D-polyacrylamide gel electrophoresis. This technique allows the identification of the proteins that adsorbed onto the nanoparticle surface. To evaluate modifications of the composition of the adsorbed protein with time, a faster method based on capillary electrophoresis can also be used. Finally, the activation of the complement produced by nano- particles can be evaluated either by a global technique or by a specific method measuring the specific activation of the component C3. In the global technique, nano- particles are incubated with serum and, after the incubation, the remaining non-activated complement in the serum is evaluated using a red blood cell lysis test.

The concentration of nanoparticle in the dispersion can be deduced from gravimetric determination or by turbidimetric measurements based on the application of the Mie's law. Density of the nanoparticles is evaluated either by pycnometry or by isopycnic centrifugation.

Pharmaceutical Applications of Nanoparticles

Nanoparticles were first developed in the mid-seventies by Birrenbach and Speiser. Later on, their application for the design of drug delivery systems was made available by the use of biodegradable polymers that were considered to be highly suitable for human applications. At that time, the research on colloidal carriers was mainly focusing on liposomes, but no one was able to produce stable lipid vesicles suitable for clinical applications. In some cases, nanoparticles have been shown to be more active than liposomes due to their better stability. This is the reason why in the last decades many drugs (e.g., antibiotics, antiviral and antiparasitic drugs, cytostatics, protein and peptides) were associated to nanoparticles.

Intravenous administration

Fate of nanoparticles and their content after intravenous administration

The main interest of nanoparticles is their ability to achieve tissue targeting and enhance the intracellular penetration of drugs. After intravenous administration, nanoparticules are taken up by the liver, spleen and to a lower extent the bone marrow. Within these tissues, nanoparticles are mainly taken up by cells of the mononuclear phagocyte system (MPS). The uptake occurs through an endocytosis process after which the particles end up in the lysosomal compartment where they are degraded producing low molecular weight soluble compounds that are eliminated from the body by renal excretion. As a result of the MPS site specific targeting, avoidance of some organs was made possible, thus reducing the side effects and toxicity of some active compounds. Due to their strong lysosomal localization, one could imagine that nanoparticles are not suitable to target to the cytoplasm. To avoid their trapping within the lysosomal compartment, several compounds able to destabilize the lysosomal membrane were added to the nanoparticulate systems (e.g., cationic surfactant) allowing some drugs to be delivered to the cytoplasm. Recently, to avoid MPS uptake, several groups have developed a strategy consisting of the linkage to the nanoparticles of poly(ethylene glycol) derivatives. This linkage results in a lower uptake of nanoparticles by the MPS and in a longer circulation time. As a consequence, these so-called stealth nanoparticles would be able to extravasate across endothelium that becomes permeable due to the presence of solid tumors.

Application to the treatment of intracellular infections

Intracellular infections were found to be a field of interest for drug delivery by means of nanospheres. Indeed. infected cells may constitute a "reservoir" for micro organisms, which are protected from antibiotics inside lysosomes. The resistance of intracellular infections to chemotherapy is often related to the low uptake of commonly used antibiotics or to their reduced activity at the acidic pH of lysosomes. To overcome these effects, the use of ampicillin, a β lactam antibiotic, bound to nanospheres was proposed as endocytozable formulation. The effectiveness of polyisohexylcyanoacrylate (PIHCA) nanospheres was tested in the treatment of two experimental intracellular infections.

Firstly, ampicillin-loaded nanospheres were tested in the treatment of experimental *Listeria monocytogenes* infection in congenitally athymic nude mice, a model involving a chronic infection of both liver and spleen macrophages. After adsorption of ampicillin onto nanospheres, the therapeutic activity of ampicillin was found to increase dramatically over that of the free drug. Bacterial counts in the liver were at least 20-fold reduced after linkage of ampicillin to PIHCA nano- spheres. In addition, nanoparticulate ampicillin was capable of ensuring liver sterilization after two injections of 0.8 mg of nanospheres bound drug, whereas no such sterilization was ever observed with any of other regimens tested. Reappearance of living bacteria in the liver after the end of the treatment was probably due to a secondary infection derived from other organs such as the spleen, which was not completely sterilized by the treatment.

Secondly, nanosphere-bound ampicillin was tested in the treatment of experimental salmonellosis in C57/BL6 mice, a model involving an acute fatal infection. All mice treated with a single injection of nanoparticle-bound ampicillin survived, whereas all control mice and all those treated with unloaded nano- spheres died within 10 days postinfection. With free ampicillin, an effective-curative effect required three doses of 32 mg each. Lower doses (3×0.8 mg and 3×16 mg) delayed but did not reduce mortality. Thus, the therapeutic index of ampicillin, calculated on the basis of mice mortality, was increased by 120-fold when the drug was bound to nanospheres.

In order to clarify the mechanism by which nano- spheres improved the antimicrobial efficacy of ampicillin, Forestier et al. have compared in vitro the efficacy of ampicillin bound to poly(isobutylcyanoacrylate) (PIBCA) nanospheres with that of free ampicillin in terms of survival of *L. monocytogenes* in mouse peritoneal macrophages. After 30 h of incubation, nanospheres-bound ampicillin decreased the number of viable bacteria by 99% as compared to the controls whereas with free ampicillin, the number of bacteria was slightly lower than in the controls. Nanoparticle-ampicillin thus appeared to be much more effective than free ampicillin for inhibiting intracellular growth of *L. monocytogenes*. With in vitro *Salmonella typhimurium* infected macrophages, the situation was a little bit more complicated since the bactericidal effect of ampicillin-bound PIHCA nanospheres was poor although the intracellular capture of ampicillin was dramatically increased and its efflux in the extra- cellular medium reduced. In another study, confocal microscopy and transmission electron microscopy were used to establish the intracellular traffic of ampicillin-bound PIHCA nanospheres and its relation with the bacteria within the subcellular compartments. The data obtained clearly demonstrated the active uptake by phagocytosis of ampicillin-bound PIHCA nano-spheres by murine macrophages and their localization in the same vacuoles as the infecting bacteria, but in a restrictive way. Thus, it was difficult to understand the limited bactericidal effect of ampicillin-bound nanospheres. The most probable explanation is to be found in the resistance mechanism of S. typhimurium involving the inhibition of the phagosome–lysosome fusion, which lets some bacteria in phagosomes free of nanospheres. If this proposed hypothesis (inhibition of phagosome–lysosome fusion) is correct, the dramatic efficiency observed in vivo should rather be due to the specific targeting of the infected tissues (rich in reticulo-endothelial cells), than to an efficient intracellular targeting as it could be supposed.

In order to eliminate both dividing and non-dividing bacteria, a fluoroquinolone antibiotic, ciprofloxacin, has been associated with PIBCA and PIHCA nano-spheres. In an animal model of persisting Salmonella infection, although an effect on the early phase of the infection was observed, neither free nor nanosphere-bound ciprofloxacin was able to eradicate truly persisting bacteria.

Since they accumulate in the MPS, nanospheres hold promise as drug carriers for the treatment of vis-ceral leishmaniosis. Thus, it has been shown that PIHCA nanospheres can be used as a carrier of primaquine whose activity was increased 21-fold against intracellular *Leishmania donovani* when associated with nanospheres. A part of the activity was attributed to the fact that phagocytosis of nanospheres led to the induction of a respiratory burst, which was more pronounced in infected than in non-infected macrophages. Dehydroemetine is also one of the drug candidates for this treatment but has some side effects involving the heart, which were reduced after linkage with nanospheres.

Application to the treatment of cancer

When given intravenously, anticancer drugs are distributed throughout the body as a function of the physicochemical properties of the molecule. A pharmacologically active concentration is reached in the tumor tissue at the expense of massive contamination of the rest of the body. For cytostatic compounds, this poor specificity raises a toxicological problem, which presents a serious obstacle to effective therapy. The use of colloidal drug carriers could represent a more rational approach to specific cancer therapy. In addition, the possibility of overcoming multidrug resistance might be achieved by using cytostatics-loaded nanospheres.

The antitumor efficacy of doxorubicin-loaded nano- spheres was first tested using the lymphoid leukemia L-1210 as a tumor model. In this study, one intravenous injection of doxorubicin-loaded PIBCA nanospheres was found to be more effective against L1210 leukemia than when the drug was administered in its free form following the same dosing schedule. Although the increased life span (ILS %) of mice injected with doxorubicin-loaded PIBCA nanospheres was twice as high as the ILS % for free doxorubicin, there were no long-term survivors.

The effectiveness of doxorubicin-loaded PIHCA nanospheres against L1210 leukemia was even more pronounced than that of doxorubicin loaded onto PIBCA nanospheres. The drug toxicity was markedly decreased when it was bound to this sort of nano- spheres, so that impressive results were obtained with this formulation at doses for which the therapeutic efficiency of free doxorubicin was completely masked by the overpowering toxicity of the drug. Furthermore, preliminary experiments suggested that one i.v. bolus injection of doxorubicin-loaded nanospheres was more active, in L1210-bearing mice, than perfusion of the free drug for 24 h.

The superiority of doxorubicin targeted with the aid of poly(alkylcyanoacrylate) nanospheres was later confirmed in a murine hepatic metastases model (M5076 reticulosarcoma). Irrespective of the dose and the administration schedule, the reduction in the number of metastases was much greater with doxorubicin-loaded nanospheres than with free doxorubicin, particularly if treatment was given only when the metastases were well established. The improved efficacy of the targeted drug, as clearly confirmed by histological examinations, shows that both the number and the size of the tumor nodules were lower when doxorubicin was administered in its nanoparticulate form. Furthermore, liver biopsies of animals treated with the nanosphere-targeted drug showed a lower cancer cell density inside tumor tissue. Necrosis was often less widespread with the nanosphere-associated drug than in the control group and the group treated with free doxorubicin.

Studies performed on total homogenates of livers from both healthy and metastases-bearing mice showed extensive capture of nanoparticulate doxorubicin by the liver; no difference in hepatic concentrations was noted between healthy and tumor-bearing animals. In order to elucidate the mechanism behind the enhanced efficiency of doxorubicin-loaded nano- spheres, doxorubicin measurements were made in both metastatic nodules and neighboring healthy hepatic tissue. This provided quantitative information concerning the drug distribution within these tissues. During the first 6 h after administration, the exposure of the liver to doxorubicin was 18 times greater for nanosphere-associated doxorubicin. However, no special affinity for the tumor tissue was detected and the nanospheres were seen by electron microscopy to be located within Kupffer cells (macrophages). However, at later time-points, the amount of drug in the tumor tissue increased in nanosphere-treated animals to 2.5 times the level found in animals given free doxorubicin. Since uptake of nanospheres by neoplastic tissue is unlikely, this increase in the doxorubicin concentration in tumor tissue probably resulted from doxorubicin released from healthy tissue, in particular Kupffer cells. Hepatic tissue could play the role of drug reservoir from which prolonged diffusion of the free drug (from nanospheres entrapped in Kupffer cell lysosomes) toward the neighboring malignant cells occurs.

This hypothesis raises the question of the long-term effect of an 18-fold increase of doxorubicin concentration in the liver. Although toxicological data have shown that doxorubicin-loaded nanospheres were not significantly or unexpectedly toxic to the liver in terms of survival rate at high doses, body weight loss, and histological appearance, this possibility should be borne in mind, especially since a temporary depletion in the number of Kupffer cells, and hence the ability to clear bacteria, was observed in rats treated with doxorubicin-loaded liposomes. A systematic study using unloaded poly(alkyl-cyanoacrylate) nanoparticles confirmed a reversible decline in the phagocytic capacity of the liver after repeated dosing, as well as a slight inflammatory response.

Nanoparticle-associated doxorubicin also accumulated in bone marrow, leading to a myelosuppressive effect. However, this tropism of carriers might be useful to deliver myelostimulating compounds such as granulocyte colony stimulating factor to reverse the suppressive effects of intense chemotherapy. Nanospheres are also captured by splenic macrophages. In this study, the spleen architecture was shown to play a role in the localization of the nanospheres: in mice, uptake was mainly observed in metallophilic macrophages of the marginal zone whereas in rats, which have sinusoidal spleens similar to that of humans, particles were found in the red pulp macrophages. On the other hand, alteration of the drug distribution profile by linkage to nanospheres can, in some cases, considerably reduce the toxicity of a drug because of reduced accumulation in organs where the most acute toxic effects are exerted. This concept was indeed illustrated with doxorubicin, which displays severe acute and chronic cardiomyopathy. After intravenous administration to mice, plasma levels of doxorubicin were higher when the drug was adsorbed onto nanospheres and at the same time the cardiac concentration of the drug was dramatically reduced. In accordance with the observed distribution profile, doxorubicin associated with nanospheres was found to be less toxic than free doxorubicin.

The ability of tumor cells to develop simultaneous resistance to multiple lipophilic compounds represents a major problem in cancer chemotherapy. Cellular resistance to anthracyclines has been attributed to an active drug efflux from resistant cells linked to the presence of transmembrane P-glycoprotein, which was not detectable in the parental drug-sensitive cell line. Drugs, such as doxorubicin, appear to enter the cell by passive diffusion through the lipid bilayer.

Upon entering the cell, these drugs bind to P-glycoprotein, which forms transmembrane channels and uses energy from ATP hydrolysis to pump these compounds out of the cell. To solve this problem, many authors have proposed the use of competitive P-glycoprotein inhibitors, such as the calcium channel blocker verapamil, which are able to bind to P-glycoprotein and to overcome pleiotropic resistance. However, since the adverse effects of verapamil are serious, its clinical use to overcome multidrug resistance is limited.

During the past few years, many studies have been devoted to evaluating the antitumor potential of carrier-drug complexes. The effect of nanospheres loaded with doxorubicin, resistance to which is known to be related to the presence of P-glycoprotein, was evaluated. The cytotoxicity of free-doxorubicin, doxorubicin-loaded PIHCA nanospheres (NP-Doxorubicin) (mean diameter 300 nm), and nanospheres without drug (NP), against sensitive (MCF7) and multidrug resistant (Doxorubicin R MCF7) human breast cancer cell lines was compared. MCF7 cells were more sensitive to free-doxorubicin than Doxorubicin R MCF7 cells with a 150-fold difference in the IC_{50}. No significant difference was observed in the survival rate of MCF7 treated with free-Doxorubicin or NP-doxorubicin. In contrast, for doxorubicin R MCF7, the IC_{50} for doxorubicin was 130-fold lower when NP-doxorubicin were used instead of free-doxorubicin. These results indicated that nanospheres provided an effective carrier for introducing a cytotoxic dose of doxorubicin into the pleiotropic resistant human cancer cell line Doxorubicin R MCF7.

Complementary experiments, conducted with other sensitive and resistant cell lines, have confirmed this efficacy of nanospheres. Doxorubicin resistance was circumvented in the majority of the cell lines tested, and some encouraging results were obtained in vivo in a P388 model growing as ascites. Further studies were undertaken to elucidate the mechanism of action of polyalkylcyanoacrylate nanospheres. The incubation time and number of particles per cell were important factors and, when PIBCA nanospheres were used, doxorubicin accumulation within P388/ADR resistant leukemic cells was increased compared with free drug, although no endocytosis of nano- spheres occurred.

On the other hand, when the less rapidly degradable PIHCA nanospheres were used, reversion was observed in the absence of increased intracellular drug. The degradation products of poly (alkylcyanoacrylate) nanospheres [mainly poly(cyanoacrylic acid)] were also able to increase both accumulation and cytotoxicity of doxorubicin, although they were soluble in the culture medium. Hence, the reversion of resistance seems to be due both to the adsorption of nanospheres on the cell surface and to the formation of a doxorubicin-poly(cyanoacrylic acid) ion pair, which facilitates the transport of the drug across the cell membrane.

In the light of the results obtained with doxorubicin-loaded nanospheres in the liver metastases model described earlier, the role of macrophages as a reservoir for doxorubicin was tested in a two-compartment coculture system in vitro with both resistant and sensitive P388 cells. Even after prior uptake by macrophages, doxorubicin-loaded PIBCA nanospheres were able to overcome resistance. However, this reversion was only partial. It was decided to take advantage of the particulate drug carrier offers to associate an anticancer drug and a compound capable of inhibiting the P-glycoprotein. This approach was tested with doxorubicin and cyclosporin A bound to the same nano-spheres and was found to be extremely effective in reversing P388 resistance. The association of cyclosporin A with nanospheres would ensure that it reaches the same sites as the anticancer drug at the same time and would also reduce its toxic side effects.

As early as 1986. al Khouri et al. observed that like other colloidal carriers, nanocapsules, administered by the IV route in rabbits, were taken up rapidly by organs of the mononuclear phagocyte system. One application that takes advantage of this uptake concerns nanocapsules of (muramyl tripeptide cholesterol) (MTP-Chol). This immunostimulating agent is able to activate macrophages and induce toxicity toward tumor cells, and would therefore be a useful agent to treat metastatic cancer. The mechanisms by which activated macrophages arrest tumor proliferation include production of nitric oxide and TNF-α. It was showed in in vitro models of rat alveolar macrophages and RAW 264.7 mouse monocyte macrophage line that nanocapsules based on poly(D,L-lactide) containing MTP-Chol are more efficient activators than the free drug. This action could be due to an intracellular delivery of the immunomodulator encapsulated in nanocapsules after phagocytosis and to an intermediate transfer of the drug to serum proteins. This system has also demonstrated its efficiency in vivo; in fact, Barratt et al. reported that antimetastatic effects of nanocapsules contained MTP-Chol in a model of liver metastases. Some antimetastatic activity was also seen after oral administration.

Nanospheres for oligonucleotide delivery

Oligodeoxynucleotides are potentially powerful new drugs because of their selectivity for particular gene products in both sense and antisense strategies. However, using antisense oligonucleotides in therapeutics is a challenge to pharmaceutical technology because of their susceptibility to enzymatic degradation and their poor penetration across biological membranes. Nanoparticulate preparations might be an interesting alternative because of better stability in the presence of biological fluids. In the case of nanospheres made of synthetic polymers [poly(alkylcyanoacrylate), poly (lactic acid)], since oligonucleotides have no affinity for the polymeric matrix, association with nanoparticles has been achieved by ion pairing with a cationic surfactant, cetyltimethylammonium bromide (CTAB) adsorbed onto the nanoparticle surface. Oligonucleotides bound to poly(alkylcyanoacrylate) nano- spheres in this way were protected from nucleases in vitro and their intracellular uptake was increased. In addition, nanospheres were able to concentrate intact oligonucleotides in the liver and in the spleen. Antisense oligonucleotides formulated in this way were able to specifically inhibit mutated Ha-ras-mediated cell proliferation and tumorigenicity in nude mice.

This approach has recently been applied to the association of a phosphodiester antisense oligonucleotide directed against the 3′ non-translated region of the PKCα gene with nanospheres prepared from PIBCA. These nanospheres were able to inhibit PKCα neoexpression in cultured Hep G6 cells.

Nanospheres containing oligonucleotides have also been formulated from a naturally occurring polysaccharide, alginate, which forms a gel in the presence of calcium ions. In this case, the oligonucleotides penetrate into the gel matrix by reptation, thus providing a high loading yield and good protection against nucleases.

Subcutaneous/intramuscular administration

Subcutaneous administration of nanoparticles was achieved mainly for the delivery of peptides and vaccines. It allows slow release of the entrapped drugs therefore reducing the number of administrations, increasing blood half-life of the active drug, and finally, in some cases, reducing side effects. PIBCA nanospheres were injected subcutaneously to rats. Autoradiographic pictures obtained after using radiolabelled polymer have shown a progressive staining reduction in the muscular tissue suggesting that nanospheres were slowly biodegraded. In the same study, nanospheres were found to release a peptide (GRF) in a sustained manner. Comparison of the AUC of free GRF and GRF-loaded nanospheres showed that in addition to the slow release process nanospheres were able to improve the bioavailability of the peptide. This improvement could be attributed to the fact that free administered GRF is very quickly metabolized at the injection site, whereas it is partly protected from massive enzymatic degradation when it is administered associated with nanospheres.

A few examples of the use of nanospheres as adjuvant for antigens/allergens delivery were described in the literature. The main advantage of this approach is to design single shot vaccine. In this case the drug carrier has to remain at the site of administration and deliver either continuously or pulsatively the antigen. The use of slowly degradable polymers (PLA, PMMA) is suitable for this application, since peptide or protein release is more adequate. Poly(methyl methacrylate) were first investigated as adjuvants for injectable vaccines.

These nanospheres were claimed to be biodegradable after subcutaneous or intramuscular injection and shown to exhibit very powerful adjuvant properties for a number of antigens. However, the adjuvant properties were shown to be better when the antigen was incorporated during the polymerization process than when adsorbed onto nanospheres. When comparing the effect of PMMA with other polymers (polystyrene and 2-hydroxyethyl methacrylate/methyl methacrylate copolymer, HEMA: MMA), it was also demonstrated that a decrease in particle size and an increase in the hydrophobicity of nanospheres increased the antibody response after immunization against influenza whole and split virus, bovine serum albumin, and HIV2 split virus.

Oral route

There are numerous reports showing that uptake and translocation of nanoparticles and microparticles take place after oral administration to animals. Different mechanisms have been proposed to explain the translocation of particulate material across the intestine: (i) uptake via Peyer's patches or isolated lymphoid follicles; (ii) intracellular uptake; and (iii) intracellular/paracellular passage. The uptake of poly(alkylcyanoacrylate) nanocapsules by Peyer's patches has been shown by Damge et al. When administered in the lumen of an isolated ileal segment of the rat, polylalkylcyanoacrylate nanocapsules were found preferentially over Peyer's patches through which they passed massively and rapidly. Nanocapsules were clearly visible in M-cells and in intercellular spaces around the lymph cells. Intracellular uptake of nanospheres has been proposed by Kreuter, Muller, and Munz based on electron-microscopic autoradiographic investigations showing radioactivity into epithelial and goblet cells after oral administration of poly(hexylcyanoacrylate) (PHCA) nanospheres labeled with ^{14}C. The translocation of particles by a paracellular pathway has been evidenced in a study done by Aprahamian et al. using PIBCA nanocapsules.

Nanocapsules were filled with an iodinized oil (lipiodol) in order to render them detectable using a scanning electron microscope equipped with an energy-dispersive X-ray spectrometer. When they were administered in an isolated segment of a dog jejunum, they appeared as vesicles associated with intraluminal mucus. Subsequently, they were observed in intravillus capillaries in close contact with red cells or adsorbed to the inner wall of endothelial cells. Among these three mechanisms and according to many studies involving nanoparticles made of other biodegradable and nondegradable polymers, translocation via the uptake in Peyer's patches seems to be the major pathway for a rapid and substantial passage after oral administration of nanoparticles. Although it might exist in certain situations, the passage of particles between the absorptive cells is rather less likely if the barrier of tight junctions has not been disrupted. Although there are abundant reports from various independent workers showing evidence of absorption of particulate systems by the gastrointestinal tract, the oral absorption of nanoparticles remains a controversial issue. However, even if a more clear estimation of the quantity of absorbed particles is needed as well as a better under-standing of the factors affecting particles uptake, it must be concluded that translocation of small sized particles like poly(alkylcyano-acrylate) nanoparticles is possible. The question remains if the extent of particle translocation is compatible with a strategy of drug administration with therapeutic perspectives.

Oral delivery of peptides and proteins and vaccines

Poly(isobutylcyanoacrylate) nanocapsules were shown 10 years ago to be able to encapsulate insulin and to increase its activity as assessed by a reduction of glycemia. Several aspects of this phenomenon are surprising: encapsulation of a hydrophilic drug in the oily core of nanocapsules; reduction of glycemia was only obtained with diabetic animals; hypoglycemia appeared two days after a single administration and was maintained for up to 20 days depending on the insulin doses, although the amplitude of the pharmacological effect (minimum level of blood glucose) did not depend on the insulin dose. Damgé et al. and Lowe and Temple suggested that nanocapsules could protect insulin from proteolytic degradation in intestinal fluids, based on the protection of encapsulated insulin, observed in the presence of different enzymes in vitro. Later studies showed that insulin did not react with the alkylcyanoacrylate monomer during the formation of nanocapsules and was located within the oily core rather than adsorbed on their surface.

The capacity of insulin nanocapsules to reduce glycemia could be explained by their translocation through the intestinal barrier, as suggested by Damge et al. for example by paracellular pathway or via M cells in Peyer's patches. Recently, the use of Texas Red-labeled insulin allowed this translocation to be visualized more readily. One hour after oral administration, nanocapsules reached the ileum. The presence of fluorescent areas within the mucosa and even in the lamina propria suggested that insulin-loaded nanocapsules could cross the intestinal epithelium. Although this passage is certainly an important factor, it does not explain the duration of the hypoglycemia. This prolonged action could be due to the retention of a part of the colloidal system in the gastrointestinal tract.

Interestingly, a prolonged hypoglycemic effect was also observed with insulin entrapped in poly(alkylcyanoacrylate) nanospheres when these were dispersed in an oily phase containing surfactant. This suggests that some components of nanocapsules could act as promoters of absorption.

Recently, Damge et al. showed that the incorporation of octreotide, a somatostatin analogue, in poly(alkylcyanoacrylate) nanocapsules also improved and prolonged the therapeutic effect of this peptide, after administration by the oral route.

Even if the main limitation to oral administration of poly(alkylcyanoacrylate) nanoparticles is that their passage through the intestinal barrier is probably restricted and sometimes erratic, they represent an interesting tool for oral delivery of antigens. Indeed, M-cells appear to be the main site for the uptake of poly(alkylcyanoacrylate) nanoparticles after oral administration. and, furthermore, it is generally accepted that limited doses of antigen are sufficient for a mucous immunization. In fact, oral delivery of antigens may be considered as the most convenient means of producing an IgA antibody response. However, it is importantly limited by enzymatic degradation of antigens in the GI tract and, additionally by their poor absorption.

Thus, it has been postulated that the use of micro- or nanoparticles for the oral delivery of antigens should be efficient if those systems are able to achieve the protection of the antigenic molecule. Poly(alkylcyanoacrylate) nanoparticles have been shown to enhance the secretory immune response after their oral administration in association with ovalbumin. This result was not fully reproduced in the case of poly(acrylamide) nanoparticles loaded with the same antigen. It was postulated that in the case of poly(acrylamide) nanospheres, much of the antigen was located at the surface of the polymer and could have been degraded during its passage through the gut. The relatively high surface concentration of ovalbumin adsorbed onto poly(butylcyanoacrylate) nanospheres may have reduced the ability of the proteolytic enzymes in the gut to gain access to and to degrade the antigen, resulting in a greater antigen availability.

Ocular delivery

The anatomical structure and the protective physiological process of the eye exert a strong defense against ocular drug delivery. This is the reason why conventional ocular dosage forms exhibit extremely low bioavailability. Limited absorption of the drug through the lipophilic corneal barrier is mainly because of short precorneal residence time due to the tear turn-over, rapid nasolacrimal drainage of instilled drug from the tear fluid, and non-productive absorption through the conjonctiva. Only a small proportion (1–3%) of the applied drug penetrates the cornea and reaches intraocular tissues. For these reasons, it is necessary to develop efficient and more acceptable ocular therapeutic systems.

Different strategies can be carried out to improve the precorneal residence time and/or penetration ability of the active ingredient. Among them, one approach consists of using colloidal drug delivery systems such as nanoparticles. Initial studies carried out with nanocapsules, as ocular drug carriers, attempted to increase the penetration of lipophilic drugs into the eye by prolonging the precorneal residence time, as observed with other colloidal systems, liposomes and nanospheres. These studies, which concerned anti-glaucomatous agents, such as betaxolol, carteolol, and metipranolol encapsulated in nanocapsules, only showed a reduction of the non-corneal absorption (systemic circulation) leading to reduced side-effects as compared with the free drug.

These systemic side-effects are due to a poor ocular retention of drugs that are directly absorbed into the systemic circulation by conjunctival and nasal blood vessels. In two cases (carteolol and betaxolol), encapsulation in nanocapsules produced an improved pharmacological effect (reduction of intraocular pressure) than produced by free drug and nanospheres (although the penetration of nanocapsules was not tested) and reduced cardiovascular systemic side-effects. Metipranolol showed the same activity alone and associated with nanocapsules but, as in the case of carteolol and betaxolol, its side-effects were reduced. When betaxolol was used, the nature of the polymer making up the nanocapsule wall was found to be important, and poly (ε-caprolactone) was more efficient than PIBCA or poly(lactic-co-glycolic acid).

Calvo et al. explored the mechanisms of interaction of nanocapsules with ocular tissues to better understand the pharmacological responses obtained with antiglaucomatous agents. By confocal microscopy, they showed that poly(ε-caprolactone) nanocapsules could specifically penetrate the corneal epithelium by an endocytic process without causing any damage to the cells, in contrast with PIBCA nanoparticles, the uptake of which was associated with cellular lysis. These results explained the improved therapeutic effect and the reduction of systemic side-effects as a result of drug loss through the conjunctiva provided by poly(ε-caprolactone) nanocapsules by increasing corneal epithelium penetration of lipophilic drugs.

Calvo et al. also excluded the influence of the oily inner structure in the activity of the nanocapsules, in the light of the absence of differences in penetration between nanospheres and nanocapsules, in contrast with Marchal Heussler et al. who observed a better therapeutic effect with nanocapsules than with nano-spheres. Moreover, Calvo et al. demonstrated with indomethacin-loaded nanocapsules that the colloidal nature of the carrier was the main factor influencing its ocular bioavailability. The same authors were also interested in the influence of the nature and the charge of the surface of nanocapsules on their physical stability and on their ocular bioavailability.

They found that coating the negatively charged surface of poly(ε-caprolactone) nanocapsules with cationic polymers could prevent their degradation caused by the adsorption of lysozyme, a positively charged enzyme found in tear fluid. Moreover, they noticed that a cationic polymer, chitosan, adsorbed on the surface of nanocapsules was able to provide the best corneal drug penetration without any local intolerance as compared to another positively charged polymer. This was achieved by a combination of effects: Penetration of particles into the corneal epithelial cells, mucoadhesion of positively charged particles onto negatively charged membranes, and a specific effect on the tight junctions.

This effect of improvement of ocular absorption was also reported by Calvo et al. with the immunosuppressive peptide cyclosporin A. The corneal level of the drug was increased fivefold as compared with an oily solution of the drug owing to a highly loaded nanocapsule preparation, also containing poly (ε-caprolactone). The efficacy of this topical formulation has also been observed on a penetrating keratoplasty rejection model in the rat. Le Bourlais et al. also proposed an alternative preparation of cyclosporin nano-capsules based on poly(alkylcyanoacrylate) dispersed in poly(acrylic acid) gel able to drastically reduce toxicity of poly(alkylcyanocrylates) on the cornea and to promote absorption of the drug.

12

Dressings in Wound Management

Throughout history, diverse materials of animal, vegetable, and mineral origin ranging from hot oils and waxes reported in the Ebers papyru through animal membranes and faeces of the Middle Ages to the picked oakum of the 19th century; have been used to treat wounds. Moist poultices are described on Sumerian tablets inscribed as early as 2100 B.C. Mediaeval manuscripts illustrate examples of both "moist" environment and biological "healing" with the practice of using dogs to lick wounds, particularly postsurgery, to moisten, cleanse, and stimulate healing thus relying on the now recognized, but at that time unknown, presence of antibacterial agents and growth factors in the saliva. Ambroise Pare (1510–1590), the "father" of wound management, used a semiocclusive, oil impregnated dressing in the 16th Century to obtain "a softness of the tissues." A Diachylon plaster consisting of a mucilaginous, moist mass made from linseed and marshmallow was originally described by Galen (130–201). In 1819, Abraham Rees, in his treatise on the use of lynette, emphasized the need to prevent "scab" formation by keeping the wound edges apart with oil soaked dossils. In the 19th Century, wet compresses or cataplasma kaolini were applied to wounds and covered in waterproof fabrics such as jaconet, batiste, or oiled silk to maintain humidity. The 20th century saw the production of leno gauze impregnated with soft paraffin, Tulle Gras.

The first authoritative monographs related to wound dressing materials appeared in early London and Edinburgh hospital dispensatories and later in the British Pharmaceutical Codices. The development of wound management products can be traced by examining these Codices together with the British Pharmacopoeia. The information is reflected in similar publications in the United States Pharmacopoeia and other national standards. Advances in the design and efficacy of wound management products was spasmodic and limited to the adaptation of available materials until 1960. Up to that date, the products were primarily of the "plug and conceal" variety exemplified by lint, gauze, cotton wool, and tow that were considered to be passive products which took no part in the healing process.

The new generation of products was a rejection of the traditional passive "cover all" dressing philosophy and was potentiated by advances in knowledge of the humoral and cellular factors associated with the healing process and the realization that a controlled microenvironment is necessary if wound healing is to progress at the optimum level, such environmental control dressings could be classified as *interactive*.

It is recognized that both the acellular and cellular activities involved in the healing cascade are optimized by a wound microenvironment that allows the free movement of cells and effective response to *bioactive* compounds. This optimal response can be expected where environmental factors such as temperature and humidity are at subdermal levels.

Performance Criteria

The concept of moist wound healing is generally attributed to George Winter after his much cited 1962 publication in Nature, although Bull, Squire, and Tophey in 1948 published results showing enhancement of healing under a "film" dressing. Turner in 1979 identified the performance criteria for a wound dressing product that would successfully contribute to an acceptable microenvironment. These were to:

1. Maintain a high humidity at wound/dressing interface
2. Remove excess exudate and toxic components
3. Allow gaseous exchange
4. Provide thermal insulation
5. Afford protection from secondary infection
6. Be free from particulate or toxic contaminants
7. Allow removal without trauma at dressing change

These criteria are still valid. An additional requirement with the advance in our knowledge of the growth factors involved in the healing process is: To be compatible with the humoral and cellular factors involved in healing.

Humidity Levels and Removal of Exudate

Partial or full thickness wounds exposed to the air will demonstrate a lower temperature than ambient due to the latent heat lost through tissue fluid evaporation. The clotting process and fibril development produces an occlusive dry eschar or scab which effectively seals and insulates the wound thereby limiting moisture and gaseous transmission and restricting the migration of epithelial cells to the moist subscab tissue. The result is slow healing with a high contamination and infection risk together with possible excessive scarring in an excised wound from closure without full cavity granulation. The maintenance of a high humidity between the wound and the dressing is therefore a requirement for rapid epidermal healing.

The absorption of excess exudate not only avoids tissue maceration but also removes exotoxins or cell debris that may retard growth or extend the inflammatory phase of the healing process. The balance between humidity and absorption is critical and excessive wicking must be avoided to prevent drying and necrosis.

Gaseous Exchange

Gaseous permeability will allow water vapor transmission which may be particularly important in a high exudate wound such as a burn, sacral, or leg ulcer. Of equal significance will be the effect of gaseous exchange on oxygen (pO_2) and hydrogen ion (pH) levels. Epithelization of the wound is greatly accelerated by the availability of atmospheric oxygen, which dissolves in the serous exudate to supplement that oxygen transported to the wound area by hemoglobin and subsequently directly utilized by the migrating epidermal cells.

Thermal Insulation

Thermal insulation will assist in maintaining the wound temperature at a level as close to body core temperature as possible. Phagocytic and mitotic activity are particularly susceptible to temperatures below 28°C. Thermal insulation and "warm" dressing change conditions are very important if the optimum healing rate is to be maintained. Long exposure of wet wounds may reduce the surface temperature to the point where mitotic activity ceases. Recovery of that tissue may take up to 3 hr. Temperatures of 30°C and above may be found beneath a good insulating dressing, and this will result in high mitotic activity with rapid epithelization and improved granulation.

Impermeability to Micro-organisms

Bacterial impermeability has a dual role. The wound will not heal if it is heavily infected. The inflammatory phase will be extended, and, unless topical or systemic antibacterial agents are used, a more general infection could result. However, a limited number of microorganisms are tolerated by most wounds, and the destructive or cleansing phase produced by phagocytic activity should result in a self-sterilized environment. The wound should be protected from secondary infection or, if still contaminated, be prevented from transmitting the infective organisms

A dressing should, therefore, be impermeable to airborne micro-organisms, which may fall on its surface and penetrate to and infect the wound. It should also act as a barrier to any organisms that may be transmitted from the wound to the dressing surface and become airborne to thus cause cross-infection. Organism transmission occurs most frequently in dressings that exhibit "strike through" of the exudate to the wound surface, providing a wet pathway to or from the wound surface. The passage of organisms can take as little as 6 hr from the time of "*strike through.*"

Freedom from Particulate and Toxic Wound Contaminants

Both particles and toxic compounds that may contaminate a wound will be responsible for disrupting the healing pattern. The incorporation of fibrous particles into a wound may result in a granuloma that could subsequently reduce the wound strength and induce keloid scarring. It is well documented that particulate contamination can also reduce the infection resistance levels by a factor of 1.0×10^{-6}.

Trauma During Dressing Change

The wound environment may be optimally maintained with a product that has the preferred performance parameters but, nevertheless, is disrupted during the dressing change. The hazards of temperature change and secondary infection may be accompanied by a secondary trauma caused by the dressing adhering to the wound and, on removal, stripping newly formed tissue.

This adhesion is normally caused by the adhesiveness of the drying exudate and the trauma can be exaggerated on removal by the destruction of capillary loops that have penetrated the dressing material.

Although not associated with the production of an acceptable microenvironment, there are certain physical characteristics required to assist in the overall dressing procedure. The dressing should have:

1. A size range to match the wounds
2. An absorption range for dry and heavy exudate wounds
3. Good conformability and good handle when both dry and wet
4. Sterility and be stable in storage
5. Be easily disposable

These parameters stimulated the development of functional products using the advances that had accrued in the technology of materials. This development was closely followed by products derived from the advances in the development of synthetic polymers. A statement of required performance could now be considered a possible specification for a polymeric product.

The range of polymeric products manufactured as surgical dressings has included:

1. Vapor permeable films
2. Polymeric foams
3. Particulate and fibrous polymers
4. Hydrogels and xerogels
5. Hydrocolloids

The above materials mark the progression towards the production of an "*ideal wound dressing.*" It should, however, be emphasized that no single dressing will produce the optimum microenvironment for all wounds or for all of the healing stages of one wound. The spectrum of performance requires that the wound is diagnosed and the treatment progressed by prescribing the most suitable dressing at each stage of the healing process. This entry will now examine the range of dressings currently available, identify their principal chemical and physical characteristics, and indicate their recommended clinical usage.

ABSORBENTS

The overall function of surgical absorbents is self-explanatory. They are available in a number of forms:

1. Fibrous (staple) absorbents
2. Fabric absorbents
3. Fiber plus fabric absorbents
4. Wound dressing pads

Fibrous Absorbents

These are made from cotton staple or from the fibers of viscose or cellulose; viscose and cotton may be admixed.

Absorbent cotton

Absorbent cotton is available in different qualities varying with the length and diameter of the cotton staple. It is available in the form of rolls and balls and is used for cleansing and swabbing wounds, preoperative skin preparation, and the application of topical medicaments to the skin.

Absorbent viscose

The absorption performance and physical character of absorbent viscose varies markedly with the manufacturing process. It is available in the bright or "dull" form, the latter containing a particulate material such as titanium dioxide within the fiber. The fibers are, in general, a continuous staple with a crenate trans-sectional profile but smooth and laminated forms are available which show different degrees of absorptive capacity and wet tensile strength.

Some fibrous absorbents contain a proportion of acrylamide or other synthetic polymeric fiber. They frequently enhance the absorptive performance and give "body" to the fleece thus improving fluid retention and avoiding "squeeze" out which is caused by fleece collapse after wetting.

Cellulose wadding

Cellulose wadding is produced from delignified wood pulp and manufactured in a multiple laminate material form. It is used in large pieces to absorb large volumes of fluid in incontinence but is not used in contact with a wound unless enclosed in an outer fabric sleeve to prevent fiber loss to the wound.

Fabric Absorbents

Absorbent lint

Absorbent lint is a close weave cotton cloth with a raised nap on one side that offers a large surface area for evaporation when placed with the nap upwards on an exuding wound. Its use generally unacceptable in modern wound management.

Absorbent gauze

Absorbent gauze is the most widely used absorbent and consists of a cotton cloth of plain weave bleached to a good white, clean and reasonably free from weaving defects, cotton leaf, and shell. It may be slightly off-white if sterilized. It absorbs water readily but its performance may be reduced by prolonged storage or exposure to heat.

Gauze products are primarily absorbents when used preoperatively, perioperatively, and post-operatively, but perioperatively, they are also required to perform other functions, including the protection of tissue and organs by occluding areas not involved in the procedure, to assist the application of wet heat, which may establish the viability of doubtful tissue and to assist in blunt dissection where fascias are separated along the lines of cleavage, thus avoiding unnecessary cutting. The gauze fabric may contain a proportion of viscose incorporated with the cotton either in the warp and the weft or exclusively in the weft. A maximum level of 45% viscose is widely accepted. A range of gauze fabrics exist graded according to the number of threads per 10 cm width of gauze.

Gauze products fall into two broad categories—the "swab" or "sponge" type produced by folding and stitching the cloth and those consisting of plain cloth. The "swab" type includes swabs, strips, pads, and pledgets. The "plain" types include packs and ribbon. Gauze swabs or sponges are commercially available as gauze folded into rectangles or squares to give various sizes or ply. They are folded in such a way that no cut edges are visible and the edges may be stitched. For use in an operating theatre, they are available with and without a radiopaque (X-ray detectable) mono- or multifilament thread containing barium sulfate woven into or heat bonded to the fabric. The commercial product can vary in size from 5 cm × 5 cm to 10 cm × 15 cm with a variation in ply from 4 to 32. Some are colored with a suitable fast, non-toxic dye.

Absorbent muslin

Absorbent muslin is a bleached cotton cloth of open weave used infrequently for the treatment of extensive burns and as a wet dressing.

Non-Woven Fabrics

Non-woven fabrics include a wide range of products manufactured from synthetic and semisynthetic fibers.

Non-woven swabs

Non-woven swabs consist of a non-woven viscose fabric and are available in folded pieces of various dimensions. They have a lower total absorbent capacity than gauze but absorb more quickly because of the random orientation of the viscose fibers. As fabrics, they constitute the outer layer on a number of wound dressing pads sometimes suitably coated with a polymer to reduce adherence at dressing change.

The types as defined in the above table are derived from the European Pharmacopoeia and the designation of type numbers is one-tenth of the sum of the threads in warp and weft.

Cellulose sponge

Cellulose sponge is a cavity foam cellulose-based sponge available in sheets and thin bands, used to absorb at small sites in surgery. The material is not radiopaque and has a tendency to lose particles; additional precautions must therefore be taken if such surgical use is contemplated.

Neuropatties

Neuropatties are small squares or strips of non-woven absorbent viscose with thread stitched through the non-woven fabric and left long. These are used as spot absorbents particularly in neurosurgery. Products vary in size and shape and there may also be a device for attaching the ends of all the threads thus producing a mini count rack.

Fibrous and Fabric Absorbents

Gauze and cellulose wadding

Gauze and cellulose wadding consists of a thick layer of cellulose wadding enclosed in a tubular form gauze. The properties of the two separate materials have already been described. Combined, the gauze and cellulose wadding tissue is used as an absorbent and protective pad. It should only be used as a wound dressing with a non-adherent layer placed between the pad and the wound. On a highly exuding surface, there is a tendency for the cellulose wadding element to collapse when wet and become a semisolid wet mass. This may cause difficulty in practice.

Gauze and cotton tissue (Gamgee tissue)

Gauze and cotton tissue (Gamgee tissue) is a thick layer of absorbent cotton enclosed in a tubular gauze. It has the same uses as gauze and cellulose wadding tissue but has the advantage of a higher absorbent capacity and less wet collapse. It is also softer in use and thus conforms more readily to the wound surface. It should be used in place of gauze and cellulose wadding tissue on high exudating surfaces such as burns but should not be used in direct contact with the wound surface.

Wound Dressing Pads

These products are widely available in a number of formulations including the fibrous and fabric absorbents previously described, plus other materials combined to meet some aspects of the acceptable performance profile.

The pads can be subdivided into:

1. Absorbents and filmated products
2. Sleeved pads with a single layer core
3. Sleeved pads with a multiple layer core
5. Low adherence pads

The absorbents and filmated products have been described. The simplest sleeved pads contain cotton, viscose, or cellulose fiber with an outer sleeve of gauze or non-woven material. Those with a multilayer core have an outer sleeve of cotton, viscose, or non-woven fabric that may have been treated with a polymer such as polypropylene to reduce adherence. Delayed "strike through" is facilitated by using a fluid retardant layer within the upper and outer sleeve that encourages lateral movement of fluid within the pad.

Low Adherence Pads

Low adherence pads have wound contact faces designed to be of low adherence. They vary from aluminum-coated fabrics to perforated polymeric films or heat bonded polyethylene films. The wound contact film may be attached to an absorbent fibrous mat and an outer woven or non-woven fabric. In some products, the polymeric film forms a continuous sleeve on both dressing surfaces. They are dressings for low exudate and drying wounds where high adherence can be expected. These low adherence, low absorptive capacity dressings are sometimes centered on an adhesive backing to produce an "island" dressing used as a postoperative adhesive dressing or, more familiarly, as a "first aid" island or strip dressing for superficial injuries.

Low Adherence Primary Dressings

These dressings consist of a partially open cell structured nylon or viscose fabric that may be finished with a silicone coating. The open cell structure allows fluid transmission to a superimposed absorbent dressing pad. This pad is changed when necessary and without disturbing the primary contact layer.

Deodorizing Dressings

These dressings have been formulated from the high gaseous sorptive material, activated charcoal presented as a woven fabric or a fibrous mat backed by a nylon sleeve, a vapor permeable film or a polyurethane foam. In each formulation, the objective is to reduce odor and the dressings must therefore be large enough to cover the entire malodorous area. One product encourages direct contact of the carbon layer with the wound exudate, and whilst this will limit gaseous absorption it is claimed that the incorporation of bound silver into the charcoal cloth inactivates bacteria adsorbed onto the fabric surface, thereby reducing the infective level and leading to a reduction of odor.

Polymeric Dressings

Vapor permeable adhesive films

Vapor permeable adhesive films are of use in those wounds in which granulation tissue is established and wound exudate is declining. These products were developed as materials that would, in part, mimic the performance of skin. The resultant products were transparent, synthetic adhesive films generically described as vapor permeable adhesive membranes, and comprised of transparent polyurethane or other synthetic films of low reflectance, evenly coated on one side with a synthetic adhesive mass. The adhesive is cohesive and inactivated by contact with moisture and will not therefore stick to moist skin or the wound bed. The films are permeable to water vapor, oxygen, and carbon dioxide but occlusive to water and bacteria and have highly elastomeric and extensible properties. They are conformable, resistant to shear and tear, sterile and particle free.

Removal of the stratum corneum results in a water vapor loss from tissues of between 3000 and 5000 g m^2 over a period of 24 hr. This loss will result in progressive dehydration; of great significance, particularly in a full thickness burn. The water vapor loss through a positioned vapor permeable membrane is reduced to 2500 gm^2 over 24hr—or less, depending upon the structure of the membrane. Excess fluid is lost by water vapor transmission through the membrane; dehydration is minimized and a moist wound interface is maintained. Where the volume of exudate produced is significantly greater than the volume removed as vapor, the water impermeability will result in serous effusion accumulating below the film. Impermeability to water prevents wetting from external sources.

The importance of a moist interface to wound healing is now well recognized. It allows the rapid migration of new epithelium across the wound surface, precludes trauma due to adherence at dressing change and contributes to gaseous diffusion in the damaged tissue. Oxygen and carbon dioxide transfer are accomplished by intramolecular diffusion through the membrane and by solution in the wound surface moisture. The oxygen permeability of the films is variously described as 4000–10,000 cm^3/m^2 over 24 hr at ambient atmospheric pressure. The pO_2 and pH levels of the wound surface are directly related to the gaseous permeability and contribute to cellular activity. The wound is protected against secondary infection by the bacterial impermeability of the film to such organisms as *Pseudomonas* sp., *S. aureus* and *E. coli*.

Film dressings are used in the treatment of a wide range of conditions, including pressure ulcers, burns, abrasions, and donor sites. In a dermabrasion, hemostasis must first be obtained and the margin of the wound dried before the film is applied. In its application for the treatment of burns, careful disinfection must precede the positioning of the film and it is only recommended for application to superficial and clinically clean burns. The use of films is contraindicated for deep burns as they retard the separation of necrotic tissue.

Decubitus ulcers and pressure sores can be covered with a vapor permeable film. The films' resistance to shear and low frictional surface properties protect the dermal layers from additional physical abrasion while producing the minimal barrier to normal skin function which allows them to be used as a prophylactic in areas that are traumatized by pressure but not ulcerated.

Film dressings can also be used for the retention of cannulae and tubes in both ward and theatre. Specific products have now been produced with a variable water vapor permeability to reduce the build up of moisture beneath the film and the resultant infective hazard.

Recently, film dressings impregnated with an antibacterial (silver) for the management of infected wounds or a deodorizer (charcoal) for malodorous wounds have been introduced.

Polymeric foams

Polymeric foam dressings are a diverse group of products with a wide range of properties. At their simplest, they are foamed polymers that have been made into sheets. The wound contact layer is often heat treated and pressure modified to produce a hydrophilic porous membrane about 0.5 mm thick to give a smooth, non- adherent wound contact surface that absorbs fluids by capillarity. The outer surface of the dressing is comprised of a layer of relatively large cells of approximately 5mm thick that remain hydrophobic. Their absorbency and water vapor permeability are varied either by a physical modification to the foam or by combining the foam with an additional sheet component.

Foaming the polymer creates small, open cells that are able to hold fluids and the cell size may be controlled during the foaming process. The most common polymer used is polyurethane. Their structure and softness also provide a cushion that protects and contributes to thermal insulation of the wound. They also may be tailored for particular applications such as tracheostomy dressing without particle loss to the wound and with the retention of their conformable characteristics. The non-adhesive foams will require a secondary dressing. The dressings are also available as in situ formed foams, adhesive island dressings, and cavity filler and are suitable for wounds with moderate to heavy exudation.

Absorption of serous exudate is limited to the wound/ dressing interface. In use, the absorptive capacity of the hydrophobic portion will be exceeded in a high exudate wound and, although moisture vapor transmission occurs through the dressing, frequent changes may be required until the exudate level diminishes. The dressing combines the function of absorbency with that of producing an acceptable microenvironment to allow healing to take place at the fastest rate concomitant with the total clinical condition of the patient. Polyurethane foam dressings of this type are recommended for the management of dry sutured wounds, minor lacerations, early pressure ulcers, and venous ulcers.

Foams have been formulated with differing absorbencies designed specifically for the management of stasis ulcers and burns. The foam designed for the management of burns has dressing as the prime function of absorbency. It consists of a highly absorbent hydrophilic polyurethane foam backed with a moisture permeable polyurethane membrane and bonded to an apertured polyurethane net on the wound contact face. The backing whilst permeable to water vapor is impermeable to water thus avoiding strike through. As the exudate level decreases, the membrane retains moisture and prevents the drying of the wound. The apertured polyurethane net interface reduces adherence to the wound surface.

Low absorptive capacity primary foam dressings have been produced from a carboxylated styrene butadiene rubber latex foam. The foam is bonded to a nonwoven fabric coated with a polyethylene film which has been vacuum ruptured. The basic foam is naturally hydrophobic and a surface active agent is incorporated to facilitate the uptake of wound exudate. The dressing is recommended for minor wounds and abrasions where exudate levels are low and adhesion is a prominent hazard at dressing change.

In situ foam

This foam has been indicated for the management of pilonidal sinus, hydradenitis suppurativa, perianal, and perineal wounds and in the management of dehisced abdominal wounds. It is necessary to occlude the cavity by packing to absorb excess exudate and to stimulate the production of granulation tissue, neovascularization, and collagen deposition. An in situ formed foam was originally designed by Dow Corning and found to be clinically superior to ribbon gauze for cavity wound packing. Its status in cytotoxic terms was in dispute but it is now available and its exclusion would be to the detriment of this entry.

The cavity foam dressing is a two-part foam composed of a filled polydimethylsiloxane base and a stannous octoate catalyst. The two components are mixed together immediately prior to use. The reaction is slightly exothermic, and over a period of 2–3 min the dressing expands to approximately four times its original volume and sets to a soft, spongy foam accurately conforming to the contours of the wound cavity. The stent is normally removed twice daily, soaked in a mild antiseptic (0.5% aqueous chlorhexidine) rinsed in cold running water, squeezed dry, and replaced. A new dressing is formed after a week or more to match the reduction in size of the cavity. The product does not adhere to granulation tissue whilst maintaining free drainage around the wound, and it has a low, but significant, absorptive capacity at the dressing surface.

Hydropolymer

This material appears visually as a foam but is described as a foamed gel designed to expand into the contours of the wound as it absorbs fluid. It is used in an island configuration with a unique adhesive portion. It has the ability to readhere once lifted enabling manipulation of the product for fit or assessment of the wound without dressing change. The hydropolymer wicks fluid into the upper layers of the dressing where it escapes through the backing.

Hydrogels

Hydrogels, or water polymer gels, are modified, cross-linked polymeric formulations which form three-dimensional networks of hydrophilic polymers prepared from materials such as gelatin, polysaccharides, cross-linked polyacrylamide polymers, poly- electrolyte complexes, and polymers or copolymers derived from methacrylate esters. These interact with aqueous solutions by swelling to an equilibrium value and retain a significant proportion of water within their structure. They are insoluble in water and are available in dry or hydrated sheets or as a hydrated gel in delivery systems designed for single use.

The physical properties of bulk polymers are directly influenced by a number of factors including the nature of monomers, copolymers, the cross-linkers and degree of cross-linking, and the polymerization initiators and processing parameters. The availability of hydrophilic and hydrophobic sites is influenced by the chain of configuration and conformation and could determine the degree of hydrophilicity and oxygen permeability. By varying the nature of the polymer backbone, a range of water binding behavior and thus mechanical, surface, and permeability properties can be obtained. The expanded nature of the hydrogel structure and its permeability allows the extraction and polymerization of initiator molecules, initiator decomposition products, and other extraneous materials from the gel network before the hydrogel is placed in contact with the living system. The tissue-like structure of most hydrogels will contribute to their biocompatibility by minimizing mechanical irritation to surrounding cells and tissues. They possess low interfacial free energies with aqueous solutions and only a weak tendency to absorb biological species such as proteins or cells. Their high moisture content (up to 96% w/w when hydrated) maintains a desirable moist interface which facilitates cell migration and prevents dressing adherence. Water can be transmitted through the saturated gel whilst the unsaturated gel will have water vapor permeability comparable with the water vapor permeability of vapor permeable membranes.

The absorption, transmission, and permeability performance result in the maintenance of a moist wound with a continuous moisture flux across the dressing and a sorption gradient that assists in the removal of toxic components from the wound area. The high moisture content allows dissolved oxygen permeability (which varies between products) to ensure the continuation of aerobic function at the wound/dressing interface and have an effect upon both epithelization and bacterial growth. It has been observed that the positioning of a hydrogel frequently results in a marked reduction in pain response in patients. It is suggested that the high humidity protects the exposed neurones from dehydration and also produces acceptable changes in pH. A secondary effect, which may contribute to this response, is the property of the gels to immediately cool the wound surface and maintain a lower temperature for up to 6 hr.

Sheet hydrogels

These dressings are sheets of three-dimensional networks of cross-linked hydrophilic polymers (polyethylene oxide, polyacrylamides, polyvinylpyrrolidone, carboxymethylcellulose, modified corn starch). Their formulation may incorporate up to 96% bound water, but they are insoluble in water and they interact by three-dimensional swelling with aqueous solutions. The polymer physically entraps water to form a solid sheet and they have a thermal capacity that provides initial cooling to the wound surface. A secondary dressing is required.

The recommendation for use of these products includes the management of donor sites and superficial operation sites and also the treatment of freshly damaged epithelium such as that seen with thermal and other painful wounds and dermatitic skin where the avoidance of topical agents is indicated. In chronic ulcers, they are used to encourage granulation and formation of cellular tissue.

Amorphous hydrogels

Many of these hydrogels have additional ingredients such as alginate, collagen, or complex carbohydrates besides water and a polymer. They are similar in composition to sheet hydrogels but the polymer has not been cross-linked. These amorphous preparations do not have the cooling properties of the sheet dressings and a secondary dressing is required. Their recommended use includes hydration of dry, sloughy, or necrotic wounds and autolytic debridement.

A primary hydrogel dressing has been produced from a colloidal suspension of radiation cross-linked polyethylene oxide and water with an equilibrium water content of 96%. The gel is sandwiched between polyethylene films. The wound contact film is routinely removed and the outer film is used to control evaporation from the surface of the gel. A novel hydrogel was developed by the Max Plank Institute for Immunobiology and Dermatology consisting of an insoluble cross-linked polyacrylamdie agarose polymer containing 95% water as the dispersion phase. This gel is available in hydrated and dehydrated forms and as granules that, with their increased surface area, absorb larger amounts of exudate. The granules can be used to fill a cavity wound with the gel sheet superimposed to produce a continuous hydrogel dressing.

An alternative to the acrylamide-based composite hydrogel dressing is an acrylamide grafted to a polyurethane film to give a transparent, flexible gel with an equilibrium water content of approximately 50%. The hydrated gel has a low modulus of elasticity and a high water permeability that facilitates the adherence of the gel to the wound surface. The permeability characteristics allow penetration of antimicrobial agents that can be applied topically to the dressing surface in situ.

Particulate and Fibrous Polymers

This group of dressings includes synthetic, semisynthetic, and naturally occurring products embracing a range of polysaccharide materials.

Xerogels

The xerogel dressings may be regarded as a subgroup of products within the larger group of polysaccharide dressings. The latter contains the well known cellulosic dressing products such as gauze and absorbent cotton but the products which consist of dextranomer beads, dehydrated hydrogels of the agar/acrylamide group, calcium alginate fibers, and dehydrated granulated Graft T starch polymers are identified specifically as xerogels, the material remaining after the removal of most or all of the water from a hydrogel (or the disperse phase from any type of simple gel). These materials have no water in their formulation but swell to form a gel when in contact with aqueous solutions.

Particulate Polymers

Dextranomer

This xerogel is a polymer of the polysaccharide dextran, a naturally derived polymer of glucose produced by cultures of a micro-organism, *Leuconostoc mesenteroides*. The gel is formed when the dextran molecules comprising the disperse phase of the hydrocolloid are cross-linked by a chemical process utilizing epichlorohydrin and sodium hydroxide. Dextranomer is available as beads or paste. The material requires a secondary dressing.

The dextranomer is supplied in beads of 100–300 *m*m diameter containing poloxamer 187, polyethylene glycol 300, and some water. A paste formulation is also available which is the dextranomer in polyethylene glycol 600 (PEG 600). The beads are offered as a discrete particle or enclosed in a low adherence pouch for insertion into a cavity wound. One company (Pfizer) offers a polymeric net which can be placed into a cavity wound before the addition of either granules or paste and facilitates removal and also a vapor permeable film which is superimposed on the dextranomer dressing to control evaporation and retard drying in a low exudating wound.

Dextranomer has a pore size that produces an exclusion limit of 1000–8000 Da, which precludes the sorption of viruses and bacteria. Micro-organisms are removed from the wound by the capillary action between the beads, a function that is absent from the paste formulation, which however demonstrates a marked increase in absorbing capacity for malodorous elements and pain producing compounds released during the inflammatory response.

It is used primarily as a debriding agent on sloughy and exuding wounds, whether clean or infected, and on small area burns where the objective is to produce a clean tissue bed for the production of a granulating tissue. It is not a product that should be used beyond this phase, as its continued application will impair epithelization. Dextranomer is not biodegradable and both granules and paste must be carefully removed with Normal saline before drying to avoid particulate residues and the subsequent development of granulomas.

Fibrous Polymers

Alginate dressings

Alginic acid is a polyuronic acid composed of residues of D-mannuronic acid and L-guluronic acid and is obtained chiefly from algae belonging to the Phaeophyceae, mainly species of *Laminaria*.

Calcium alginate dressings are flat, non-woven pads of either calcium sodium alginate fiber or pure calcium alginate fiber. The alginate wound contact layer may be bonded to a secondary absorbent viscose pad. Alginate hanks and ribbon are also available as packing for deeper cavity wounds and sinuses. Alginates have been shown to be effective in the management of injuries where there has been substantial tissue loss. The non-adhesive formulations require a secondary dressing.

Gel formation is via ion exchange of sodium in serum for calcium within the alginate dressing. A biodegradable gel is formed when the fiber is in contact with exudate, and the released calcium contributes to the clotting mechanism. The gel may be firm or soft depending upon the proportions of calcium and sodium in the fiber. It is removed with saline.

The isomeric acids are present in varying proportions depending upon the seaweed source. The guluronic acid forms an association with calcium providing the stimulus to produce the continuous disperse phase of a hydrogel. Calcium ions and a phospholipid surface promote the activation of prothrombin in the clotting cascade. Calcium alginate products are used as the source of these ions to arrest bleeding, both in superficial injuries and as an absorbable hemostat in surgery. The rate of biodegradation is related to the sodium/calcium balance in the preparation.

The dressings may be removed with a sterile 3% sodium citrate solution followed by washing with sterile water or they may be removed with sterile Normal saline. The "wet" integrity of the dressing which facilitates removal from the wound may be improved by incorporating fibers of greater strength such as viscose (rayon) staple fiber or fibers which interact with the alginate fibers when wet such as chitosan staple fibers. The primary hemostatic usage of calcium alginate is in the packing of sinuses, fistulae, and bleeding tooth sockets. The alginate dressings have recently become widely used as soluble wound packing for a number of additional wound types. They have been used as useful non-adherents for lacerations and abrasions and are effective in the management of hypergranulation tissue (proud flesh), interdigital maceration, and heloma molle. Their hospital and community use includes intractable skin ulcers and pressure ulcers, where they would appear to accelerate healing; and in the successful management of diabetic ulcers, venous ulcers, burns, and infected surgical wounds.

Alginates have proved to be useful debriding agents. When applied to these injury types, the alginate must be covered by a secondary dressing of foam or film. Some proprietary products bond calcium alginate to a secondary backing such as absorbent viscose pad or semipermeable adhesive foam to produce an island dressing.

Hydrocolloids

Hydrocolloid dressings consist of composite products based on naturally occurring hydrophilic polymers. Generally, these dressings are flexible, highly absorbent, occlusive or semiocclusive adhesive pads formulated from biocompatible, hydrophilic polymers such as sodium carboxymethylcellulose, hydroxyethylcellulose pectins, and gelatin incorporated into a hydrophobic adhesive. The dressings may be backed by a polymeric film and may be contoured to fit difficult areas. Hydrocolloids are also available as pastes or powders or gels. The pads do not require a secondary dressing.

In general, they consist of a pressure sensitive adhesive layer which is composed of a so-called "*hydrocolloid*" dispersed with the aid of a tackifier in an elastomer and secondly a film coating composed of a gas permeable but water impermeable, flexible, elastomeric material. A currently available hydrocolloid dressing is a flexible mass with an adherent inner face and an outer semipermeable polyurethane foam.

The formulation is:

Sodium carboxymethylcellulose	20%
Polyisobutylene	40%
Gelatin	30%
Pectin	20%

The product is also available as granules of similar formulation, which allows larger cavity wounds and heavily exuding wounds to be treated with a continuous hydrocolloid system. Other hydrocolloid dressings with formulations consisting of sodium carboxymethylcellulose combined with karaya gum or sodium carboxymethylcellulose on its own are also available.

The adhesive formulation of hydrocolloids gives an initial adhesion higher than some surgical adhesive tapes. After application, the absorption of trans- epidermal water vapor modifies the adhesive flow to maintain a high tack performance throughout the period of use. In situ the dressings provide a gaseous and moisture proof environmental chamber strongly attached to the area surrounding the wound and offering protection against contamination from incontinence or other sources. In the wound contact area, the exudate is absorbed to form a gel that swells in a linear fashion with higher moisture retention at the contact surface. This results in an expansion of the gel into the wound cavity with the continued support and increasing pressure from the remainder of the elastomeric dressing. The advantage of this is that a firm pressure is applied to the floor of a deep ulcer, a basic surgical maxim for the production of healthy granulating tissue. It is this function that contributes to the recommended usage for venous leg ulcers.

The formed *"colloidal"* gel also produces a sorption gradient for soluble components within the serous exudate thereby allowing the removal of toxic compounds arising from bacterial or cellular destruction. However, during use, the dressing in contact with the wound liquefies to produce a pus-like liquid with a somewhat strong odor.

Hydrocolloids are suitable for desloughing and for light to medium exuding wounds—but are contraindicated if an anaerobic infection is present. They have been used successfully in the treatment of chronic leg ulcers, pressure ulcers, minor burns, granulating wounds, and wounds exhibiting slough or necrotic tissue or wounds with moderate exudate, as well as skin barriers in the management of stoma.

Superabsorbents

Superabsorbent hydrocolloid dressings have a highly absorbent capacity and entrap exudate so that it cannot be squeezed out once absorbed. One product incorporates the highly absorbent material into an island pad covered by a non-woven absorbent and surrounded by an extra thin hydrocolloid as the adhesive portion. The covering acts as a transfer layer while its surface stays dry. This is used for heavily exuding ulcers.

Hydrofibers

Hydrofibers are fibers of carboxymethylcellulose formed into flat, non-woven pads. It is produced as a textile fiber and presented in the form of a fleece held together by a needle bonding process, and is available both as a "ribbon" for packing cavities, and as a flat non-woven pad for application to larger open wounds. The dressing absorbs and interacts with wound exudate to form a soft, hydrophilic, gas-permeable gel that traps bacteria and conforms to the contours of the wound whilst providing a microenvironment that is believed to facilitate healing. The resultant gel is similar to a sheet hydrogel but it does not dry out or wick laterally. Therefore, there is no maceration of the skin surrounding the wound. The high absorbent capacity reduces the frequency of dressing changes.

Sheet formulations may be applied to exuding lesions including leg ulcers, pressure areas, donor sites, and most other granulating wounds, but for deeper cavity wounds and sinuses the ribbon packing is generally preferred. The dressing is easy to remove without causing pain or trauma, and leaves minimal residue on the surface of the wound.

Impregnated Dressings

Originally, these materials were formulated to coat the area of the wound with hydrophobic paraffin spread on an open mesh gauze thereby providing both insulation and partial occlusion but allowing excess exudate to be absorbed by a superimposed absorbent pad. The products had the advantage of low adherence and allowed gaseous diffusion, but the disadvantages included the incorporation of the soft paraffin or loose cotton fibers into the healing wound thereby leading to an extended inflammatory phase with consequent delayed wound healing. These products also, when used excessively, retained wound exudate causing maceration to the surrounding, otherwise healthy, tissue.

Paraffin Gauze (Tulle) Dressing

Paraffin gauze is bleached cotton or combined cotton and rayon cloth impregnated with yellow or white soft paraffin. It is available as sterile single pieces or multi-packs. The paraffin is present to prevent the dressing adhering to a wound. The gauze that may be leno in nature is coated so that all the threads of the fabric are impregnated but the spaces between the threads are free of paraffin. The material is used primarily in the treatment of wounds such as burns and scalds where the protective function of the stratum corneum is lost and water vapor can escape. Paraffin gauze dressing functions by reducing the fluid loss whilst the water barrier layer is reforming. In addition to burns and scalds, the dressing is used as a wound contact layer in lacerations, abrasions, and in ulcers where it is used as a packing material to promote granulation. Postoperatively, it is used as a vaginal or penial dressing and for sinus packing. Povidone iodine 10%, chlorhexidine 0.5% w/w, sodium fusidate 2%w/w, and 1% framycetin sulfate are examples of available gauze impregnations and are recommended for the reduction of wound infection. However, diffusion of the antibacterial agent into or onto an infected and exuding wound has been shown to be minimal and the possibility of development of resistant strains of infective organisms has reduced the usage of these products.

Silver Dressings

Advanced wound management products containing silver have been developed to treat difficult-to-heal wounds, chronic ulcers, and extensive burns. Nano- crystalline silver represents a new format of the metal for use in wound management. Silver is a broad-spectrum antibiotic active against such organisms as *Pseudomonas* sp., *S. aureus*, *E. coli*, and *Candida albicans* and to which there has been little reported evidence of resistance. Although silver is an efficient antimicrobial, its use has been limited because of the difficulty of delivering it to the tissues. Nanotechnology has overcome this as it allows for the building of chemical compounds one atom at a time. A nanocrystalline structure gives a greater surface area for, in this instance, silver release.

Free silver ions are the active components of antimicrobial silvers, and it has been shown that as little as one part per million of elemental silver in solution is an effective antimicrobial. Materials such as polymers, charcoal, and hydrocolloids when formulated with silver not only aid wound management and healing but also regulate its release into the wound environment and surrounding tissues. Silver ions kill micro-organisms by inhibiting cellular respiration and cellular function. It is known that their mode of action is exerted by binding cysteine residues on the cell walls of yeasts such as *C. albicans* thereby inhibiting the enzyme phosphomannose isomerase (PMI). This enzyme is essential for the synthesis of the cell wall and without it phosphate, glutamine, and other nutrients are released from the cells. Phosphomannose isomerase was not inhibited by silver in *E. coli* cultures. In a wound environment, silver combines with proteins, cell surface receptors, and wound debris.

It has been suggested that some nanocrystalline silver products release a cluster of silver ions and radicals, which are highly antibacterial because of unpaired electrons in outer orbitals. Silver and silver radicals released from these products are reported to act by impairing electron transport, inactivating bacterial DNA, cell membrane damage, and binding and precipitation of insoluble complexes.

Advanced wound management products containing silver have been developed to treat difficult-to-heal wounds, chronic ulcers, and extensive burns. Odor absorbing dressings adsorb polarized bacteria onto the surface of the charcoal cloth used in the formulation. The silver present in the dressing exerts a bactericidal effect that gradually diminishes as wound exudate saturates the material.

Silicones

Silicones are long chain polymers comprised of alternate atoms of silicone and oxygen with organic groups attached to the silicon atoms. The degree of polymerization determines the physical form of the silicone. Soft silicones are a particular family of solid silicones that are soft and tacky. These properties enable them to adhere to dry surfaces. A soft silicone dressing is coated with soft silicone as an adhesive or wound contact layer and may be removed without trauma to the wound or surrounding skin. Silicone dressings have been used clinically as an alternative to paraffin gauze for the fixation of pediatric skin grafts where it was found that changing the outer absorbent dressing was painless as was the removal of the silicone dressing itself so that no analgesia or anesthesia was required.

Generally, silicone dressings have a porous, semitransparent wound contact layer consisting of a flexible, polyamide net that is coated with silicone. The dressing is non-absorbent but the pores within its matrix allow the passage of exudate from the wound to the secondary dressing. Its use is limited to minor skin grafts because the dressing requires a margin of healthy skin for application of at least 2 cm surrounding the wound.

Silicone dressings have also been used to manage wounds generated by radiotherapy, fingertip injuries, severe mycosis fungoides, and epidermolysis bullosa. The silicone material needs to be kept in intimate contact with the surface of the wound to function effectively which means that wounds in convex areas present few problems whereas those on concave, jointed, or contoured areas need adequate padding to be applied to exclude voids beneath the dressing where exudate could accumulate. As silicone is an inert material, it has been shown that, where clinically indicated, topical steroids or antimicrobial agents can be applied either over or under the silicone material without diminishing their efficacy.

There have been reports indicating that use of silicone dressings leads to improvements in the appearance (scar size, erythema, elasticity) and symptoms (pruritis, burning pain) after application to hypertrophic scars and keloids. Silicone dressings are thought to effect this by promoting hydration of the scar and applying pressure, thereby flattening scar tissue, increasing wound elasticity, and reducing discoloration.

Tissue Adhesives

Tissue adhesives are formulated from cyanoacrylate compounds such as bucrylate, enbucrilate, or mecrylate which polymerize in an exothermic reaction on contact with a fluid or basic substance to form a strong, flexible, and waterproof bond. They are synthesized by reacting formaldehyde with alkyl cyanoacetate to obtain a prepolymer, which may be depolarized to a liquid monomer by heat. This monomer may then be modified by altering the alkoxycarbonyl (-COOR) group of the molecule to give compounds of different chain lengths.

Tissue adhesives are generally applied to simple lacerations where they give similar cosmetic results to suturing. It is essential that the wound edges are accurately apposed to ensure that no adhesive passes between them. There have been no reports of carcinogenicity or toxicity when they are used topically. They should not be used over joints as repetitive movement will cause the adhesive to peel off.

BIODRESSINGS

Biodressings are composed of materials almost exclusively originating from living tissue and are said to "participate actively and beneficially in the biochemistry and cellular activity of wound "healing." They can be identified as biological dressings and biosynthetic dressings and the biological dressings can be further subdivided into natural or cultured—depending upon their origin.

Collagen Dressings (Biosynthetic Dressings)

These dressings are formed from denatured collagen peptides derived from pigskin and purified bovine hide collagen cross-linked with the glycosaminoglycan, chondroitin-6-sulfate, and freeze dried. When applied to damaged tissue, the dressings stimulate the production of fibroblasts and endothelial cells whilst accelerating the migration of epithelial cells. These biological components are combined with silicone elastomers to control moisture vapor loss during the accelerated growth period.

The bovine material used for the extraction of the Type 1 collagen used in these dressings is non-antigenic due to enzymatic purification. The bovine Type 1 collagen is in a triple helical form and may be combined with oxidized, regenerated cellulose. The collagen helix may be attached to a non-adherent backing and, therefore, these materials require a secondary dressing. Addition of collagen to a wound bed may accelerate wound repair by the provision of a matrix for cellular migration.

They are available as sheets, particles, pastes, or gels and the dry materials absorb exudate to form a gel. One manufacturer has incorporated 10% alginate in the dressing formulation. These dressings are recommended for use on any recalcitrant wound free from necrotic tissue and showing no signs of infection.

"Natural" Biological Dressings

Autologous (self) skin is harvested from a healthy area of the patient's body and transferred to the wound, generally a burn. The procedure leaves a second injury or donor site. The advantages of non-allergenicity, non-toxicity, non-pyrogenicity, and direct incorporation into the healed area with the overall performance parameters of intact skin make this the dressing of choice.

Skin harvested from fresh cadavers and used as an allograft is a possible alternative to autologous skin. This skin undergoes processing to remove fibroblasts, endothelial cells, and epidermis, which would stimulate an immune response. The resulting product is an acellular, dermal collagen matrix which is immunologically inert but retains elastin, proteoglycans, and the basement membrane complex.

Porcine Skin

Sterile, denatured lyophilized skin of porcine origin is produced and consists of the dermal and/or epidermal layers. The material is reconstituted by immersion in sterile water or saline before being applied dermal side to the wound. It is used as a temporary dressing in burns and ulcers, particularly where a site is being prepared for grafting.

"Cultured" Biological Dressings

Cultured biological dressings are derived from mammalian cell culture procedures which facilitate the development of sheets of cells derived from a few of the patients' own epidermal cells. Cultured human keratinocytes form cultured epithelial grafts that are not bioengineered tissues but are cultured cell products with limited use. These cultures may be regarded as a precursor which has led to the development of other products through bioengineering.

Bilayered Skin Equivalent

A bilayered composite skin equivalent has been developed with a viable dermis and epidermis. The epidermis is composed from cornified differentiated keratinocytes and a dermal matrix composed of a collagen lattice containing viable fibroblasts. Its cellular components assist with wound closure through stimulation of the wound bed. The outer layer of the differentiated bilayered skin equivalent, the stratum corneum, acts as a specialized vapor permeable membrane and protective outer barrier.

Human Dermal Replacement

This material requires cultivation of human diploid fibroblasts on a three-dimensional polymer scaffold. The cells are derived from newborn foreskin and are living cells which are metabolically active following implantation into the wound bed.

Hyaluronic Acid

Vapor permeable adhesive films derived from materials found in some tissues are being used more commonly in wound management. Most of the available films are composed of industrially manufactured and purified benzyl ester derivatives of hyaluronic acid and may be used for direct application to wounds such as diabetic foot ulcers or venous leg ulcers or as scaffolds for the cultivation of fibroblasts and keratinocytes for further transplantation.

Bioactive Dressings

The introduction described the performance parameters of *interactive* dressings that distinguished them from the *passive* products. Current developments have confirmed that the next generation of products will participate "actively" in the wound healing process by contributing growth hormones, chemotactic agents, angiogenic agents, and other growth factors either in a depot release mode or as sequentially released compound as well as controlling the microenvironment surrounding the wound.

Each wound management product will eventually be designed to meet the environmental, nutritional, and growth requirements of particular wound types and will probably be based on those "*biodressings*" described above. The group will be designated bioactive wound management products. Bioactive dressings already include such materials as antimicrobial dressings, single component products of biological origin, and combinations of both these. These "*biodressings*" must be the precursors for the development of many more exciting products that will improve the morbidity of wound healing to the advantage of both patient and clinician. The content of this entry has been restricted to products in direct contact with the wound. There are many other products outside this limitation used successfully for wound management. These include surgical adhesive tapes and non-extensible, conforming, and elastic net bandages, used to retain dressings in position, and the extensible bandages which may vary from the light support and compression products for the management of sprains and strains and the prevention of edema, to the high compression bandages used either alone or superimposed on various dressings to apply pressure to a limb.

13

Intrathecal Chemotherapy

The central nervous system (CNS) is an increasingly recognized site of tumor recurrence. Tumor spread to the CNS, manifest as either neoplastic meningitis or intraparenchymal metastases, is in part due to the pharmacologic sanctuary created by the blood–brain (BBB) and blood–cerebrospinal fluid (CSF) barriers. As a result, tumor cells within the CNS are protected from the cytotoxic effects of systemically administered chemotherapy. Leukemias and lymphomas remain the most common cancers with a predilection for leptomeningeal spread. However, there are many solid tumors that may also disseminate within the CNS including breast and small-cell lung cancer; primary CNS tumors such as medulloblastoma and glioma; and childhood tumors such as neuroblastoma, retinoblastoma, and rhabdomyosarcoma.

Strategies to treat metastatic CNS disease include intrathecal (IT) chemotherapy, radiation therapy, and high-dose systemic chemotherapy. These therapeutic strategies have been used successfully for the prevention and treatment of CNS leukemia. In fact, IT chemotherapy is currently incorporated into all front-line leukemia treatment protocols, and is the primary therapeutic modality for the prevention of leptomeningeal dissemination. Unfortunately, for most patients with neoplastic meningitis from underlying solid tumors or for patients with recurrent/refractory CNS leukemias, there is no effective therapy. Ongoing challenges to the successful treatment of these high-risk patients include the limited spectrum of antineoplastic agents that are currently available for IT administration as well as the lack of effective IT combination chemotherapy regimens.

The primary focus of this chapter is to describe the role of IT therapy in the treatment and/ or prevention of neoplastic meningitis, including a brief review of the limitations of systemically administered chemotherapy in the treatment of neoplastic meningitis, an overview of important pharmacologic principles that are relevant to intrathecal administration of anticancer agents, and a review of the pharmacokinetics and toxicities of the most commonly administered intrathecal agents. In addition, we provide an overview of new agents for IT administration that are in early stages of preclinical or clinical evaluation.

IT Chemotherapy

Rationale

The BBB and the blood–CSF barrier are natural membrane barriers that, among other physiologic functions, regulate drug delivery and egress from the central nervous system. The BBB, located at the level of the CNS endothelial cell, and the blood–CSF barrier, located in the epithelium of the tiny organs surrounding the ventricles (e.g., choroid plexus, median eminence, area postrema), effectively limit the CNS penetration of toxic substances, including most hydrophilic anticancer agents, from the bloodstream. Drug egress from the CSF generally occurs via passive diffusion. However, in contrast to non-CNS endothelial cells, there are metabolic enzymes and transporters (e.g., P-glycoprotein [Pgp], multidrug-resistance associated proteins [MRPs], and organic acid transporters [OATs]), in the blood–brain and blood–CSF barriers that play an important role in the clearance or egress of specific drugs from the CSF.

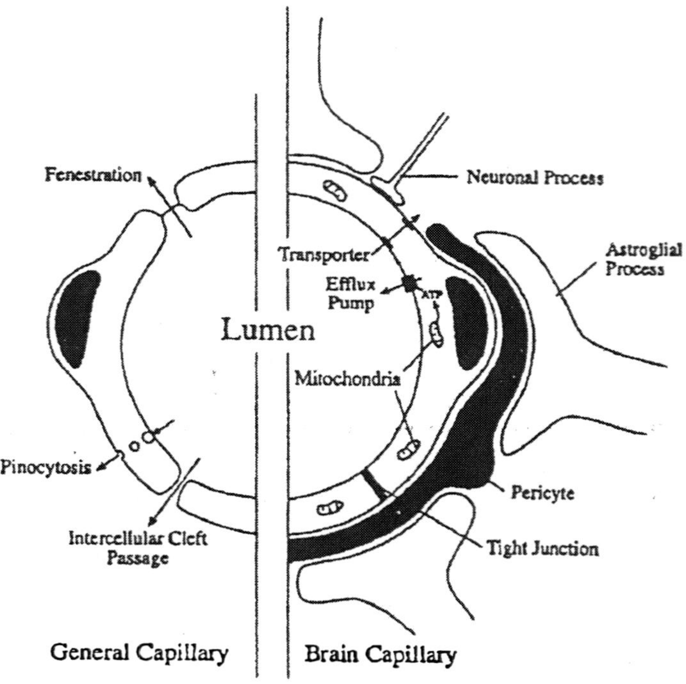

Fig. 13.1. Differences between brain capillary endothelial cells and endothelial cells in other organs.

CSF drug exposure is often used as a surrogate for drug exposure in the brain interstitial space. Since the cytotoxic activity of many anticancer agents is best correlated with exposure, an estimate of CSF drug exposure following systemic drug administration provides insight into whether or not an agent has potential utility in the treatment or prevention of CNS disease. CSF drug exposure is most accurately determined by comparing the ratio of steady-state concentrations in plasma and CSF or the ratio of the area under the plasma and CSF concentration–time curves (AUC_{CSF}/AUC_{plasma}). CSF exposure data are frequently derived from preclinical models, as it is neither practical nor feasible to routinely obtain serial CSF and plasma

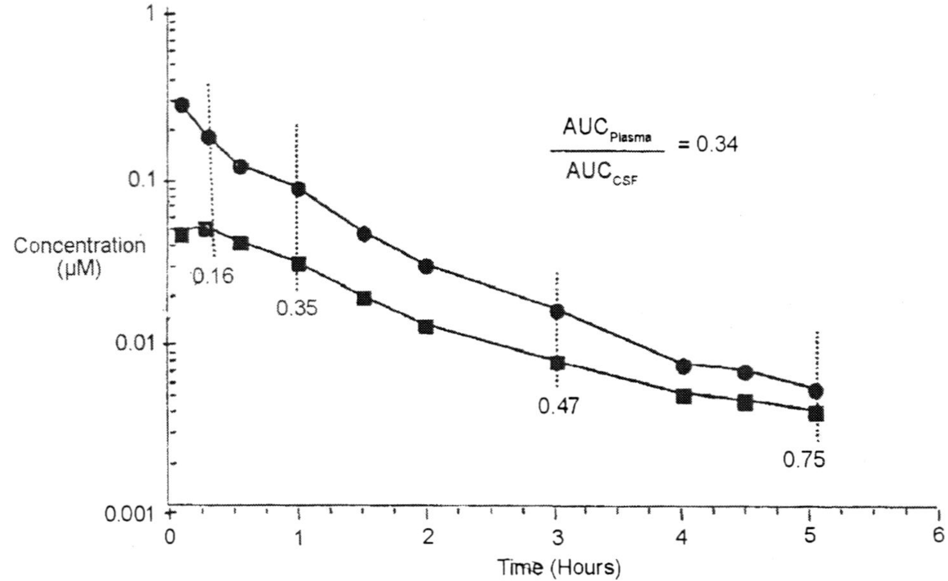

Fig. 13.2. Plasma and CSF concentration of topotecan in nonhuman primates after an intravenous dose.

drug levels after systemic administration in humans. The CSF exposure for the most commonly used anticancer agents is < 10% of the plasma exposure. As a result of this limited exposure, other approaches, such as high-dose chemotherapy and IT drug delivery, were developed to circumvent the blood-brain and blood–CSF barriers.

Table 13.1. Central nervous system penetration of commonly used anticancer drugs

Agent	*CSF/Plasma ratio (%)*
Alkylating agents	
Cyclophosphamide	
Total drug	50
Active metabolite	15
Ifosfamide	
Total drug	30
Active metabolite	15
Thiotepa	>95
Carmustine	>90
Cisplatin	
Free platinum	40
Total platinum	<5
Carboplatin	
Free platinum	30
Total platinum	<5
Antimetabolites	
Methotrexate	3
6-Mercaptopurine	25
Cytarabine	15
5-Fluorouracil	
Bolus	50
Infusion	15
Gemcitabine	7
Antitumor antibiotics	
Anthracyclines	ND
Dactinomycin	ND
Plant alkaloids	
Vinca alkaloids	5
Epipodophyllotoxins	<5
Topoisomerase I inhibitors	
Topotecan	32
Irinotecan	
CPT-11 lactone	14
SN-38 lactone	<8
Miscellaneous	
Prednisolone	<10
Dexamethasone	15
l-Asparaginase	ND

Systemic Chemotherapy

The primary advantages of systemic therapy compared with IT chemotherapy are that it is technically easier to administer and that it provides more uniform drug distribution throughout the neuraxis. In addition, there is the potential for prolonged CNS drug exposure after protracted infusions, which is of critical importance for cell-cycle specific cytotoxic agents. The primary disadvantage of systemic chemotherapy is that there is limited penetration of most hydrophilic agents into the CSF. Therefore, to attain cytotoxic levels of drug in the CSF after systemic dosing, very high doses of drug may be required.

Although a high-dose strategy has been employed effectively with methotrexate, an agent for which calcium leucovorin provides adequate rescue from systemic toxicities, this approach is generally not feasible because specific rescue agents or treatment strategies are not available for most antineoplastic agents. As a result, systemic toxicities, specifically the potential for severe or life-threatening myelosuppression, preclude the widespread use of high-dose chemotherapy without stem cell rescue.

Intrathecal Drug Delivery

IT chemotherapy is usually administered via lumbar puncture or via an indwelling ventricular access device (e.g., Ommaya reservoir). The primary advantage of intrathecally administered therapy is that it facilitates direct delivery of drug to the principal target tumor site, that is, the CSF and leptomeninges, using a relatively small drug dose. This is possible because the CSF volume of distribution is relatively small compared to the plasma volume of distribution (150 cm^3 vs 3500 cm^3). Therefore, high CSF drug exposure can be achieved using a relatively small drug dose, which minimizes the potential for systemic toxicity. In addition, because CSF drug clearance is often slower than systemic clearance, there is the potential for more prolonged drug exposure at the target site following bolus intrathecal drug administration.

Although there are pharmacokinetic advantages associated with IT drug delivery, there are also disadvantages. Intralumbar drug administration may be associated with pain or suboptimal delivery to the subarachnoid space, owing to leakage or inadvertent injection into the subdural or epidural space. In addition, there is heterogeneous drug distribution throughout the neuraxis after IT dosing due to the cephalo-caudad flow of CSF. As a result, after intralumbar dosing some agents may undergo metabolic inactivation or clearance via active transport or bulk flow prior to reaching the ventricles and cerebral convexities. Finally, there is limited drug penetration (2–3 mm) from the CSF into the surrounding tissue, thereby limiting potential efficacy in patients with bulky leptomeningeal disease. This is of particular concern for solid tumor metastases that may frequently include isolated or disseminated nodular tumor deposits, ranging in size from millimeters to centimeters, within the subarachnoid space or on the cranial or spinal nerve roots.

Lumbar puncture is the most common method of IT drug delivery. Children with leukemia routinely receive intralumbar methotrexate, either as a single agent or in combination with cytarabine and hydrocortisone, in addition to their frontline systemic chemotherapy. Although lumbar punctures may cause local pain or discomfort, the procedure is generally well tolerated with the use of local anesthesia. In infants and very young children, the potential for pain and discomfort is reduced further by the use of either conscious or general sedation. Some investigators have attempted to use indwelling lumbar access devices to minimize procedural pain and to ensure drug delivery to the subarachnoid space. However, there is limited oncologic experience with intralumbar access devices. Such devices have inherent risks including bleeding and infection plus additional risks such as catheter breakage or leakage. These devices are not recommended for routine IT drug administration for patients receiving preventative IT therapy.

Many of the limitations associated with intralumbar drug delivery can be overcome by the use of an intraventricular access device such as an Ommaya reservoir. Ommaya reservoirs are frequently used in adults with leptomeningeal cancer because of technical difficulties in performing repeated lumbar punctures in patients with spinal stenosis. Ommaya reservoirs are also routinely used in children with nonleukemic neoplastic meningitis or refractory CNS leukemia. An obvious advantage to an Ommaya reservoir is that it facilitates reliable drug delivery to the subarachnoid space. In addition, Ommaya reservoir injections are more convenient and less painful than intralumbar injections. In fact, the relative ease of intra-Ommaya drug delivery facilitates more effective, less toxic dosing schedules. Finally, CSF drug distribution throughout the neuraxis is theoretically faster and more uniform after intraventricular injection, as CSF flow is not against gravity. The obvious disadvantage of an Ommaya reservoir is that it requires a neurosurgical procedure for placement. There is also the associated inherent risk of infection.

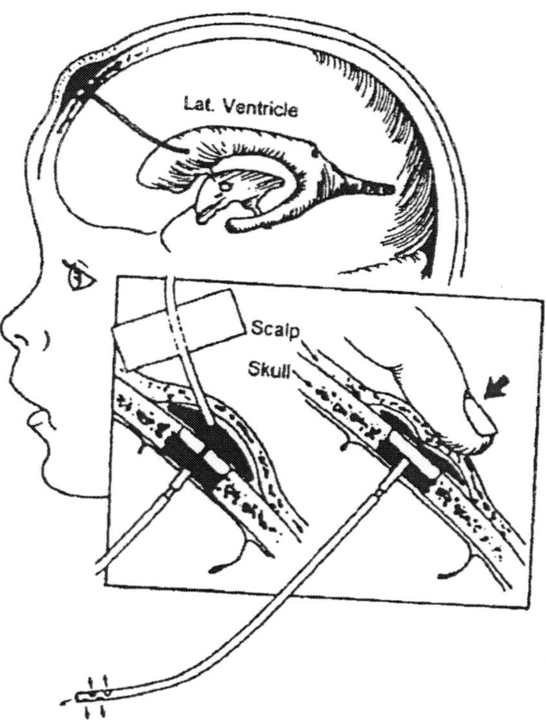

Fig. 13.3. Diagram of an intraventricular drug delivery system consisting of a subcutaneously implanted ommaya reservoir attached to a catheter, the tip of which sits in the lateral ventricle.

The classic example of an IT dosing approach facilitated by the placement of an Ommaya reservoir is the "concentration times time" ("$C \times T$") dosing schedule which involves administration of relatively small but frequent consecutive doses (daily $\times$ 3) of methotrexate or cytarabine. The goal of "$C \times T$" dosing is to maximize efficacy, by attaining drug levels above a cytotoxic threshold level for a prolonged period of time, while minimizing toxicity, by avoiding high peak concentration-associated neurotoxicity. Several studies of the "$C \times T$" approach have suggested improved therapeutic results for intraventricular vs intralumbar chemotherapy in patients with recurrent CNS leukemia or lymphoma. The "$C \times T$" regimen was found to be as efficacious as the standard regimen and was associated with less neurotoxicity in a study of 19 patients with meningeal leukemia who were randomized to receive 12 mg/m^2 of intrathecal methotrexate twice weekly vs "$C \times T$" methotrexate (1 mg every 12 h for six doses). In another study, the complete response duration following "$C \times T$" dosing was 15 mo for 14 of 15 patients (93%) with refractory meningeal leukemia or lymphoma.

Factors Affecting Drug Exposure and Distribution After IT Administration

Other unique considerations to IT drug administration that greatly affect CSF drug exposure and distribution include: relative changes in CSF volume of distribution with age; alterations in drug distribution due to alterations in CSF flow that directly or indirectly result from the underlying disease process; and alterations in drug distribution based on site of administration, that is, intraventricular or intralumbar; as well as on patient position following drug administration

Age-Based Dosing Recommendations for IT Agents

Whereas most systemically administered anticancer agents are dosed based on body surface area (BSA) or weight, dosing for IT anticancer agents is based on patient age. This is because the CSF

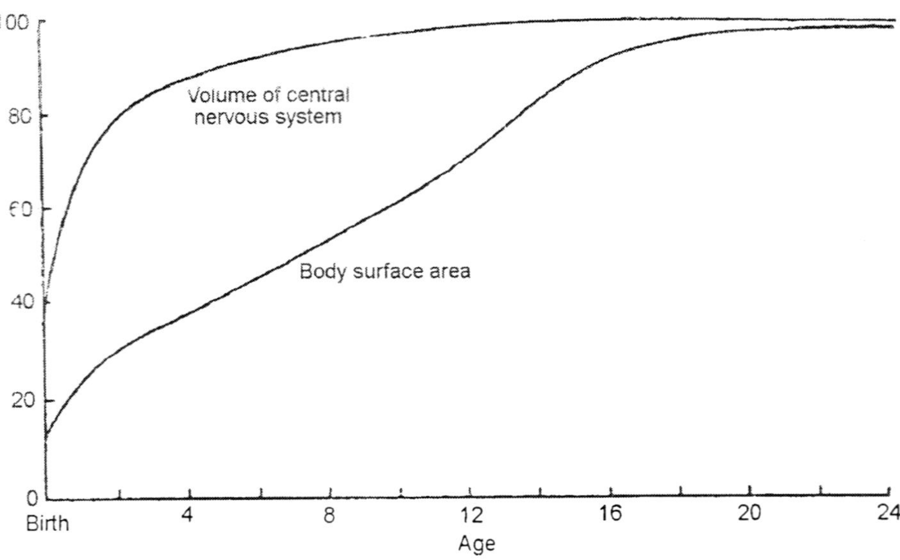

Fig. 13.4. Relationship between body surface area and CNS volume as a function of age.

volume of infants and young children increases at a proportionally greater rate than BSA. As a result, the CSF volume of infants and children is large relative to their BSA. In fact, by 3 yr of age the CSF volumes of adults and children are essentially the same. Thus, dosing practices based on age rather than BSA avoid "*underdosing*" infants and avoid "*overdosing*" adolescents and adults. As a result, age- based dosing recommendations for the commonly used IT agents are standard. The direct advantages of age-based dosing for IT agents in children with CNS leukemia included less neurotoxicity, less variability in drug concentrations, and a reduction in the incidence of CNS relapse.

Table 13.2. Dosage regimens for intralumbar methotrexate and cytarabine based on patient age

Patient age (yr)	*Methotrexate dose (mg)*	*Cytarabine dose (mg)*
< 1	6	12
1	8	16
> 2	10	20
≥ 3–9	12	24
≥ 10	15	30

Alterations in IT Drug Distribution

Unobstructed physiologic CSF flow and normal rates of CSF production and resorption are required for optimal drug distribution following IT administration. Nonuniform drug distribution throughout the neuraxis may compromise efficacy, as a result of inadequate drug exposure, or may increase the risk of local or delayed toxicities, owing to increased local drug exposure. Even in the absence of bulky leptomeningeal or parenchymal CNS disease, patients with neoplastic meningitis may have significant alterations in obstruction to normal CSF flow. Neuroimaging modalities, such as computed tomography (CT) or magnetic resonance imaging (MRI), are less sensitive in evaluating alterations in or obstruction to CSF flow than radionuclide CSF flow studies. Therefore, strong consideration should be given to obtaining a radionuclide CSF flow study, such as 111-DTPA or ^{99m}Tc-DTPA scan, prior to the initiation of IT chemotherapy, especially in patients with nonhematologic neoplastic meningitis. In some circumstances, focal CSF flow abnormalities can be readily restored through the use of local radiation to relieve the obstruction. IT chemotherapy should not be administered to patients with significant abnormalities in or obstruction to CSF flow.

Patient Position After IT Drug Administration

Patient position after IT drug administration may also have a major impact on CSF drug distribution, especially after intralumbar drug dosing. This has been confirmed in nonhuman primates that were maintained in either an upright or prone position for 1 h after intralumbar methotrexate dosing. Peak ventricular methotrexate concentrations and ventricular drug exposure were up to 10-fold greater in animals that remained prone. In addition, there was less variability in ventricular methotrexate levels when the animals were prone.

Pharmacology of Standard Anticancer Agents for IT Administration

Methotrexate

Intralumbar methotrexate

Intralumbar methotrexate is the most commonly used drug for IT administration. Interval administration of IT methotrexate for presymptomatic treatment of leptomeningeal leukemia, a standard component of front-line protocols for acute lymphocytic leukemias (ALL) and many lymphomas, has been instrumental in significantly decreasing the risk of CNS relapse in these settings. IT methotrexate is also effective in inducing CNS remissions in patients with overt CNS leukemia and is commonly used for palliative treatment in the treatment of solid tumor neoplastic meningitis. Nevertheless, the utility of methotrexate for most solid tumors is limited or has not been demonstrated due to its restricted spectrum of antitumor activity.

The initial detailed pharmacokinetic studies of methotrexate were performed prior to the development and routine implementation of age-based dosing guidelines. These studies revealed that after an intralumbar dose of 12 mg/m^2, CSF methotrexate elimination is biphasic with terminal half-lives of 4.5 and 14 h. Average methotrexate levels in lumbar CSF exceed 10 μM at 6 h and fall to 0.1 μM by 48 h, while ventricular CSF levels averaged only 10% of simultaneous lumbar levels. Drug elimination occurs primarily via bulk CSF resorption, although a nonspecific transport mechanism exists.

As was previously discussed, intraventricular methotrexate administration may overcome many of the limitations associated with intralumbar dosing. Pharmacokinetic studies following an intraventricular methotrexate dose of 6.25 mg/m^2 reveal that peak ventricular methotrexate concentrations exceed 200 μM and remain above 0.2 μM for 48 h. In addition, there is good distribution throughout the neuraxis; lumbar CSF methotrexate is detected within 1 h and lumbar CSF levels exceed ventricular levels within 4 h after intraventricular dosing.

Toxicities of IT Methotrexate

The neurological toxicities associated with IT methotrexate can be characterized as acute, subacute, or delayed. Acute toxicities are not uncommon and occur within several hours to a few days after drug administration. Commonly observed toxicities include headache, stiff neck, back pain, vomiting, fever, and lethargy. These adverse events may occur in isolation or may be associated with a CSF pleocytosis, indicative of a chemical arachnoiditis. Subacute toxicities, occurring days to weeks after administration are relatively uncommon and are not always reversible. Subacute toxicities include paraplegia, myelopathy, or encephalopathy, with concomitant symptoms of weakness, ataxia, cranial nerve palsies, seizures, depression of mental status, or coma. Leukoencephalopathy, a chronic progressive, demyelinating process, is a late neurotoxicity that may occur months to years after treatment. Leukoencephalopathy has most commonly been observed patients who received IT methotrexate combined with craniospinal irradiation.

Plasma drug exposure after IT methotrexate is approx 100 times less than CSF exposure. However, plasma levels of methotrexate exceed 0.01 μM for twice as long as following a systemic equivalent dose. Nonetheless, systemic toxicity is minimal, demonstrating one of the advantages of regional chemotherapy.

An unfortunate, albeit rare, event is the occurrence of an accidental overdose of IT methotrexate. This has most often occurred when a patient inadvertently receives the dose of methotrexate that was intended for intravenous administration. If untreated, the resultant overdose causes overwhelming acute neurotoxicity with subsequent severe morbidity or death. Treatment for such an overdose should include immediate CSF drainage, ventriculolumbar perfusion, and administration of systemic leucovorin and steroids. In addition, carboxypeptidase-G2, a more specific antidote that converts methotrexate to an inactive metabolite, has recently been developed by Adamson and Widemann. Evaluation of carboxypeptidase-G2 in a preclinical nonhuman primate model demonstrated that after a methotrexate overdose of 50 mg (equivalent to 500 mg in humans), carboxypeptidase-G2 successfully reduced CSF methotrexate concentrations 400-fold within 5 min of administration. Widemann et al. recently confirmed these observations in six patients who received accidental intrathecal methotrexate overdoses (median dose 482 mg). CSF methotrexate concentrations decreased in all but one patient by >95% following carboxypeptidase administration. Furthermore, all patients recovered completely with the exception of impaired short-term memory in one. This potentially life-saving antidote is available to all Children's Oncology Group institutions in the United States. It should be available for immediate use in pharmacies of any hospital that routinely administers IT methotrexate.

Cytosine Arabinoside

Cytosine arabinoside (cytarabine, or ara-C) is the second most commonly used intrathecal agent. Similar to methotrexate, cytarabine is primarily used in the treatment and prevention of leptomeningeal leukemias and lymphomas. The disposition of cytarabine in the CSF after IT dosing is very different than plasma disposition after intravenous dosing owing to relative differences in cytidine deaminase levels between these two sites. Cytidine deaminase, a ubiquitous enzyme in the liver and blood, rapidly converts systemically administered cytarabine to an inactive metabolite, ara-U. However, cytidine deaminase levels in human CSF are markedly lower than plasma levels. As a result, there is minimal conversion of cytarabine to ara-U following IT dosing. Thus, there is a marked reduction in cytarabine clearance after IT vs systemic dosing. Cytarabine clearance after IT dosing is essentially that of CSF bulk flow, that is, 0.4 mL/min, vs plasma clearance after intravenous dosing which approximates 1000–3600 mL/min/m^2. Thus, there is a tremendous pharmacokinetic advantage for IT cytarabine administration. As with methotrexate, the duration of neoplastic cell exposure to cytotoxic concentrations of cytarabine is an important determinant of response. After intraventricular administration of a 30-mg cytarabine dose, elimination from CSF is biphasic with terminal half-lives of 1 and 3.4 h. Peak CSF concentrations are > 2 mM and exceed 1 μM for more than 24 h. Plasma concentrations after a dose of IT cytarabine are undetectable. In a simulated schedule of ara-C administered using a "$C \times T$" dosing approach, 30 mg daily for 3 d, cytotoxic concentrations were achieved for more than 72 h compared with approx 24 h after a single larger dose of 70 mg. Thus, a "$C \times T$" approach is the preferred approach for attaining sustained CSF levels when the standard cytarabine formulation is utilized. Another alternative is use of a sustained-release cytarabine formulation, DTC101, that has recently been approved for use in the treatment of lymphomatous meningitis.

Toxicities

The most common toxicity of cytarabine after IT administration is chemical arachnoiditis. Less commonly, seizures, paraplegia, peripheral neuropathy, and encephalopathy have been reported. Leukoencephalopathy has been reported with combined IT therapy and radiation.

DTC101

DTC101 (DepoCyt), a sustained-release formulation of cytarabine for intrathecal administration, was specifically developed to maximize the therapeutic efficacy of this S-phase-specific agent. Pharmacokinetic studies after a single dose of DTC101 demonstrate that this novel formulation improves drug distribution throughout the neuraxis. Within 6 h of intraventricular delivery, lumbar CSF concentrations are equivalent to ventricular concentrations. In addition, DTC101 increases the terminal CSF half- life, vs that of standard cytarabine, by approx 40-fold (3.4–141 h). Thus, an obvious advantage of DTC101 is that it can be administered less frequently than standard cytarabine. Randomized multicenter trials comparing DTC101 vs methotrexate in adults with lymphomatous meningitis demonstrated that there was a trend to improvement in neurologic progression and median survival in the DTC101 arm. Likewise, in adults with neoplastic meningitis due to solid tumors, there was a trend toward increased time to neurological progression in the DTC101-treated patients.

Studies in children demonstrate that despite equivalent CSF volumes, pediatric patients ≥ 3 yr of age appear to tolerate a somewhat lower dose of DTC101 than adults. The recommended treatment dose for adults is 50 mg while in the Phase I pediatric study the maximum tolerated dose (MTD) was 35 mg. At higher doses, children experience protracted headaches. Despite the lower dosage recommendation, DTC101 appears to be an active agent in children with refractory leptomeningeal leukemia with seven of nine patients experiencing an objective response. Pharmacokinetic studies at the pediatric recommended Phase II dose of 35 mg demonstrated that 8 d after DTC101 administration, four of five patients still had free cytarabine CSF levels ≥ 0.4 *μM*. The primary disadvantage of DTC101 vs standard cytarabine is the toxicity profile. DTC101 must be given with concomitant oral dexamethasone for approx 5 d to prevent chemical meningitis. Otherwise, the toxicity profile of intrathecal DTC101 plus dexamethasone is very similar to that of the standard cytarabine formulation. Acute toxicities include fever, headache, back pain, nausea, and encephalopathy.

Thiotepa

Thiotepa is a lipid-soluble alkylating agent that has been administered by the IT route to children and adults with neoplastic meningitis. Thiotepa is rapidly converted to an active metabolite, TEPA, after intravenous administration; and both thiotepa and TEPA readily and extensively penetrate into the CSF after systemic dosing. In contrast, after IT administration there is no intra-CSF conversion to TEPA, and CSF clearance exceeds bulk flow by almost ninefold. Therefore, there is not a pharmacokinetic advantage for this lipophilic agent after regional drug administration. Clinical studies of IT thiotepa have failed to provide compelling evidence for its use. In a randomized prospective study evaluating IT methotrexate vs IT thiotepa in adults with neoplastic meningitis, the overall toxicity and efficacy of these agents were essentially identical and overall quite dismal. The median survival for the methotrexate group was 15.9 wk vs 14.1 wk for the thiotepa group. Likewise, in a retrospective study of 15 children with neoplastic meningitis who received IT thiotepa in combination with other therapy the median survival was only 15.1 wk.

New Agents for IT Administration

The limited number and spectrum of antineoplastic agents that significantly penetrate the blood–brain and blood–CSF barriers and the paucity of agents that are available for IT administration impose significant limitations on the development of strategies to successfully prevent or treat solid tumor neoplastic meningitis or refractory CNS leukemia. Combination chemotherapy regimens are an integral component of successful treatment regimens for many systemic cancers. However, similar strategies cannot be employed for neoplastic meningitis because, with the exception of IT, combination regimens are not available. Therefore, we must identify additional agents suitable for IT administration or agents with favorable toxicity profiles and high CSF/plasma exposure ratios. We have used a nonhuman primate model to identify several candidate agents for IT administration. In this section we summarize the current status of ongoing clinical trials with these novel agents that hold promise for future widespread study.

Mafosfamide

Cyclophosphamide is a widely used alkylating agent that has a broad spectrum of antitumor activity against many pediatric and adult cancers. However, cyclophosphamide requires oxidation by hepatic microsomal enzymes to express activity and thus is not a candidate for IT or other regional therapeutic approaches. Mafosfamide is a cyclophosphamide derivative that does not require hepatic activation for tumoricidal effect. The spectrums of antitumor activity for mafosfamide and cyclophosphamide are essentially identical. Thus, mafosfamide was deemed an excellent candidate for further study.

Preclinical in vitro studies, using a representative panel of tumor cell lines with a predilection for leptomeningeal spread, were performed to define an optimal cytotoxic exposure. Preclinical studies in a nonhuman primate demonstrated the feasibility of this dosing approach and provided data for a safe starting dose. A Phase I study of IT mafosfamide as a single agent is ongoing. Initial results demonstrate that headache and pain during or shortly after drug administration are dose limiting at the 6.5-mg dose level. Unfortunately, pharmacokinetic studies at this dose level showed there was not adequate drug exposure throughout the neuraxis for optimal cytotoxicity. Therefore, strategies to facilitate dosage escalation, including decreasing the dose rate of administration and prophylactic treatment with analgesics, have been employed. Patients are currently being enrolled at the 12-mg dose level with a plan to continue dose escalations until, in the absence of neurotoxicity, exposure is deemed to be adequate in both the ventricular and lumbar CSF. IT mafosfamide has also been incorporated into a Pediatric Brain Tumor Consortium front-line treatment protocol for infants and young children (< 3 yr of age) with embryonal CNS tumors. The rationale for this front-line treatment approach is that infants and young children with primary CNS tumors frequently have leptomeningeal tumor involvement either at diagnosis or at time of tumor progression. In addition, they have a very poor overall prognosis. Therefore, we are evaluating the feasibility of a regional therapy approach using IT mafosfamide during the first 20 wk of systemic therapy, followed by conformal radiotherapy, and 20 more wk of systemic therapy. The ultimate goal of this approach is to improve leptomeningeal disease control and to minimize or eliminate the need for radiation therapy and its inherent morbidity.

Topotecan

Topotecan is a water-soluble topoisomerase I poison that has demonstrated objective antitumor activity against a variety of adult and pediatric malignancies including non-small-cell lung cancer, ovarian carcinoma, leukemias, and rhabdomyosarcomas. This spectrum of antitumor activity and lack of neurologic toxicity after systemic administration led to a series of preclinical studies that demonstrated the feasibility of IT drug delivery. A Phase I study of IT topotecan was recently completed. Arachnoiditis characterized by fever, nausea, vomiting, and headache with or without back pain was the dose-limiting toxicity in two of four patients enrolled at the 0.7-mg dose level. The MTD was subsequently defined as 0.4 mg. Six of the 23 evaluable patients had evidence of benefit manifested as prolonged disease stabilization or response. A pediatric Phase II trial of IT toptecan was subsequently initiated by the Children's Oncology Group. The primary study endpoints of this ongoing study are response rate in patients with CNS leukemia in second or greater relapse and response rate and progression-free survival in children with leptomeningeal medulloblastoma.

Busulfan

Busulfan is a dimethanesulfonyloxyalkane that functions as a cell-cycle nonspecific alkylating agent. Clinical busulfan use is generally restricted to preparative regimens for bone-marrow transplant owing to profound systemic toxicities, including severe myelosuppression and pulmonary fibrosis. Historically, regional busulfan administration was limited by its poor solubility in aqueous solutions. However, a microcrystalline formulation of busulfan with greatly enhanced aqueous solubility, Spartaject busulfan, was recently developed. This formulation was specifically developed for IT administration based on preclinical studies demonstrating antitumor activity against medulloblastoma cell lines and xenografts. Subsequent studies in a nude rat model of neoplastic meningitis demonstrated antitumor activity, although toxicity studies suggested that there may be a very narrow therapeutic window. Phase I studies to evaluate the safety and feasibility and to identify a dose of intrathecal busulfan for subsequent evaluation of efficacy are currently in progress.

Gemcitabine

Gemcitabine (2', 2'-difluorodeoxycytidine or dFdC), a deoxycytidine analog, has a broad spectrum of clinical antitumor activity against a variety of tumors with potential for leptomeningeal spread. Similar to cytarabine, gemcitabine is rapidly deaminated to an inactive metabolite following intravenous administration, thereby limiting CSF gemcitabine exposure. Studies in the nonhuman primate model were thus performed to evaluate the feasibility and toxicity of IT administration of gemcitabine. After a 5-mg IT gemcitabine dose (equivalent to 50 mg in humans), CSF drug exposure (measured by AUC) was eight times that in plasma after a 400-fold higher intravenous dose. A Phase I study of IT gemcitabine for neoplastic meningitis has recently been initiated. Significant advances in the treatment and prevention of CNS leukemias and lymphomas have been a direct result of a better understanding of CNS pharmacology and the development of effective therapeutic strategies to circumvent the limitations imposed by the blood- brain and blood-CSF barriers. Unfortunately, the treatment and prevention of leptomeningeal metastases from solid tumors and the treatment of recurrent CNS leukemia remain unsatisfactory. Further advancements in the treatment of this devastating disease require continued preclinical and clinical research efforts to identify new agents and combination regimens for IT administration and to evaluate new treatment strategies such as IT delivery of monoclonal antibodies or immunotherapies. Furthermore, correlative clinical pharmacology studies to maximize efficacy and minimize toxicity are of paramount importance in ensuring that optimal dosing strategies are developed.

14

TREATMENT OF PRIMARY TUMOR

There were about 1.2 million nonskin cancers diagnosed in North America in 2002. Conventional cancer therapeutic regimens include surgery, chemotherapy, and radiotherapy. Modern oncology has brought immunotherapy, hyperthermia, cryotherapy, radiofrequency ablation, and molecularly targeted drug therapy to the investigational front. Historically, these therapies have been focused on tumor cell kill. More recently, however, cancer research has begun to examine the permissive environment in which the cancer cell survives. This has led to extensive research in the fields of invasion and metastases, extracellular matrix biology, and angiogenesis. Some of the most powerful antitumor agents include molecules in that inhibit angiogenesis. It is the objective of this chapter to review the evidence and rationale for treating primary tumors with a combined regimen of angiogenesis inhibitors and radiotherapy.

TWO-CELL COMPARTMENT MODEL OF TUMORS

Angiogenesis is the growth of blood vessels that are necessary for the progression and survival of tumors. Most solid tumors begin as an avascular nodule, and remain < 1–2 mm in diameter. Nutrients are supplied and wastes are removed by passive diffusion. A permissive environment allows an angiogenic "switch," whereby a previously dormant tumor becomes vascularized by undergoing this process termed angiogenesis. The newly vascularized tumor can be conceptualized as a two-compartment model. The tumor cells receive nutrients and survival factors from the vasculature, and the endothelium receives stimulus from the tumor, for example, vascular endothelial growth factor (VEGF), for endothelial proliferation and migration. To achieve tumor "*cure*" one of two things must happen: either the tumor cells or the supporting stromal cells must be targeted. Endothelial cell kill can lead to tumor cell death through starvation. Combination therapy directed against either compartment theoretically should lead to more successful cure rates.

This two-compartment model, in which the endothelial cell supports the tumor cell, led to the discovery of a class of compounds called angiogenesis inhibitors. There are multiple subclasses of antiangiogenic agents including growth factor inhibitors such as VEGF blockers, small molecules including thalidomide and TNP-470, and natural protein fragments such as angiostatin. Many naturally produced angiogenesis inhibitors are fragments of larger proteins that are normally intimately involved with the vasculature. For example, angiostatin is a fragment of plasminogen, endostatin is a fragment of collagen XVIII, and antiangiogenic antithrombin III is a fragment of antithrombin III. These drugs are highly potent, work against a variety of tumor types, and are minimally toxic in preclinical animal trials.

Changing Views of the Radiotherapy Target

Radiation therapy has been used for more than 100 yr in the treatment of cancer. The "*radiation effect*" against tumor cells is conventionally thought to occur through DNA damage caused by ionizing radiation, resulting in reproductive cell death. With fractionated regimens, tumor cells are more sensitive to radiation than normal tissues. Radiation-induced side effects and complications are thought to result from unrepaired DNA damage within normal cells. For example, acute radiation damage to the small intestine is thought to result from DNA damage in epithelial stem cells located in the intestinal crypts of Lieberkuhn.

A recent article by Paris et al. challenges this hypothesis. By using supratherapeutic doses of radiotherapy, they demonstrated that endothelial apoptosis leads to secondary gut stem cell apoptosis. Therefore, the target for radiation-induced small bowel toxicity was the gut endothelium and not the gut epithelial stem cell. This effect could be abrogated by the administration of basic fibroblast growth factor, acting as an endothelial survival factor, which prevented endothelial cell apoptosis. The authors also demonstrated that in a transgenic knockout mouse model of acid sphingomyelinase, in which the endothelium is resistant to radiation-induced apoptosis, the gut epithelial stem cells survived a larger dose of radiation before undergoing apoptosis. In this transgenic mouse model, in which the normal signaling pathways in endothelial cells were altered, the gut endothelium and not the intestinal epithelial stem cell pool was the primary target for acute radiation- induced gastrointestinal syndrome.

Targeting of the endothelium with radiotherapy is not a new idea. In 1982 Denekamp described the differential proliferation rates between the endothelial cells found in tumors and those found in normal tissues. The tumor endothelium had a proliferation rate 20 times greater than the proliferation rate of the normal vasculature. The proliferating endothelium seemed to be a perfect target for an emerging technology at the time, radiolabeled monoclonal antibodies (MAbs). MAbs against antigens found on proliferating endothelial cells would allow a very high dose of radiation to be selectively targeted to the tumor endothelium. As yet, MAbs have had limited success in the clinic in part due to their large size and heterogeneous distribution. Modern techniques utilizing phage display technology are now being used to the discover receptors or antigens that might be differentially expressed between tumor endothelium and normal endothelium. The identification of such a differential expression could lead to novel molecular therapeutic strategies specifically targeted to tumor endothelial cells.

Endothelium as a Target for Angiogenesis Inhibitors

As early as 1971, publications by Folkman emphasized that tumors need a constant blood supply to survive. Early work was successful at finding a stimulator of angiogenesis, termed tumor angiogenesis factor (TAF), but much effort was spent on isolating and characterizing a tumor-derived inhibitor of angiogenesis. The key to finding this inhibitor was the observation of a unique clinical pattern of metastases in 10–15% of all surgical patients. A patient with this pattern of metastases would have a primary tumor without evidence of metastases but following surgery would demonstrate an immediate and rapid growth of previously undetectable metastases. If the primary tumor was producing an inhibitor of angiogenesis, and the removal of the primary tumor resulted in the growth of metastases, then the inhibitor should be detectable in either urine or blood.

It was this model that O'Reilly and colleagues studied with the Lewis lung carcinoma cell line. By selecting a tumor cell line variant that suppressed growth of its own metastases, they had selected a tumor cell line that was producing an inhibitor of angiogenesis. After many years of work and laboratory analysis from hundreds of liters of mouse urine, a protein was purified that could inhibit endothelial cell proliferation in vitro and prevent the growth of the metastases in vivo when given exogenously. This protein was called angiostatin, a fragment of the larger molecule plasminogen. The unique and significant feature of this molecule was its ability to inhibit endothelial cell proliferation (in three different endothelial cell lines) without inhibiting the proliferation of nonendothelial cells (nine different cell lines tested).

Finding an inhibitor of angiogenesis that was a fragment of a larger molecule already found within the vasculature gave credence to the hypothesis that angiogenesis, even in tumors, is a highly regulated process. This process is also quite complex, as demonstrated in attempts to elucidate the mechanism of angiostatin production from plasminogen. Other molecules, which were thought to be strictly involved in cellular invasion and metastases, such as metalloelastase and matrix metalloproteinase-2, have now been implicated in the production of angiostatin.

It is with a similar experimental method, in this case using a hemangioendothelioma cell line that suppressed the growth of its own metastases, that O'Reilly was able to purify another inhibitor of angiogenesis, endostatin. Endostatin, a fragment of collagen XVIII, is a specific inhibitor of endothelial cell proliferation and has little effect on the proliferation of six other nonendothelial cell lines. The production of endostatin from its precursor molecule can be regulated by either elastase or cathepsin-L. A wide range of other molecules have now been identified as having antiangiogenic properties. To be classified in this category, a molecule must inhibit endothelial proliferation in more than one of the standard assays: endothelial cell proliferation, chick chorioallantoic membrane assay, matrigel migration assay, or corneal micropocket assay, while not inhibiting the proliferation of other nonendothelial cell lines.

Combination of Radiation and Antiangiogenic Therapy: Impact on Local Control of Primary Tumors

The oxygen effect on the radioresistance of hypoxic tumor cells has been well demonstrated. It may be counterintuitive to some that the use of antiangiogenic therapy may augment local control with radiotherapy. Classic dogma teaches that if the tumor bed is rendered more hypoxic with antiangiogenic therapy, then the tumor cells must be less radiosensitive. Generating hypoxia with antiangiogenic therapies may select cancer cells that have acquired hypoxia resistance and have a higher metastatic and invasive potential. Paradoxically, three preclinical studies have shown that the treatment of tumors with antiangiogenic drugs actually increases the tumor partial pressure of oxygen (pO_2).

In 1992, Teicher published the seminal paper describing a combination of antiangiogenic therapy and radiotherapy against a primary tumor. She demonstrated, in a tumor growth delay study, that the combination of minocycline (a weak metalloproteinase inhibitor), TNP-470, and radiotherapy was superadditive against Lewis lung carcinoma cells in mice. The growth delay observed with radiotherapy alone was 4.4 d while the delay with combination therapy was 12.6 d ($p < 0.0001$). These results triggered a paradigm shift in the rationale for combining antiangiogenic therapy with radiotherapy.

Why do we see this greater than additive effect? Radiotherapy can reduce the number of 5–15 μm diameter vessels in a dose-dependent fashion with no change in the tumor volume. Yet, the numbers of 20–50 μm diameter vessels are unchanged. This has led to speculation that although the quantity of the vessels has decreased, the quality, as measured by oxygen carrying capacity, has actually increased. Anti-VEGF therapy has also been shown to decrease microvessel density and tumor interstitial fluid pressure, yet increase the measured pO_2. Therefore, the combination of radiotherapy and antiangiogenic therapy may result in more oxygenated and radiosensitive tumors.

Angiostatin or Endostatin and Radiotherapy

The surprising results presented by Teicher, combined with the high potency and low toxicity of naturally occurring antiangiogenic protein fragments, led to the experimental combination of radiotherapy and angiostatin by Weichselbaum' s group at the University of Chicago. They treated four different tumor cell lines, one mouse and three human, with a dose of angiostatin that reduced the tumor volume by 38%. When they combined angiostatin with radiotherapy, they observed an additive effect. Tumor volume reduction was greater than with either angiostatin or radiotherapy alone. When the tumors were examined histologically, microvessel density was lower in tumors treated with combination therapy, compared to either angiostatin or radiation treatments alone. They concluded that radiotherapy and angiostatin both targeted the tumor endothelium in an additive fashion.

The same group followed up on this early work by looking at the timing of angiostatin administration when used in combination with radiotherapy. In this case, they gave angiostatin in three different combination schedules with radiotherapy. Radiotherapy was given on d 0 and 1 and angiostatin was given on d 0 and 1, d 0–13, or d 2–13. They were able to demonstrate that concurrent schedules resulted in a greater effect than sequential administrations. It was also interesting to note that in the two groups that received concurrent angiostatin administrations, similar tumor growth inhibition was observed. Adjuvant administration of angiostatin alone had no effect, consistent with a radio sensitizing mechanism of action.

Later experiments with recombinant endostatin confirmed a significant benefit to combination therapy compared to either modality alone. It was also demonstrated, similar to their results with angiostatin, that the microvessel density in endostatin-treated mice was 40 vessels/area vs 14 vessels/area in endostatin plus radiotherapy treated mice.

VEGF Inhibition and Radiotherapy

VEGF, or vascular permeability factor, is a heparin binding angiogenic growth factor that was first discovered by Dvorak in 1983. VEGF can stimulate endothelial cells to proliferate or migrate through its interaction with VEFGR-1 (flt-1) or VEGFR-2 (KDR/flk-1) and is up-regulated by hypoxia. This VEGF up-regulation by hypoxia is mediated through an up-regulation of hypoxia-inducible factor 1 (HIF-1), which binds upstream of the VEGF promoter.

The first study using an anti-VEGF drug in combination with radiotherapy was published in 1999, in this case with a soluble antibody against VEGF-165. VEGF levels in irradiated tumors were three- to fourfold higher than in nonirradiated controls as measured by enzyme-linked immunosorbent assay (ELISA) and Northern blotting. In four separate tumor model experiments, the investigators were able to demonstrate a more significant tumor growth delay with combined therapy compared to either anti-VEGF therapy or radiotherapy alone. This group concluded that radiation up-regulates endothelial cell production of VEGF which in turn acts as a survival factor, and that VEGF inhibition counters this survival effect.

Another group of investigators were able to demonstrate a similar effect in 2000. Using a MAb against human VEGF, they measured several interesting tumor parameters including microvessel density (MVD), pO_2, and interstitial fluid pressure (IFP). They hypothesized that anti-VEGF therapy should decrease IFP resulting in radiosensitization. Results indeed showed a significant reduction in MVD (36–60%) and IFP (approx 75%), and an increase in pO_2 with anti- VEGF therapy compared to controls. The increase in pO_2 may have been due to an improvement in the quality of oxygen delivery, partly owing to a decreased IFP.

Their subsequent work investigated the effects of a VEGF-receptor blocking peptide, DC 101, on tumor control probability in combination with radiotherapy. For each cell line tested, they observed an additive effect. Surprisingly, tumor oxygen levels measured with an Eppendorf polarographic probe did not reveal a change in pO_2. One should note that although both studies were performed by the same group of investigators, different experimental techniques were employed, which could account for the difference seen in pO_2 measurements. It is interesting to speculate that inhibition of VEGF receptor binding with a peptide and antibody binding of the VEGF-R may result in different physiological effects.

A second and possibly more appealing method of inhibiting VEGF-R is to block the tyrosine kinase (TK) portion of the receptor with a small molecule such as SU-5416, SU-6668, or PTK787/ZK222548. These small molecules have been shown in mouse tumor models to have significant antitumor effect. They have also been found to act synergistically with radiotherapy. The first paper addressing this question tested SU54 16, a TK inhibitor specific for flk- 1 (K_i of 0.16 μM) in combination with radiotherapy. Several parameters were measured, including vascular ultrasound (US) measurements, tumor window measurements, and tumor growth delay. They found that combined therapy with SU5416 decreased the number and length of vessels measured in the dorsal chamber window, which correlated with the drop in US flow measurements. They also found a greater than additive effect in tumor growth delay with combined therapy compared to either SU5416 or radiotherapy alone.

These results were confirmed by two additional groups, using both SU54 16 and SU6668, a broader TK antagonist of VEGF, fibroblast growth factor (FGF), and platelet-derived growth factor (PDGF). Both groups found a greater than additive effect on tumor growth delay with combined therapy using SU6668, and one group confirmed an increase in pO_2 after treatment with SU6668. Furthermore, SU6668 was found to have a greater therapeutic effect than SU5416 by almost doubling the tumor growth delay from 6.5 d to 11.9 d. The authors speculated that this more pronounced effect might be due to the inhibition of multiple growth factor receptors with SU6668 compared to the more specific inhibition of VEGF-R with SU5416.

By examining the entire anti-VEGF strategy, several general conclusions can be drawn. The first is that combination therapy with VEGF inhibitors is more effective than radiotherapy alone. The second is that the effect appears to be at least partly due to an elevation in pO_2, which may be mediated through a change in MVD and/or IFP. As VEGF is a growth factor that is up-regulated by radiotherapy and acting as a survival factor for endothelial cells, it is plausible that VEGF-R inhibition results in blockade of this survival signal, leading to a greater radiation effect.

Combination Therapy to Address Micrometastatic Disease Outisde the Radiation Field

Angiostatin and endostatin cure tumors in mice, and early Phase I clinical trials demonstrate little toxicity; however, they also demonstrate little efficacy. It is currently felt by the oncology community that antiangiogenic agents, as a class, are cytostatic and not cytotoxic. This accounts for the very low toxicity observed thus far. Therefore, to reap the most benefit from a cytostatic agent, one needs to combine these compounds with cytotoxic agents such as radiotherapy.

An alternate explanation for the lack of efficacy in the early trials is that cytostatic agents are not effective in a widely metastatic setting, which is the cohort of patients so far recruited to Phase I trials. Another patient cohort theoretically worthy of investigation would be locally controlled patients who have a high risk of distant failure. For example, a patient with limited stage small-cell lung cancer has a 30% risk of brain metastasis after complete regression of his or her thoracic disease. In such a patient, antiangiogenic agents could be administered following successful primary therapy and followed for a change in the incidence of growth of already metastatic microscopic disease.

Imaging Angiogenesis

The rapidly proliferating endothelium is an appealing target for antiangiogenic therapy and for molecular imaging techniques. As the number of compounds targeting the endothelium continues to increase, the need for noninvasively monitoring tumor microvasculature is becoming more critical. Multiple modalities including US, computed tomography (CT), magnetic resonance imaging (MRI), and radionuclide imaging such as positron emission tomography (PET) are currently being investigated to image the tumor microvasculature and the endothelium. US, CT, and MRI make use of the differences in vascular flow and permeability between normal and tumor tissues utilizing Doppler color images and/or contrast materials. MRI and PET scanning can potentially image very specific molecules engineered to bind to endothelial cells. Clinical trials that investigate antiangiogenic treatments should consider incorporating a detailed imaging protocol as part of the evaluation process, especially in the context of radiation therapy which is always designed and delivered with image reference.

Classic tumor biology has focused on a method of damaging malignant cells to eradicate tumors. As the fields of angiogenesis and vascular biology mature, new drugs with new targets can be investigated in combination with classical therapies. Antiangiogenic strategies focus on inhibiting the proliferation of endothelial cells, while antivascular strategies target more mature vascular structures. Each field perceives the support structure of a tumor as a potential site of intervention. It should be remembered that antiangiogenic and antivascular treatments are not mutually exclusive and will likely be used in combination in the future.

A thorough review of the literature has shown that many antiangiogenic agents administered concurrently with radiotherapy result in synergistic cell killing. Early warnings of a theoretical disadvantage to this combined approach due to hypoxia have been disproved. However, much still needs to be learned in both preclinical and clinical trials. For example, timing of drug administration, duration of drug exposure, and combination antiangiogenic drug therapies must be investigated. Of concern is that there are no data concerning the late effects in normal tissues of antiangiogenic agents alone or in combination with radiotherapy. Future clinical studies should address this important issue and closely monitor untoward normal tissue late effects.

15

TREATMENT OF CANCER

Since the initial confirmation that genetic alterations cause disease, the pervasive outlook has been that the future for gene therapy is very promising, but curing diseases by the transfer of specific nucleic acid sequences has been problematic. It should be recognized, however, that the hurdles facing investigators in the field of gene therapy can be defined and are likely not insurmountable. The major limitations facing gene therapy investigators are the inability to genetically modify sufficient numbers of target cells and the inability to express the transferred gene(s) over prolonged periods. With respect to the application of gene therapy for the treatment of cancer, in many aspects the fundamental cause of these hurdles is not different than those faced by pioneers of other treatments, for example, in the development of chemotherapy agents, which is mainly a lack of understanding of the biological systems being manipulated. Even so, great strides and accomplishments have been achieved during the last decade, not only with respect to the physical transfer of genes into target cells but also in the clinical practice of gene therapy. The purpose of this chapter is to provide a general background on how genes are transferred as well as a specific example focusing on the translation of a gene therapy study from inception through a completed Phase III clinical trial.

Although it was initially envisioned that gene therapy would be used to cure monogenetic inherited disorders, numerous ingenious applications have been developed to treat a wide variety of diseases. As of September 2001, there are more than 600 gene therapy clinical trials registered worldwide. Of these more than 60% are focused on cancer as the target illness and have enrolled more than 2300 patients. Classic gene therapy strategies seeking to reprogram tumor cells in vivo by direct transgene delivery are now being complemented by a growing array of studies exploring the use of engineered autologous immunocompetent cells, engineered oncolytic viruses, cancer vaccines, and others, as biopharmaceuticals. When compared with mature fields of cancer clinical research, gene

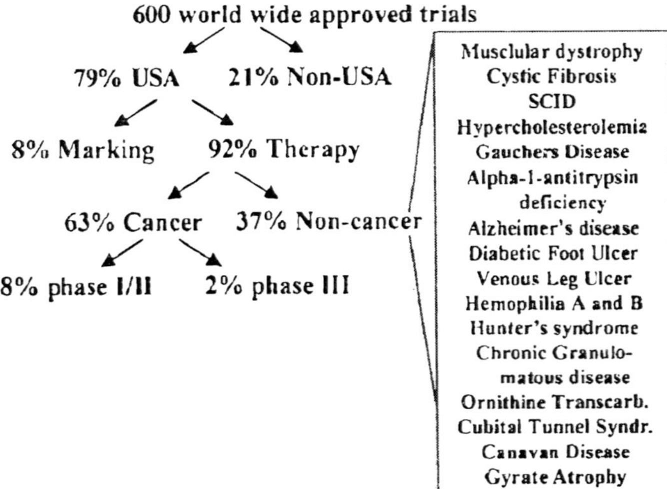

Fig. 15.1. Summary of gene therapy clinical trails.

therapy is rich in potential but weak in accomplishments. This is reflected by the very high proportion of Phase I and Phase II studies (>550) underway worldwide, with fewer than 2% of all trials being Phase III. Interestingly, the first human gene therapy trial, performed in May of 1989, involved the treatment of melanoma; a year later a second trial was initiated that was designed to treat the genetic defect of adenosine deaminase deficiency.

Gene Transfer Techniques

A hope for gene therapy is to be able to supply a physician with a vial containing material that can easily be administered and that efficiently alters cellular functions by incorporating new genetic sequences. Although this scenario is far from reality, the transfer of genetic material is currently accomplished using a variety of techniques, with the majority of transfer techniques being classified as either viral or nonviral delivery systems, both of which are being developed for the treatment of cancer. There are also many strategies that are under development to target specific cells for genetic modification, which can be classified as (1) systemic in vivo administration of the genetic delivery system; (2) *in situ* delivery, in which the material is delivered only to a local area, such as a tumor; and (3) ex vivo delivery, in which target cells are removed from the affected patient or from a suitable donor and genetically modified before reinfusion into the patient. The number of ideas conceived to treat cancer using gene transfer techniques is astounding. The majority of these investigations can be grouped into one of the following categories:

1. Transfer of genes into target cells that affect drug sensitivity:
   - (a) Confer protection to chemotherapy-sensitive noncancerous tissues by transferring genes that encode drug-resistance proteins. The encoded proteins serve to protect the sensitive tissues and thereby allow for altered dosing, and possibly more aggressive treatment, of chemotherapy agents.
   - (b) Transfer of genes into cancerous tissues that confer drug sensitivity to the modified cells. The encoded proteins serve to sensitize cancer cells to specific drugs that increase the selectivity of chemotherapy.
2. Transfer of genes into cancer cells that inhibit or alter specific cellular functions:
   - (a) Transfer of genes that encode complementary nucleic acid sequences that can hybridize to specific RNA sequences and block the expression of cancer-promoting gene products.
   - (b) Transfer of genes that encode antibodies that specifically recognize proteins critical to tumor cell proliferation.
   - (c) Transfer of genes that encode proteins that replace or augment missing gene products of tumor suppressor genes.
3. Transfer of genes that affect the immune response against cancer cells:
   - (a) Transfer of genes that encode missing or down-regulated costimulatory molecules into cancer cells for the purpose of increasing the immune recognition of cancer cells.
   - (b) Transfer of genes that encode proteins uniquely expressed or overexpressed in cancer cells into antigen-presenting cells to activate cytotoxic T cells against the cancer.
   - (c) Transfer of genes that encode specific cytokines that stimulate an immune response against cancerous cells.

Nonviral Gene Transfer

Depending on the specific requirements of the gene transfer vehicle, the physical transfer of nucleic acid sequences can be achieved by several methods. The use of nonviral gene transfer is very attractive because the components of the delivery system can be chemically synthesized and can be very well regulated. A well-regulated system is certainly more appealing for FDA approval compared to the use of viral transfer systems that, as discussed below, require a number of components that are more difficult to standardize. But compared to viral gene transfer, the use of nonviral gene transfer reagents is very inefficient. It is anticipated, however, that studies aimed at understanding the mechanisms involved in the entry of nucleic acids into cells will result in the generation of improved compounds. Indeed, the use of cationic liposomes has shown some promise and has been used clinically. In general, the formation of a liposome/DNA delivery vehicle requires a synthetic cationic amphiphile such as DOTMA or GL67, and a neutral lipid, such as dioleoyl L-α-phosphatidylethanolamine (DOPE). The key to efficient gene transfer is to determine the exact molar ratio of each component that will allow the greatest amount of DNA to be transfected into the target cells. In addition to liposome/DNA delivery systems, cationic polymers such as poly-L-lysine and various peptide complexes have been used to deliver plasmid DNA. The gene being transferred is typically contained in a plasmid, and its expression can be driven by a variety of promoters. Because large quantities of highly purified plasmid DNA can be obtained by growing relatively small bacterial cultures, the isolation of the genetic material to be transferred is relatively straightforward. The success of many of these new agents is encouraging in the fact that several have mediated high-level gene transfer in vitro, but the lack of in vivo success has been discouraging.

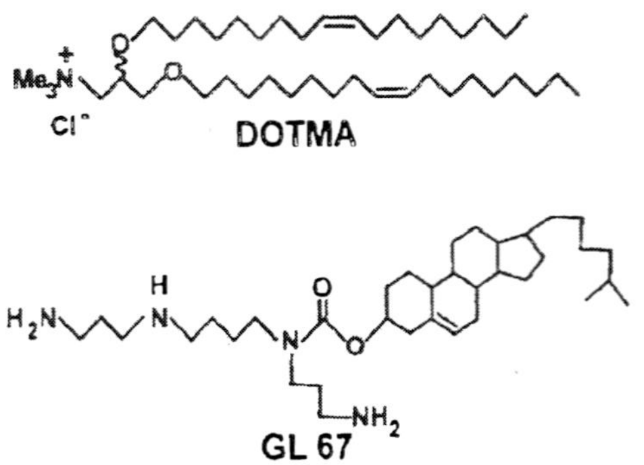

$Me_3\overset{+}{N}$ Cl^- DOTMA

H_2N H N O N O NH_2 GL 67

Fig. 15.2. Structures of two cationic liposomes used in nonviral gene transfer.

Viral Gene Transfer

Although it is hoped that the efficiency of gene transfer using synthetically derived compounds can be sufficiently increased for general use, if high transduction efficiencies are needed recombinant viruses are typically used. Because of the early success and high transduction levels achieved with viral transfer systems, vast amounts of resources have been expended to develop novel viral delivery systems as well as to understand better the basic biology of viral gene transfer. In general, a basic concept for creating recombinant viruses is the use of a viral-packaging cell line. Recombinant retroviral packaging cell lines are derived by specifically controlling the expression of wild-type viral sequences. The virus contains two long-terminal-repeat (LTR) regions, the 5' and 3'-LTRs. The 5'-LTR contains an enhancer region and a promoter that drives the expression of the viral RNA transcript. From the processed RNA transcript the proteins necessary for the assembly of an infectious viral particle are translated from the *gag*, *pol*, and *env* sequences. The *gag* gene translates a single polyprotein that is subsequently cleaved into three proteins—the matrix, capsid, and nucleic acid-binding protein. The *pol* gene encodes both the reverse transcriptase and integrase proteins. Importantly, the ψ region of the preprocessed RNA transcript is recognized by and incorporated into the viral particle. So the genome of the viral particle contains the full-length RNA transcript. The viral particle is then released by budding from the cell membrane. The envelope proteins are encoded by *env* and recognize specific cell surface proteins on target cells, which dictate viral tropism. On recognizing specific cellular receptors, the viral particles bind to the target cells and the RNA transcript is deposited into the cell. The RNA is reverse transcribed into DNA and then incorporated into the genome of the target cell. Once the viral sequence becomes part of the genome of the target cell (or proviral sequence), more infectious virus can be generated. Because the viral sequence integrates into the genome of the target cell, as the host cell divides the viral sequence is also replicated and the genome of both resulting cells contains the viral sequence.

To produce recombinant viruses that can be used in gene therapy applications, the generation of packaging cells was paramount. Packaging cells are generated from cell lines that are easily grown in the laboratory, such as NIH 3T3 or 293T cells. To generate a packing cell that produces replication incompetent virus, that is, viruses that can infect target cells but do not contain the necessary elements to make more virus, specific sequences of a wild-type virus were cloned into expression cassettes and transferred into tissue culture cell lines. Safe packaging cells have been generated by expressing the *gag* and *pol* sequences from one promoter and *env* by a separate promoter on a second expression cassette. Expression of these sequences is sufficient to generate a viral particle. However, because the ψ region is eliminated from these expression constructs there is no viral RNA transcript packaged into the viral particle. The packaging cell line is, therefore, capable of producing viral particles but the particles being produced are void of RNA. The RNA to be packaged is supplied by retroviral vectors. Retroviral vectors contain 5'- and 3'-LTRs, the ψ region, and the cDNA sequence necessary to encode a therapeutic protein. By transfecting the retroviral vector into a packaging cell-line, the 5'-LTR drives the production of the retroviral vector RNA. Because the retroviral vector RNA contains the ψ region, the RNA sequence will be recognized by the viral particle and packaged, generating a recombinant virus. The recombinant virus is composed of all the protein components of the wild-type virus but the packaged RNA sequence is supplied by the retroviral vector. The recombinant virus can be collected from the supernatant of the packaging cells and used to infect target cells. Using the cellular entry mechanisms of a wild-type virus, the RNA sequence is introduced into the target cell, is reverse-transcribed into DNA, and integrates into the genome of the infected cell. The only nucleic acid sequence transferred is the sequence that encodes the therapeutic protein. Because the viral genome is not transferred, the targeted cells do not produce infectious virus. Noncompetent recombinant retroviruses can therefore be used to introduce specific gene sequences safely into target cells.

A useful feature of the murine leukemia virus transfer system is the ability to switch easily the *env* sequences to produce pseudotyped virus. Pseudotyped viruses have altered receptor usage owing to the expression of the different envelope proteins. For example, if the gene encoding the gp70 envelope is used, ecotropic virus is produced that will infect only mouse and rat cells because this envelope recognizes the mCAT1 receptor specific for mice and rats. But if the A2070A envelope is expressed, amphotropic virus is produced that can infect many mammalian cell types because this envelope recognizes the PIT-2 receptor that is present on many types of cells. Recent studies have shown that the degree of PIT-2 expression on target cells determines the efficiency of viral transduction. Cells that have low-level amphotropic receptor RNA expression, such as human hematopoietic stem and progenitor cells, are inefficiently transduced with amphotropic pseudotyped virus, whereas subpopulations of cells with high amphotropic receptor RNA expression are more efficiently transduced. The G-protein from the vesicular stomatitis virus (VSV-G) is also used for viral pseudotyping because this envelope protein mediates viral entry through association with anionic phospholipids. VSV-G pseudotyped viral particles have the added advantage of being more physically stable, which allows the virus to be concentrated by centrifugation. More recently, the envelope of the RD1 14/type D retrovirus, which recognizes a neutral amino acid transporter, has been used for gene transfer into human and nonhuman primates with relatively high efficiency.

In addition, retroviruses other than the murine leukemia virus (MLV) have also been develolped. Although much more complicated in molecular structure, lentiviruses such as the human immunodeficiency virus have been genetically altered to create safe gene packaging vehicles. A major limitation to the use of MLVs is the requirement that the target cell must proceed through at least one round of replication. Many cell types that are possible targets for gene therapy are quiescent and therefore resistant to MLV transduction. Lentiviruses can infect mitotically inactive cells, and recombinant viruses generated from the HIV genome also appear to infect nondividing cells. Pseudotyping recombinant lentivirus with VSV-G expands the viral host range and allows for targeting of a broad range of cell types. Because lentiviruses are extremely efficient gene transfer vehicles, tremendous effort has been directed at making safe transfer systems using the lentiviral genome. In addition to lentiviruses, ecombinant retroviruses derived from foamy viruses have also shown potential as vehicles for gene transfer. The genome of foamy viruses is similar to that of the MLV, that is, *gag*, *pol*, and *env* genes, but several accessory proteins are also encoded that are referred to as *bel* genes. Although the exact function of each *bel* gene product is unknown, packaging cells have been generated that encode the necessary proteins required for viral particle formation. Advantages of using recombinant foamy viruses are their broad host range and their ability to package large retroviral vectors.

The ability to transfer specific nucleic acid sequences reproducibly made recombinant retroviruses the choice for many investigators. However, the limelight is now being shared by viral transfer systems that are more complex and for many applications superior to retroviral transfer. DNA virus vectors such as adenovirus, adeno-associated virus, and herpes simplex virus are finding their own niches in the field of gene therapy. Adeno-associated virus type 2 (AAV) is a human parvovirus having several features that make it a very attractive vehicle for gene transfer. Although 80% of adults are seropositive for AAV-2, the wild-type virus is not associated with any disease, and unlike retroviruses that integrate randomly into the genome, recombinant adeno-associated virus can be engineered to integrate into the long arm of human chromosome 19. However, a major limitation to the development of recombinant AAV gene therapy products is the difficulty in producing highly purified virus. One reason for this is because AAV-2 is in the genus *Dependovirus*, meaning it requires a helper virus for replication. Wild-type adenovirus is its helper virus and is a major contaminant of recombinant AAV-2.

Wild-type AAV-2 is a nonenveloped virus with an icosahedral capsid composed of three proteins—VP-1, VP-2, and VP-3—in a 1:1:10 ratio. Two rep proteins, Rep 78 and Rep 68, have DNA helicase and DNA nicking activities and are required for site-specific integration of the AAV-2 genome. The wild-type genome of AAV-2 is a 4681 single DNA strand that has a 145 nucleotide inverted terminal repeat (ITR) at each end, which are required for DNA encapsulation. Between the two ITRs are the genes that encode the rep and VP proteins. Similar to the production of recombinant retroviruses, a vector plasmid was developed by removing the rep and VP sequences and replacing them with a therapeutic gene. The rep and VP sequences are expressed from a separate plasmid that does not contain the ITR packaging signal, similar to the controlled expression described above for *gag/pol* and *env* for recombinant retroviral production. To generate recombinant AAV-2 the two plasmids, that is, vector plasmid and rep-cap expressing plasmid, are cotransfected into a suitable cell line. Unlike the production of recombinant retrovirus, transfection of the AAV genome into tissue culture cells does not produce recombinant virus. Transfectants must then be infected with adenovirus to help stimulate AAV-2 expression. Recombinant AAV-2 is produced and a single strand of DNA sequence encoded by the vector plasmid is packaged. In addition, wild-type adenovirus is also produced. The wild-type virus can be heat inactivated and removed by cesium chloride density gradient centrifugation. Alternatively, affinity chromatography methods have been developed to increase the speed and purity of recombinant AAV-2 isolation. The ability to isolate purified AAV-2 has increased the feasibility of using AAV-derived vectors in gene therapy applications.

Recombinant adenovirus has also been used extensively in preclinical and clinical cancer gene therapy applications. Adenovirus virions are composed of a protein-only capsid consisting of three main proteins: the hexon, penton, and fiber. The hexon proteins compose the structural framework of the virion and the penton and fiber proteins compose the infectious machinery. The fiber proteins mediate the initial association with the membrane of the target cell, and the penton proteins mediate viral internalization by secondary interactions with specific membrane proteins such as integrins. The genome of the adenovirus is a single double-stranded DNA molecule of approx 36,000 basepairs. Once the adenovirus genome enters the nucleus of an infected cell, the viral DNA does not integrate into the cell's genome but replicates in an extrachromosomal state. A serious of "timed" transcription events occur that initiate formation of new virions. Several genes are initially transcribed, termed early genes, one of which is *E1A*. Because the function of *E1A* is to initiate transcription of other early genes, nonreplication competent recombinant adenoviruses were first generated by deleting *E1A* from the viral genome. The technology for generating recombinant adenoviruses has now advanced to the point at which most of the adenovirus genome is deleted and the genes necessary to encode a functionally infectious virion are supplied by a helper genome. By gutting the wild-type genome of all but regions necessary for replication and packaging, adenoviral vectors can accommodate extremely large nucleic acid sequences. For efficient packaging the adenoviral vector must be between 27,000 and 38,000 basepairs, which is sufficiently large for most gene transfer purposes. However, as described more fully below, the limiting aspect for using adenoviruses is the pronounced immunogenicity of the capsid proteins and the transient expression of the transferred gene. Initial administration of recombinant adenovirus generates immune responses that limit the effectiveness of subsequent virus administrations. Although not typically observed with the use of adenoviruses for the treatment of cancers, immune responses can be so significant as to result in severe complications.

There are a number of methods available to transfer therapeutic nucleic acid sequences into target cells. With respect to the clinical practice of gene therapy, although almost 20% of patients are treated using nonviral gene transfer methods, approx 35% of gene therapy protocols use recombinant retroviruses, and about 50% of patients in gene therapy trials are treated using recombinant retroviruses. Protocols using adenovirus constitute an additional 27% of gene therapy protocols, and 18% of patients in gene therapy trials receive recombinant adenovirus. Therefore, the majority of gene therapy is being conducted using recombinant viral gene transfer.

Phase III Studies in Cancer Gene Therapy

There were seven cancer gene therapy phase III studies posted worldwide as of September 2001. They can be segregated into two broad categories: (1) use of p53-expressing adenoviral vectors in combination with chemotherapy for treatment of ovarian, non-small-cell lung cancer (NSCLC) and squamous cell carcinoma of the head and neck (SCCHN) and (2) use of retroviral vectors encoding *HSVtk* for treatment of glioma. The latter strategy is the first cancer gene therapy biopharmaceutical that has completed scientific analysis and Phase III clinical trial scrutiny and will serve as a paradigm for discussion. The common denominator of all these approaches is the use of replication-defective viral vectors for tumor-targeted tumoricidal transgene delivery and sponsorship by large pharmaceutical interests.

HSVtk and Cancer Gene Therapy/HSVtk as a Tumoricidal Transgene

The "*suicide*" gene approach was originally developed to act as a fail-safe mechanism for replacement gene therapy. It was later reasoned that the same "*suicide*" gene, inserted into malignant cells, should also induce cell death when activated. The concept of suicide gene therapy is thus based on the paradigm that gene transfer can confer new properties to tumor cells, enabling them to activate a given prodrug. The best characterized and most widely used suicide gene is by far the *HSVtk* gene. It encodes a viral enzyme that converts the nontoxic guanosine analog ganciclovir (GCV) into a monophosphorylated metabolite, which is subsequently converted by cellular granylate kinases to a toxic triphosphorylated form. Because GCV is a relatively poor substrate for mammalian thymidine kinase, plasma concentrations can be achieved in vivo that are lethal to cells expressing the *HSVtk* gene but nontoxic to normal mammalian cells. Triphosphorylated GCV acts as a DNA polymerase inhibitor and a chain terminator, eventually leading to cell death. In vitro and in vivo treatment of *HSVtk*-positive tumor cells with GCV has also been shown to induce apoptosis and/or necrosis. Craperi et al. examined the molecular process leading to the in vitro cell death of C6 rat glioma expressing *HSVtk* following exposure to GCV. They demonstrated that GCV triggered cell cycle arrest in the S phase, which was followed by apoptosis. They found that this cytotoxic effect was independent of p53 and Bcl-xL expression, but associated with Bax induction. They showed that GCV treatment up-regulates the level of Bax protein. Given that Bax can antagonize the antiapoptotic protein Bcl-xL, it is conceivable that the balance between Bax and Bcl-xL may be a critical determinant. This is consistent with earlier observations that cell death could be inhibited by Bcl-2 expression.

Bystander Effect

Moolten and Wells demonstrated that tumor cells expressing the *HSVtk* gene could be killed in vitro and in vivo after administration of GCV. Freeman et al. further demonstrated that the toxic effect of GCV is not limited only to *HSVtk* gene modified tumor cells, but also affected adjacent nontransduced tumor cells. When a mixed population of tumor cells containing only 10% *HSVtk*-positive cells was exposed to GCV, the entire population was eradicated. This phenomenon, in which a minority of *HSVtk* expressing cells leads to the death and elimination of adjacent tumor cells not expressing *HS Vtk* is known as the "*bystander effect*".

Understanding the mechanism of this bystander effect is crucial because it would be almost impossible to gene modify all the cells of a tumor in vivo using available gene transfer techniques. When *HSVtk*-positive and -negative murine sarcoma cells were cultured in Transwell plates separated by a filter membrane, the bystander effect was abolished, suggesting that this phenomenon was dependent, in part, on cell--cell contact. In their autoradiography studies using [^{3}H]GCV, Bi et al. further showed in vitro the apparent cell to cell transfer of radioactivity that correlated with the observed bystander effect. Ishii- Morita et al. later demonstrated unequivocally the presence of the three phosphorylated metabolites of GCV in *HSVtk*-negative cells. Because different studies showed that phosphorylated GCV cannot pass through the cell membrane, this suggests that the bystander effect is dependent in part on intercellular communications through gap junctions. This is in accordance with other observations in different cell types that nonimmune bystander killing requires cell-to-cell contact through gap junctions.

Clearly, gap junctions play a crucial role in the bystander effect. However, it is obvious that other mechanisms are also involved in distinct cell types. There is evidence that the uptake of apoptotic vesicles by adjacent *HSVtk*-negative cells can lead to cell death. In another study, Princen et al. demonstrated that the transfer of filtered supernatant from *HSVtk*-positive DHD/K12 GCV-treated cells to *HSVtk*-negative cells killed these cells in a concentration-dependent manner, clearly evoking a gap junction independent bystander effect.

Immune bystander effect

If in vitro exposure of *HSVtk*-positive cells to GCV can induce apoptosis, several independent studies demonstrated, on the other hand, that different animal tumors expressing the *HSVtk* gene predominantly die by necrosis when GCV is administered in vivo. Vile et al. showed that in vivo GCV ablation of *HSVtk*-positive B16 murine melanoma cells converted the tumor in an immuno-stimulatory environment characterized by the induction of the cytokines interleukin-2 (IL-2), IL-12, interferon-γ (INF-γ), tumor necrosis factor-α (TNF-α), and GM-CSF accompanied by a pronounced tumor infiltrate consisting of macrophages as well as CD4$^+$ and CD8$^+$ T cells. Several other in vivo experiments with different cancer cell lines have also shown that the host immune system was implicated in the observed bystander effect. The current model is that rapid necrotic cell death of *HSVtk* cells after GCV administration can provide an initial stimulus for the recruitment of immune cells to the tumor site, leading to effective presentation of tumor antigens to immune cells infiltrating the tumor in response to the cytokines released. This immune bystander effect is not specific to *HSVtk* because it has also been described for another suicide gene, encoding for the *E. coli* cytosine deaminase, which activates 5-fluorocyto sine (5-FC). These observations suggest that "suicide" activity leads release of tumor antigens previously unrecognizable by immune cells and that these antigens are distinct from *HSVtk*. In sum, the "*bystander*" effect is dependent, in part, on: cell–cell contact; phagocytosis of gancyclovir phosphate laden cell debris; an antiangiogenic effect; cytokine-mediated hemorrhagic necrosis in local, but noncontiguous, tumor deposits; and immune recognition and rejection of tumor. $CD4^+$ lymphocytes, $CD8^+$ lymphocytes, natural killer (NK) cells, and antigen presenting cells take part in a tumor-specific immune response which is an important component of the local as well as the distant antitumor immune bystander effect.

Pros and Cons of Replication Defective Viral Vectors for Tumor-targeted Suicide Gene Delivery

As described earlier, viral vectors, such as adenoviral vectors and retroviral vectors, remain the most efficient and most studied means to introduce genetic material in tumor cells in vivo. This is usually achieved by direct intratumoral injection of viral particle suspension. Clinical trials examining the safety and utility of tumor-targeted gene delivery have been hampered by diametrically opposite problems depending on the gene vehicle used. First, as previously discussed, nonviral vectors are inefficient as tumor-targeted gene delivery vehicles in animals. Conversely, viral vectors, such as adenoviral vectors, are very potent for gene delivery. However, adenoviral vectors will efficiently modify cancer and normal tissue. This is of significant concern if toxic genes are delivered. Also, murine recombinant retroviruses modify only actively dividing cells, a characteristic of cancer cells, but their efficiency in doing so is very low. In sum, current technology for tumor-targeted gene delivery is plagued by nonspecific or inefficient gene delivery. Both scenarios may lead to either intolerable toxicity or ineffectiveness.

HSVtk Adenoviral Vectors: Trials and Tribulations

Replication-defective adenoviral vectors (AVs) are nonintegrating vectors that can infect both dividing and nondividing cells that express the coxsackie-adenoviral receptor (CAR). Among viral vector delivery platforms, adenoviruses are among the most studied because they can be concentrated to high titers ($>10^{10}$ pfu/mL), which facilitate pharmacological delivery of a large viral dose at tumor sites. AVs are very efficient at transducing normal tissue that express CAR and this can create problems when AVs encode for a toxic, "*cancer-killing*" transgene. Furthermore, first-generation AVs can evoke an early and late cellular and humoral reaction by the host that eventually leads to the elimination of all transduced cells—malignant and normal—by cytotoxic T lymphocytes and macrophages. This poses a formidable, even lethal, dose-limiting obstacle when AVs are given systemically for nonmalignant illnesses. The same problem may also arise in cancer therapy applications.

In brain cancer models, AVs can, however, disseminate and genetically modify contiguous normal brain cells. For instance, Dewey et al. have demonstrated that an adenovector coding for herpes simplex virus thymidine kinase (HSVtk) injected intratumorally in rodents with brain cancer led to regression of tumor following gancyclovir treatment. However, the "*cancer cured*" animals developed demyelinating encephalitis as a consequence of an immune reaction to AV-driven expression of HSVtk in normal neurons. Thus, the use of AVs may theoretically lead to toxicity in patients, limiting their application.

Phase I clinical trials using recombinant adenovirus to deliver the *HSVtk* gene were conducted in patients with advanced non-central nervous system (CNS) cancers revealed some systemic toxicities.

Delivery of the *HSVtk* gene by means of AVs was performed in 21 patients with malignant mesothelioma. The treatment consisted of a single intrapleural injection of AVs ranging from 1×10^9 to 1×10^{12} pfu followed by intravenous GCV twice daily for 14 d. Eleven patients out of 20 analyzed had evidence of *HSVtk* gene transfer in a dose-related fashion. Side effects reported included fever, anemia, transient liver enzyme elevations, and skin eruptions. A transient systemic inflammatory response was seen in all patients receiving the highest dosages. Three of the treated patients remained clinically stable for at least 26 mo after the trial. In a prostate cancer Phase I trial, 18 patients with local recurrence were intratumorally injected with *HSVtk* AVs ranging from 1×10^8 to 1×10^{11} pfu. Three patients were reported to have achieved an objective response (one for each of the highest dose levels). However, one patient developed reversible grade 4 thrombocytopenia and grade 3 hepatotoxicity at the highest dose level. Alvarez et al. reported the absence of dose-limiting toxicity when adenovectors encoding *HSVtk* (up to 10^{12} pfu) were injected intraperitoneally in women with recurrent ovarian cancer. It is conceivable that the peritoneal cavity is more tolerant of viral vectors compared to other closed compartments. In contrast to the above studies, Trask et al. treated 13 glioblastoma patients with a single intracranial injection of replication-defective adenoviral vectors (up to 10^{12} pfu) followed by intravenous injection of GCV. They observed a stabilization of the disease in one patient for at least 29 mo, while 11 patients died from tumor progression. Of note is that the highest dose treatment induced CNS toxicity with confusion and seizures in all patients. In sum, the use of adenovectors for in vivo gene delivery targeting normal or malignant tissue may be associated with significant side effects that can limit their clinical utility and the impetus to initiate Phase III studies.

HSVtk Retroviral Producer Cells as a Biopharmaceutical for Therapy of Gliomas

Recombinant retroviral vectors are well characterized as vehicles for tumor-targeted gene delivery. Moloney-based retroviruses can integrate only in cells undergoing mitosis. Because uncontrolled mitotic activity defines the basic nature of cancer, Moloney- based retrovectors are expected to restrict gene transfer to proliferating malignant cells when injected directly into a tumor mass. In contradistinction to adenovectors, quiescent cells—such as normal tissue adjacent to a targeted tumor deposit—will be refractory to retroviral gene transfer and spared from subsequent toxicity. The concept has been robustly validated, repeatedly, in animal models of cancer, including brain cancer. Further, experimental brain tumor implants consisting of a mixture of unmodified tumor cells with *HSVtk*-expressing cells will also regress following gancyclovir treatment without harm to adjacent normal tissue. Retroviral vectors have been extensively used in human clinical trials studying suicide gene delivery to malignant brain tumors, as discussed below. Limitations to the use of retroviruses are their inability to infect cells that do not express the retroviral receptor and the low particle concentration($< 10^6$ cfu/mL) in clinical grade viral preparations. The logistical impediment to low titer retroparticle delivery to tumor was addressed experimentally in clinical trials by injecting retroviral vector producing cells directly into glioma. The idea was that constant production of viral particles could transduce cancer cells more efficiently than low-titer, cell-free retrovector injections.

With this purpose at hand, Genetic Therapy Inc. developed a novel cancer gene therapy biopharmaceutical. The platform is based upon the PA317 retroviral packaging cell line originally designed by Miller et al. This cell line is derived from murine NIH3T3 cells transfected to express continuously the Moloney oncoretroviral gag-pol polyprotein as well as the MLV amphotropic envelope protein. These cells were subsequently transfected with a plasmid retroviral vector construct encoding for *HSVtk* within a replication-defective retroviral genome construct. A resulting retroviral producer clonal cell line (PA317/G1TkSvNa.53) was characterized and validated as a biopharmaceutical for clinical trials. This clonal vector producing cell (VPC) line was shown to generate a titer of 10^4–10^5 cfu/mL, which roughly translates to a few infectious retroviral particles generated per producer cell per day.

In 1997, Ram et al. published the results of a Phase I–II study in which 15 patients suffering from primary or metastatic brain cancer received up to 10^9 PA317/G1TkSvNa.53 VPCs intratumorally by computed tomography (CT)-guided stereotactic injections. All patients were given high-dose dexamethasone and GCV intravenously (5 mg/kg) for 2 wk following VPC injection. Four patients with radiological evidence of regression received a second treatment. Four patients had a PR that lasted from 4 to 11 wk, including one patient with apparent absence of any tumor growth for more than 2 yr after treatment. Two patients had elective resection of their VPC-injected glioma prior to GCV treatment. *In situ* hybridization for *HSVtk* mRNA on histological specimens revealed low-level gene transfer to tumor along needle tracks, especially in regions of angiogenesis where transduction of endothelial cells occurred, a phenomena also observed by others. Further, in some patients in whom a PR was noted in the injected lesion, other contemporaneous brain lesions continued to progress, suggesting that a distant bystander effect was absent. Interestingly, 10 of 15 patients developed humoral immunity to the VPCs. It was concluded that no safety hazards attributable to the use of xenogenic VPCs in brain tumor were identified.

An international Phase II study of VPCs for glioma was performed by the GLI328 European–Canadian Study Group and their results published in 1999. This group utilized an improved biopharmaceutical generated by Genetic Therapy Inc. The PA317/ G1TkSvNa.7 clonal producer (GLI-328) had a 100-fold higher titer than the VPCs used in the trial by Ram et al. An important clinical trial design distinction was the use of GLI328 immediately following surgical debulking of recurrent glioblastoma, as opposed to direct injection into unresected primary cancer. Following surgical removal of the tumor, 10^9 VPCs where injected in the resection cavity in as many as 60 distinct injection sites to ensure wide distribution of VPCs. GCV was given intravenously for 2 wk without systemic steroids. One patient remained disease-free 31 mo post-therapy; however 46 of 48 patients died of progressive disease or complications related to glioma. Interestingly, 17 patients tested polymerase chain reaction (PCR)-positive for vector sequences in peripheral blood leukocyte DNA, and all except one became negative at 12 mo post-therapy. As observed in the previous study, five patients developed an antiretrovector humoral response. The results were corroborated by the Study Group on Gene Therapy for Glioblastoma that explored the use of the conceptually related biopharmaceutical M11 HSVTK retroviral vector-producing cell line. In sum, 12 patients were enrolled in a Phase II study with a design similar to that of the GLI328 Study Group, and comparable conclusions of tolerability and a perception of improved survival was noted.

A Phase III randomized controlled trial of GLI-328 VPCs gene therapy was therefore initatied by the GLI328 International Study Group on 248 patients with previously untreated glioblastoma multiform and the results published in November 2000. Treatments consisted either of standard therapy alone—gross resection of tumor with radiation therapy—or standard therapy plus intratumoral implantation of *HSVtk* encoding VPCs followed by GCV administration. There was no severe neurological side effects during treatment, comparable to the previous Phase I–II studies. After more than 2 yr of follow-up, this extensive trial failed to show that the addition of VPC gene therapy provided any advantage in regard to tumor progression or overall survival. The median survival was 365 vs 354 d in the gene therapy and control groups, respectively. The main cause of failure of this therapeutic strategy is presumably low tumor gene transfer efficiency. A follow-up study performed on autopsy material collected from 32 patients determined that retroviral DNA was detected in 55% of brain tumor samples, albeit at a very low <0.03% transduction efficiency. As observed in the Phase II studies, vector DNA sequences were transiently detected in peripheral blood of nine patients, possibly from transduced lymphocytes at the time of implantation. Thus, the greatest impediment to retrovector VPCs suicide gene therapy seems to be the very low efficiency of in vivo gene transfer to cancer cells, possibly compounded by a specific immune response against VPCs. Although "suicide" retrovectors are "safe," implantation of VPCs as a means to deliver *HSVtk* to glioma is of limited efficacy. It remains to be seen whether the *HSVtk* gene—if it were delivered in a sufficiently high tumor fraction—will lead to a therapeutic effect following GCV administration in humans.

Failure Analysis

In a strictly formal sense, it is still unknown whether *HSVtk* gene expression in human cancer is of use or not. Until gene transfer efficiencies exceeding 10% are achieved in a tumor-restricted manner, this question will remain unanswered. Possible remedies likely lie in refinement of gene delivery platforms. Possible candidate remedies could include helper- dependent (gutless) adenoviral vectors or adeno-associated vectors that incorporate robust tumor-specific promoters; oncolytic viruses engineered to express an exogenous suicide gene, or even concentrated pseudotyped suicide retrovectors. Furthermore, the use of more potent suicide genes and clinically tolerable variants of GCV could be of use. In a sense, the issue of safe, high-efficiency and durable tumor-specific gene transfer is one that plagues the field of cancer gene therapy as a whole and is not solely an idiosyncratic problem of "*suicide*" gene therapy.

Of Mice and Men

Gene therapy readily and easily cures "*artificial*" cancers in inbred rodents. Unfortunately, the biology of spontaneous cancer in outbred mammals is very distinct, much to the regret of cancer gene therapists. The ability to deliver, the gene and the biology of the gene, once delivered, can be quite difficult to ascertain in clinical trials. Ethical considerations, such as repeated invasive biopsies and the like, markedly reduce our ability to perform failure analysis in humans suffering of cancer. Indeed, it has not always been clear which (or both) of the two has failed: inappropriate gene transfer or unsatisfactory anticancer transgene biology. Creative use of small mammals, such as cats and dogs, suffering from spontaneous malignancies may be a complementary and informative way of testing complex biopharmaceuticals such as gene therapy stratagems.

Roland Scollay, chief scientific officer of a california gene therapy company, shared his view that "...therapies going to the clinic are not always the very best available; rather, they are those for which licenses are held, another factor contributing to the high failure rate of gene therapy trials to date". Indeed, pressure to develop gene therapy for large-market indications (i.e., profitable), unrealistic appraisal of sometimes unproven intellectual property value, and the perverse effect of "*royalty stacking*" all conspire to a competitive rather than a cooperative spirit. This may, in part, explain the multiplicity of similar, ineffective and iterative early phase studies in cancer gene therapy. The societal aim of science—improvement of man's condition through reason—can be directly translated in the applied science that is gene therapy. Effective and safe cancer gene therapy biopharmaceuticals can be creatively developed only if there is ongoing cooperative arrangements between diverse interests: academic, medical, and commercial.

Vaccines for the Treatment of Cancer

The primary goal of cancer vaccines is to activate the immune system to eliminate tumor cells without affecting normal tissues. There are two major approaches to cancer immunotherapy: active immunotherapy and passive immunotherapy. Active immunotherapy involves the delivery of a substance designed to elicit an immune reaction. The host's immune system must first recognize and then respond to the target. Passive immunotherapy involves the delivery of a substance with intrinsic immunological activity such as an antibody or activated lymphocytes. This chapter focuses on the former approach. General strategies for vaccine development use either whole cell approaches or vaccines that are based on a specific tumor-associated antigen (TAA).

Cancer Vaccine Strategies

Whole Tumor Vaccines

Whole tumor cells (either autologous or allogeneic) rendered safe by radiation and often mixed with an immunological adjuvant were one of the earliest forms of active immunotherapy. Throughout the last five or more decades whole tumor cells have been used in clinical trials for a number of cancers particularly melanoma and renal and colorectal cancers.

In early studies whole tumor vaccines were often admixed with nonspecific adjuvants (e.g., bacillus Calmette-Guerin [BCG]) as initial attempts to immunize with irradiated autologous tumor cells were met with little success. Following these initial disappointments, new developments with cancer vaccines have led to a resurgence of interest. New technologies now allow for improved immunogenicity of vaccines genetically modified tumor cells to produce cytokines (interleukin [IL]-2, IL-4, tumor necrosis factor-α TNF-α), growth facto-- such as granulocyte colony-stimulating factor (G-CSF), T-cell costimulatory factors such as CD 80 and CD 86, or a combination thereof. This approach is known as ex vivo gene therapy.

Clinical trials of either autologous tumor cell preparations (from the patients own tumor cells) or allogeneic tumor cell preparations (human tumor cells from another individual or from cell lines) have been reported and results remain inconclusive.

With the scarcity of fresh autologous tumor material, a number of investigators began using allogeneic cell lines with more frequency. Despite attempts to match allogeneic cell lines in order to have the same HLA class I as autologous tumors, some studies revealed that allogeneic cell lines can confer and enhance antitumor activity compared with autologous cells. It was thought that perhaps the allogeneic cells may be inducing some form of graft vs tumor activity. A full understanding of inducing cross-reactive cytotoxic T-lymphocyte (CTL) response may lead to development of more effective allogeneic based vaccines strategy.

One major advantage to the whole tumor cell vaccine approach is that the preparations contain multiple undefined antigens and avoid the need for tumor antigen preselection. This approach increases the probability that the vaccine contains unidentified immunogenic antigens that are essential for vaccine activity. However, a major limitation to this approach is that there is a limited supply of vaccine product, limiting repeated treatments. The other disadvantage is that standardizing and characterizing the vaccine product may be problematic, expense is increased, and measuring vaccine-specific immune responses are difficult, if not impossible.

Despite these issues, there remain interesting positive clinical data and continued interest in the whole vaccine approach.

Hybrid cell fusion

Hybrid cell vaccination "*hybridoma*" is a novel approach aimed at recruiting T-cell help for the induction of tumor-specific cytolytic immunity. The patient's tumor cells are fused with allogeneic major histocompatibility class (MHC) II bearing cells. The theory is that the hybrid cells generated will display the full antigenicity of tumor cell and be highly immunogenic by the effect of those of the allogeneic MHC II and costimulatory contributed by the fusion partner cell. This concept has been tested in animal models for thymoma, hepatocellular carcinoma, and adenocarcinoma of various origins. Two small studies with metastatic melanoma and renal cell cancer patients demonstrated preliminary evidence of survival benefits with minimal toxic effects.

Dendritic cell vaccines

Antigen presentation is a crucial step in the initiation of an effective immune response, which requires antigens to be presented in order to sensitize naive T cells and to restimulate primed T cells.

The most efficient antigen presenting cell (APC) is the dendritic cell (DC). DCs are found in most tissues where they exist in an immature state, unable to stimulate T cells but possessing an exceptional ability to capture and process antigens. These captured antigens can be presented efficiently by both class I and class II MHC molecules. Antigen capture acts as a signal for the DC to mature and mobilize to regional lymph nodes. These cells undergo extensive transformation and antigen capturing decrease while T-cell stimulatory functions increase. The unique capacity of these "mature" DC cells to activate T cells is probably related to the presence of an exceptionally high number of MHC, costimulatory, and adhesion molecules.

Sufficient DCs can now be generated ex vivo using DC growth factors such as GM-CSF and flt-3 ligand. The concept of hybridomas has been applied to DC therapy whereby tumor cells have been infused with DCs to create an APC full of tumor antigens. Adoptive transfer of autologous or allogeneic DCs pulsed or loaded with tumor antigens prior to reinfusion are now entering clinical trials. In one study that was recently updated, patients with B-cell lymphoma were vaccinated with idiotype-pulsed DCs cellular and immune responses were noted.

The optimal method to load DC with antigens such as tumor-specific peptides, protein, mRNA, or apoptotic or necrotic cells is currently an area of intensive investigation. DCs can be genetically modified with genes encoding tumor antigens (and/or cytokines). Tumor antigen expression within the DCs should provide the cells with a renewable source of antigen for presentation, and, consequently, more sustained antigen presentation. Recombinant viruses, including adenoviruses and retroviruses, can be used to transduce DCs. Although transduction through this method is highly effective, the expression of viral genes may occur. These viral genes may prime antiviral immunity including cytotoxic T-cell lysis, which in turn may rapidly destroy the DCs in subsequent rounds of immunization. Several murine models have shown that preexisting immunity does not prevent successful immunization with adenoviral infected DCs. However, there are new vectors ("gutless adenovirus") that don't express viral gene products. In pilot clinical studies in patients with non-Hodgkin's lymphoma, myeloma, and melanoma, vaccination with DC vaccination induced both antitumor immune responses and tumor regression.

Tumor-Associated Antigen (TAA)

Potential advantages of vaccines that are directed against a specific TAA include immune responses that can be reliably measured, standardization in vaccine production, and minimized nonspecific immune activation. The development of TAA-directed vaccine involves identification of a target antigen and selection of a platform (e.g., proteins, peptides, carbohydrates, and DNA-or virus-based vectors) for presentation to the immune system. Potential target candidates are antigens that are expressed only on tumor cells or only those that are relatively overexpressed on tumor cells compared to normal cells. Very few antigens are truly tumor specific to a particular patient's tumor. Some may be limited in expression to a particular tumor type while others have a wide expression on a variety of different tumor types. Molecular techniques such as SERAX analysis, microarrays, serial analysis of gene expression (SAGE), and differential displays have been used recently to identify new antigen targets for vaccine targeting.

Vector-driven TAAs

TAAs are by definition either weakly immunogenic or functionally nonimmunogenic. Vaccine strategies must be developed in which the presentation of these TAAs to the immune system results in far greater activation of T cells than is being achieved naturally in the host. One way to increase the immunogenicity of a TAA is to use a viral vector to deliver the appropriate genetic material. The advantages of using a viral vector include (1) the incorporation of the entire tumor antigen gene, parts of that gene, or multiple genes (including genes for costimulatory molecules and cytokines); (2) the ability of selected vectors to infect APCs allowing them to process the antigens; and (3) the relative cost of viral vector vaccines is low compared with preparation and purification of proteins. Overcoming tolerance to carcinoembryonic antigen (CEA) in CEA transgenic mice was not accomplished with a peptide-based vaccine but was relatively easily accomplished with a vaccinia CEA construct.

Types of vectors

Viral vectors can be divided into those that are capable of replicating in mammalian species and those that can infect mammalian cells but cannot complete the replication process. There are advantages and disadvantages to each. Some of the viruses that can are replication competent have been extensively studied and have well-defined safety profile. These vectors can continue to infect additional cells, producing more TAA until eradicated by the immune system. Often vaccines associated with these cells are more immunogenic than those using replication-defective vectors. The replication-defective vectors, however, are in theory safer as they can infect mammalian cells only once and therefore cannot cause the rare but in immunocompromised individuals, the potentially life-threatening conditions associated with replication-defective vectors such as vaccinia. One group of vectors extensively studied in tumor vaccines are the pox viruses. These viruses have several advantages including the ability to make stable recombinant vectors with accurate replication and efficient posttranslational processing of the transgene. In addition, as many as seven transgenes have been expressed in a single vaccinia vector, making these potentially powerful tools for vaccine gene delivery.

Replication competent vectors

One of the most studied pox viral vectors is vaccinia. This virus has been used since 1796 to vaccinate against smallpox, with more than a billion doses given worldwide. The success of this vaccine in eradiating this disease has led to the discontinuation of the vaccination to the general population. Early of recombinant vaccinia viruses containing human immunodeficiency virus (HIV) transgenes revealed that vaccinia naïve patients had higher antigen specific T-cell responses and antibody responses to a vaccinia vaccine than patients previously vaccinated with vaccinia. Subsequent studies have demonstrated that significantly higher doses (e.g., 10^8 *plaque-forming units* [PFU]) of vaccinia vector given to patients could induce a vigorous response to the transgene. A trial with 26 patients who had advanced colon carcinoma demonstrated a recombinant vaccinia CEA (rV-CEA) vaccine given monthly for 3 mo was well tolerated by patients. While there were no clinical responses observed, this was the first demonstrate generation of a human cytolytic T-cell response to specific epitopes of CEA. Other trials with rV-CEA also showed lack of toxicity, antibody responses, and apparent equivalence of subcutaneous and intradermal injections.

These trials and pre-clinical models demonstrated that further increases in antigen specific immune responses were limited after the second and third vaccination, presumably due to the vigorous immune response to the vaccinia proteins. Avipox vectors, which do not express the late viral antigens in mammalian cells, and thus are replication defective in humans, do not have a significant immune response generated to them. Thus trials using heterologous prime and boost strategies were developed with recombinant vaccinia vectors and recombinant avipox vectors.

Replication-defective vector

Avipox vectors, which do not express the late viral antigens in mammalian cells and thus are replication defective in humans, do not have a significant immune response generated against them. Thus trials using heterologous prime and boost strategies were developed with recombinant vaccinia vectors and recombinant avipox vectors.

Avipox vectors are capable of infecting human cells and expressing their transgene for up to 3 wk before cell death ensues. Avipox vectors include fowlpox and canarypox (ALVAC). Clinical trials with these vectors have shown that these can be given numerous times with a resulting increase in

CEA-specific T-cell responses. To take advantage of the potency of vaccinia-based vaccines and the lack of immunogenicity of the avipox-based vaccines, prime and boost strategies were developed. In an effort to determine which heterologous prime and boost regimen to use, a small randomized trial was conducted looking at either giving the rV-CEA as the initial priming vaccination followed by boosting with avipox-CEA (VAAA), or giving the three vaccinations with avipox-CEA first followed by rV-CEA (AAAV). This study showed that the immune responses seen in the VAAA arm were much better than in the AAAV arm. Furthermore, continued follow-up of these patients revealed that although there were only nine patients in each arm, at the time of a recent presentation five or nine patients were alive on the VAAA arm (2-yr survival estimate 67 ± 19%) whereas in the AAAV arm zero of nine patients were alive (2-yr survival estimate 0 ± 0%). An ongoing randomized Phase II clinical trial has demonstrated that rV-prostate-specific antigen (rV-PSA) admixed with rV-B7.1 followed by monthly rF-PSA can generate PSA-specific T-cell responses and, in one patient, a sustained PSA decrease from 8.7 ng/dL at the start of the study to 0.19 ng/dL.

Pharmacodynamics: Immunological Endpoints

A number of different vaccine strategies that activate T-cell responses are now being investigated in clinical trials to evaluate the role of immunotherapy as a modality of antitumor therapy. Examples of these approaches include the use of TAAs such as CEA, PSA, and MUC-1, either as full proteins delivered in viral vectors or as peptide pulsed dendritic cells. Other well known characterized antigens used in cancer vaccine clinical trials include MART-1, gp100, MAGE-1, tyrosinase, and HER2/neu. It is crucial to evaluate the relative effects of these vaccines on the immune system, in order to develop more potent vaccines that may be used in patients with earlier stages of disease and to combine with other traditional therapeutic modalities such as chemotherapy and/or radiation therapy.

Immune activity can be evaluated by specific responses involving both cell-mediated and humoral immunity. Cell-mediated immunity in general refers to the production of CTL responses against the tumor that the vaccine specifically targets. This involves $CD8^+$ T cells along with mature $CD4^+$ T-helper cells, type 1 (Th1) cells. On the other hand, assays measuring humoral immunity involve antibody production from mature B cells along with B cells that are in part induced by mature $CD4^+$ T-helper cells, type 2 (Th2) cells.

The optimal vaccination strategy in humans using specific TAAs against tumors expressing the antigen won't be determined until large multiarm clinical trials correlating survival, disease-free interval, or tumor regression are completed. In the absence of such data, immunoassays (both T-cell-mediated immunity and antibody-based) may be useful to help define: (1) if a given vaccine can elicit any immune response and (2) the relative potency of such a response.

Delayed-Type Hypersensitivity Testing (DTH)

DTH is performed by injecting a soluble protein antigen of interest subcutaneously and measuring the area of induration 48–72 h after the antigen has been administered. It is a technically simple test that reflects the development of systemic antigen-specific immunity. Although it has been used commonly to study infectious disease models, such as tetanus toxoid, the significance of this assay is still debatable as a tool for measuring tumor-specific immune responses. It has been shown that selected cancer patients who are anergic to common immunogens by DTH can mount immunologic responses to TAAs. However, recent studies seem to suggest that the DTH response is an accurate indicator of a patient's T-cell response, at least in some populations. Disis et al. looked for the development of tumor antigen-specific DTH responses, using HER-2/neu peptides as the model antigen in patients with advanced stage cancer to test if they would correlate to in vitro measurements of systemic antigen-specific T-cell responses as measured by lymphocytic proliferation. The authors demonstrated that tumor antigen-specific DTH

responses ≥ 10 mm^2 correlate significantly to a measurable antigen-specific peripheral blood T-cell response.

Limiting Dilution Assay

Early immunologic monitoring methods to determine precursor frequency analysis of CTL to a particular immunogen were labor intensive and required numerous in vitro stimulations (IVS) of the cell lines. The limiting dilution assay (LDA) was used most frequently. In a recent CEA vaccine clinical trial described by Marshall et al., LDAs were used to determine the CTL precursor frequency to CEA peptide-1 in the prevaccination and postvaccination peripheral blood mononuclear cells (PBMCs) from HLA-A2-positive patients. However, this assay is extremely time consuming and labor intensive. Various numbers of PBMCs were seeded into 96-well flat-bottom plates, with autologous irradiated PBMCs and incubated with. At least 48 cultures were used in this study for each dilution of PBMCs. The 5 d of incubation with peptide plus the 11 d with IL-2 constituted one in vitro stimulation cycle. After two in vitro stimulation cycles, the CTL activity was tested for each well against C 1R-A2 target cells with and without incubation with CAP-1, using the procedure described earlier, with unlabeled K562 cells added to each assay at a ratio of 10 unlabeled K562 cells to one target cell, to eliminate the natural killer cell activity.

Precursor frequencies were calculated by χ^2 minimization, as described by Taswell et al. Individual counts obtained from each experimental well were compared with the mean counts from the controls on the same plate. LDAs of PBMCs were conducted to quantitate CEA-specific CTL precursors before and after each vaccination per patient. CTL activity that was greater than the mean plus three SDs of the control wells was considered significant.

Enzyme-Linked Immunosorbent Assay (ELISA)

Other methods such as cytokine production assays by ELISA measure cytokine production of mixed-cell populations. Cytokine production by T cells undergoing in vitro stimulation is considered a well accepted measure of T-cell activation. Various cytokines such as interferon-γ (IFN-γ), IL-2, and TNF-α have been used to monitor numerous tumor immunotherapy studies. Increase levels of IFN-γ and IL-2 would suggest an increase in CTL activity. However, the standard ELISA assay measures overall cytokine levels, which may vary considerably. This assay does not provide a quantitative measurement of TAA-specific T-cells.

Tetramers

Newer techniques for analysis of specific T-cell responses to vaccines include tetramers and the Fast Immune assay. Tetramers allow for the identification of a specific T-cell type. Tetramers have been widely used to quantify the number of viruses and bacteria-specific T cells in animal models. However, this technique can be cumbersome, requiring the preparation and purification of a tetramer for each peptide evaluated. Although tetramers have been developed to several epitopes of human TAAs to phenotype T-cell populations pre- and postvaccination, their sensitivity has not yet been established as an assay to evaluate cancer vaccines.

Fast Immune

The intracellular cytokine Fast Immune assay can be used to phenotype T-cell responses from vaccinated patients. This technique incorporates the use of cell flow cytometry to detect intracellular or cell-associated cytokines and allows the examination of multiple cytokines within individual cells. Careful comparison of this assay with the enzyme-linked immunospot (ELISPOT) assay has determined that the sensitivity of this assay is similar to that of the ELISPOT. However, the cost of second antibody reagents and extended fluorescence-activated cell sorter (FACS) scanning time make this assay more expensive and time consuming as compared to the ELISPOT assay.

ELISPOT Assay

The ELISPOT assay is relatively sensitive and quantitative. By measuring cytokine release on a single-cell basis, the assay can detect a peptide-specific T-cell response against specific HLA class I binding peptides. The level of cytotoxicity determined by the standard chromium release assay after in vitro expansion of specific T cells has been shown to correlate with the number of IFN-γ releasing cells measured by the ELISPOT assay in a study of both healthy donors and melanoma patients.

The ELISPOT assay without IVS has been used to monitor two different types of CEA-based cancer-vaccine trials. These trials showed that the ELISPOT assay can be performed with previously frozen PBMCs from HLA-A2–positive patients as a source of T cells. C1RA2 cells were used as APCs and were pulsed with Flu matrix peptide and a CEA 9-mer peptide.

However, most studies to date have required in vitro stimulations of PBMCs with peptide and IL-2 to monitor immune responses to TAAs. A number of variables may alter the results of the ELISPOT assay. The APCs used to conduct the assay may vary. An HLA-A2–positive, Tap-defective T2 cell line has been used by others as the APC. One of the problems reported with T2 cells is the potential for high backgrounds, possibly due to alloreactivity of residual MHC I expression. Other studies have used autologous PBMCs for peptide presentation. However, autologous PBMCs may not be the ideal APC with which to perform the ELISPOT assay in cancer patients, owing to shifts from the Thl to Th2 subset. In our previous study we used the C1RA2 cell line to circumvent the use of possible defective APCs in cancer patients. Other issues such as the weak signal 1 of the TAAs and the limited number of PBMCs also can contribute to the lack of detection of potential immune responses.

Drug Development Issues Associated with Vaccines

Schedule of Administration

Although there has been an explosion of new cancer vaccines being tested in clinical trials, there has been little focus in these trials on the schedule of administration. Because the primary goal of noncancer vaccines is prevention of disease, there is little pressure to create a rapid, powerful immune response. Instead, there is time for priming and boosting over months to years. In contrast, most of the vaccines being tested today for cancer treatment are used in patients with advanced cancer who frequently have rapidly growing, refractory disease. In this patient population, time is of the essence as these patients will have demonstrated progression of their tumors in a very short time (6–12 wk) if effective therapy is not given. By convention, if patients do progress in this time frame, they are removed from the study as treatment failures.

Conventional chemotherapy is given in "cycles," which are typically 3–4 wk long. In the case of cytotoxic agents, the treatment is given and then time away from treatment is built in to allow for recovery from the toxic effects of the treatment. The effects of the chemotherapy are seen acutely, with the antitumor responses observed during the first few treatments. If responses are not seen in the first two or three cycles, then the treatment is unlikely to be of benefit and treatments are stopped and/or changed. However, none of this applies to vaccines. First, we have a very poor understanding of the timing of an optimum immune response. There are no objective data that guide us in deciding when we have achieved an "effective" level of activity, which of course is complicated further by the various ways of measuring an immune response, different types of vaccines, and different vaccination schedules employed. What is an effective/adequate level of T cells, antibodies, and so forth when seeking an anticancer response? How does the time course of an immune response vary when using a viral vector based vaccine compared to a DC approach, and how do cytokines influence this? Should we be giving these vaccines weekly, monthly, or every 3 mo? The truth is that we have very limited insights into the answers to these quite fundamental questions.

Arguably, we do not have the answers to these questions when initially testing novel chemotherapy, but these agents commonly result in toxicity and clinical responses that guide us in designing optimum administration schedules. In the case of cancer vaccines, the absence of toxicity, objective clinical responses, and validated intermediate immune endpoints makes this very difficult. Furthermore our ignorance increases the risk of rejecting a vaccinen not because it does not have potential clinical utility, but because we do not know how to evaluate it's effects properly.

The majority of trials have used an every 2- to 4-wk vaccine administration schedule, often with vaccines given close together at first and then spreading out the subsequent boosting treatments. Some trials have given only a fixed number of vaccines and then stopped, regardless of treatment outcomes. Virtually all of these schedules were designed with regard to convenience, convention, and "best guess" and not based on a firm understanding of the immune response. Of course none of this would matter if frequent anticancer responses were observed in these trials, but unfortunately responses have not been routinely observed. Many vaccines have already been abandoned from further development owing to lack of clinical activity but without a clear understanding concerning the level at which they failed (immune response, administration schedule, dose).

Future vaccine trials must begin to address the issue of administration schedule. To do this, incorporate the best immune monitoring available, optimize the patient selection, and we must test various schedules early in the agent's development. The topic of immune monitoring is covered elsewhere in this chapter, but its importance cannot be overstated. Without the ability to measure a biologic response (specific or nonspecific), we will continue to "*fly blind*" in our trial designs and conclusions. Optimizing patient selection is critical. The current standard to test vaccines in patients with refractory, advanced cancer adds to our problems. These are not the best patients on whom to test immune-based therapies. These patients have frequently received multiple chemotherapy treatments that might interfere with the immune response, they have larger tumor burdens against which the immune response must fight, and the shortened life expectancy these patients experience limits our ability to understand the long-term effects of these therapies. While it remains extremely important to continue to test novel vaccine approaches in patients with metastatic disease in the hopes of uncovering significant anticancer activity in this patient population, it is also important to recognize that the ultimate target population for these types of therapies is likely to be a much earlier stage patient. Performing early phase clinical trials in patients such as this, however, is more expensive and in some ways riskier. Examples of patients currently being accrued to these types of trials are colon cancer patients following resection of metastases (CALGB 89903), patients with high-risk prostate cancer, and high-risk breast cancer patients (Her-2 based vaccines). Although the results of these studies take longer to mature they are extremely important and worth the wait.

Combination Therapies Utilizing Vaccines

There is a great deal of excitement about cancer vaccines in clinical trials today, we must recognize that there have only been limited positive objective clinical responses in these studies. At the same time there have been anecdotal reports of clinical activity and frequent reporting of positive immune responses. Based on this it is logical to consider combining vaccine-based approaches with other anticancer treatments in the hopes of capitalizing on the advantages of each approach. The most commonly utilized and most successful form of cancer therapy is cytotoxic chemotherapy. The rationale for combining cytotoxic chemotherapy with immune-based approaches includes evidence supporting a lessening of immune suppression with the potential for enhancing the overall immune response, and the potential that chemotherapy will add to the overall clinical response and allow for adequate disease control to enable the immune system to mount an effective response. However, this approach has been tempered by the unknown impact of chemotherapy on the ability to mount an immune response in general. Preclinical and clinical studies experiments have demonstrated that chemotherapy can modulate the immune response to include enhancement of T-cell activity, tumor vaccines, and macrophages. Machiels et al. demonstrated a positive impact of "*immune modulating doses*" of cyclophosphamide, doxorubicin, and paclitaxel on the immune response (as measured by ELISPOT and tumor rejection) independent of the cytotoxic anticancer activity of the chemotherapeutic agents alone. In another preclinical trial combining an peptide- based vaccine and 5-fluorouracil (5-FU)/leucovorin chemotherapy, Watson et al. demonstrated that the chemotherapy had no effect on the generation of vaccine-specific antibodies and the combination actually had an increased therapeutic effect on tumors in the mouse xenograft model.

A series of small clinical trials testing nonspecific immune enhancers (IFN-α, BCG, etc.) in combination with chemotherapy demonstrated no detectable inhibition of the immune responses or clinical outcomes. Several larger clinical trials have been performed combining immune-based approaches with chemotherapy. The largest of these utilized a monoclonal antibody combined with 5-FU-based chemotherapy in the adjuvant setting. This trial was negative and it is unclear whether these results are reflective of an agent that is inactive or a trial design that failed to recognize the potential negative interaction between chemotherapy and immune-based therapies. Recently a Phase II randomized trial was performed in metastatic pancreas cancer utilizing a vaccine alone compared to patients being treated with the combination of gemcitabine and vaccine. In this study the chemotherapy did not have a negative influence on the immune response as measured by the detection of target-specific antibodies. Other trials are underway combining vaccines with chemotherapy, many of which with little data to support a positive interaction between the two classes of compounds. When designing trials such as this, the importance of solid preclinical data supporting the combination cannot be underestimated. Future studies should emphasize chemotherapy doses and schedules to optimize the direct anticancer effects and immune modulatory effects of the chemotherapy–vaccine combinations.

Regulatory Issues for Vaccine-Based Clinical Trials

The last decade of clinical research has been marked by a dramatic increase in regulatory requirements for all trials involving investigational agents, and this increase may have been most dramatic for the so-called "*biologic therapies.*" These agents include viruses, gene therapies, protein therapies, and other "natural" products and, of course, virtually all immune-based therapies fall into one of these categories.

Institutional review board review

Typically, there are no unusual requirements in obtaining IRB approval for these classes of compounds. However, with a heightened awareness of and concern about these agents following a few highly publicized problems with trials using biologic therapies, IRB reviews have become more critical, requiring more safety data and tighter controls on all aspects of the trials. These issues should be accounted for in the writing and design of all trials but are particularly important for biologic agents. In specific, great attention should be focused on the consent form, eligibility criteria, drug storage and handling, and clear reviews of all the known preliminary data that exist supporting the trial and its design.

Institutional biosafety reviews

The first additional step in the review process for virus- and gene-based therapies is a review by an institution's biosafety committee. The primary purpose of this review is to focus on the proper handling of potentially hazardous biologic products, ensuring that patients and staff are adequately protected from exposure, and that proper documentation is on file detailing the agents in question. This is a frequently overlooked step by investigators and protocol administrators. Often, information requested is not found in investigators' brochures (such as vector maps) but must be obtained and provided. Obviously, different institutions require different information as they interpret the regulations provided by government agencies, so as with all regulatory steps, it is best and most efficient to discuss this early in the process.

Federal review

Protocols that include gene therapy all must be reviewed at the federal level by two institutions. As with any investigational agent, the US Food and Drug Administration (FDA) must be involved through either the filing of an Investigational New Drug Application (IND) or the cross-filing to an existing IND. In addition, the protocol must be reviewed by the Recombinant DNA Advisory Committee (RAC), a review group that is responsible for tracking all gene-based therapies in the United States. The RAC was established in 1974 and its major role is to review trials that involve the transfer of recombinant DNA to humans. Currently, the RAC reviews only those trials in which NIH funding is involved. Compliance at the institutional level is the responsibility of the Institutional Biosafety Committees. In summary, vaccines for the treatment of cancer are an attractive therapeutic adjunct to standard chemotherapy because it represents non-cross-resistant therapy that adds minimal additional toxicities. Currently there are a number of clinical trials using novel vaccine designs and administration that hold promise for the future. However, a considerable amount of work is still required to optimize vaccination regimens, combine vaccines with other cancer treatment modalities, vaccinate populations with early stage disease, and define the most intermediate endpoint assays. The FDA and the public may need to judge whether prolonged time to relapse in the absence of survival difference will justify the approval of vaccines for routine care.

16

ONCOLOGY DRUG DEVELOPMENT

Drug development and clinical trial structure functions most efficiently when based on pharmacometric (PM) knowledge. PM knowledge comes from outstanding data, and when it is interpreted in light of development goals and other knowledge, then an understanding is gained of the direction that future development ought to take. In the current drug development climate volumes of data are generated but little emphasis is placed on knowledge generation and therefore the direction that drug development should take is ambiguous. Poor decision-making is supported by the fact that the cost of introducing a drug to market in 2001 was $802 million and the time for a drug to reach market was 7–12 yr with the execution of more than 60 clinical trials. The process of knowledge discovery when applied to PM model development ensures that information embedded in the data is thoroughly understood and apporopriately applied. Modern data analysis methods and modern statistical software such as S-Plus have revolutionized the manner in which PM analyses can be performed.

PM KNOWLEDGE DISCOVERY (PHARKNOWDISC)

PM knowledge is best extracted from data when the knowledge discovery process is applied to its generation. Knowledge discovery has been defined as the search for relationships and global patterns that exist in large data sets but are "hidden" among the vast amounts of data. PM modeling, especially population PM modeling, is itself a process of knowledge discovery from the population PM data set. When applied to PM modeling, knowledge discovery incorporates all steps taken from data assembly to the development of the PM model to the reporting of the results. Knowledge discovery exists at the intersection of computer science (database, artificial intelligence, graphics, and visualization), statistics, and several application domains such as clinical pharmacology in general and PM in particular. Some modern graphical and statistical procedures useful in PHARKNOWDISC include histograms with density plots, pairs plots, multiple linear regression (MLR), generalized additive modeling (GAM), box plots, nonparametric smooth plots, and tree models. Knowledge discovery from a large PM data set is a process that can be formalized into a number of steps. In brief, these steps are as follows:

1. Defining or stating the objective of the PHARKNOWDISC process.
2. Creating a data set on which PHARKNOWDISC will be performed. (Data preparation is a very critical in the PHARKNOWDISC. Sometimes more effort can be expended in preparing data than in analysis.)
3. Data quality analysis (i.e., cleaning and processing the data.
4. Data structure analysis, exploratory examination of raw data (dose, exposure, response, and covariates) for hidden structure, and the reduction of the dimensionality of the covariate vector.

5. Determining the basic PM model that best describes the data and generating *post hoc* empiric individual Bayesian parameter estimates.
6. Searching for patterns and relationships between parameters and covariates through graphical displays and visualization.
7. Exploratory modeling using modern statistical modeling techniques such as MLR, GAM, cluster analysis, and tree-based modeling (TBM) to reveal structure in the data and initially select explanatory covariates.
8. Consolidating the discovered knowledge in item 7 into an irreducible form, that is, developing a population pharmacokinetic/pharmacodynamic model, using the nonlinear mixed effects modeling approach.
9. Determining model robustness through sensitivity analysis, examination of parametric/ nonparametric standard errors, stability checking with or without predictive performance depending on the objective of the PHARKNOWDISC.
10. Interpreting the results: the PHARKNOWDISC process prescribes that the model developedis interpreted in a relational manner. That is, do the findings of the PHARKNOWDISC make sense in the domain in which they will be used? Can the results be communicated in a manner that they can be used? Only if they make sense can the results be considered as "knowledge".
11. Applying (or utilizing) the discovered knowledge. The pragmatic view of knowledge implies that the results of the PHARKNOWDISC process must have some impact on the way individuals act. Thus, the discovered knowledge must be applied to demonstrate how it can be used.
12. Communicating the discovered knowledge.

The PM knowledge discovery process must be focused. Having a clearly defined objective for the process greatly influences the remainder of the steps. For instance, the choice of data set(s) to be used in the PM knowledge discovery process is determined by the objective that prompts the process.

LEARN: CONFIRM-LEARN APPROACH TO DRUG DEVELOPMENT

The drug development process is governed by one's philosophy of the process, which in turn will affect one's attitude and approach to both the macro-strategy and any individual study. A very useful and promising philosophy of drug development has been described by Sheiner, termed the learn–confirm approach. Sheiner contends that drug development ought to consist of alternating elements of learning from experience and then confirming what has been learned. One ought always to be interested in learning, even when confirming is the primary objective of a study; therefore, we have modified the terminology slightly by naming the second phase confirm-learn.

The earliest parts of the process of clinical drug development ought to emphasize learning but later stages will, by their nature, emphasize the confirm–learn type of study and analysis. Thus, learning and confirming become a part of each clinical trial although their relative emphasis changes as the drug progresses toward approval. Although learning and confirming can be performed to varying degrees on the same data set, their goals are quite different. Clinical trial structures that optimize confirming often impair learning. The focus of commercial drug development on confirmation is understandable, as this immediately precedes and justifies regulatory approval. However, the focus on confirming has led to a low level of learning that has in turn resulted in drug development that is most often inefficient and inadequate.

Learning has as its objective answering many questions such as the relationship among dose, prognostic variables, and outcome. Learning is often model based and focuses on building a model between outcome and many variables such as dosing strategy, exposure, patient type, and prognostic variables. The model that is built here is the defining of the response surface. The response surface can be thought of as three-dimensional. On one axis are the input variables (controllable factors) such as dosage regimen and concurrent therapies. Another axis incorporates patient characteristics, which summarizes all the important ways patients can differ that affect the benefit to toxicity ratio. The final axis represents the benefit to toxicity ratio. Sheiner has stated, "... the real surface is neither static, nor is all information about a patient conveyed by his initial prognostic status, nor are exact predictions possible. A realistically useful response ... must include the elements of variability, uncertainty and time ...". The response surface deals with a complex of relationships to answer the question of what is the relationship between input profile and dose magnitude to beneficial and harmful pharmacological effects and how does this relationship vary with individual patient characteristics and time to explain tolerance or sensitivity? For rational drug development and the optimization of individual therapy, this response surface must be mapped for the target population. These models then allow extrapolation beyond the immediate study subjects to predict the effects of competing dosing strategies, patient type selection, competing study structures, and endpoints; they therefore aid in the construction of future studies. One important feature of model-based learning is that models increase the signal-to-noise ratio because they can translate some of the noise in a data set to signal. This is important because the information content of a data set is proportional to the signal-to- noise ratio. For the learning study, which attempts to define the dose–concentration–effect model, pharmacokinetics (PK) delineates the dose–concentration component and pharmacodynamics (PD) defines the concentration–effect component of the model.

In contrast, the goal of confirming is to falsify the hypothesis that efficacy is absent and the only question that it aims to answer is, Is the null hypothesis true or false? Therefore, factors that increase learning such as administering differing dose levels and enrolling subjects who differ with regard to demographics and disease state are often eliminated from confirming studies. Confirming studies proceed by contrasting the average outcomes between two study groups.

PHARMACOMETRICS

Pharmacometrics (PM) has been defined as the science of developing and applying mathematical and statistical methods to characterize, understand, and predict a drug's pharmacokinetic and pharmacodynamic behavior; quantify uncertainty of information about that behavior; and rationalize knowledge-driven decision-making in the drug development process. PM is dependent on knowledge discovery; the application of informative graphics; and an understanding of bio-markers/surrogate endpoints. When applied to drug development, PM often involves the development or estimation of pharmaco-kinetic, pharmacodynamic, pharmaco-dynamic-outcomes linking, and disease progression models. These models can be linked and applied to competing study designs to aid in understanding the impact of varying dosing strategies, patient selection criteria, different study endpoints, varying study structure, and so forth on the final study results.

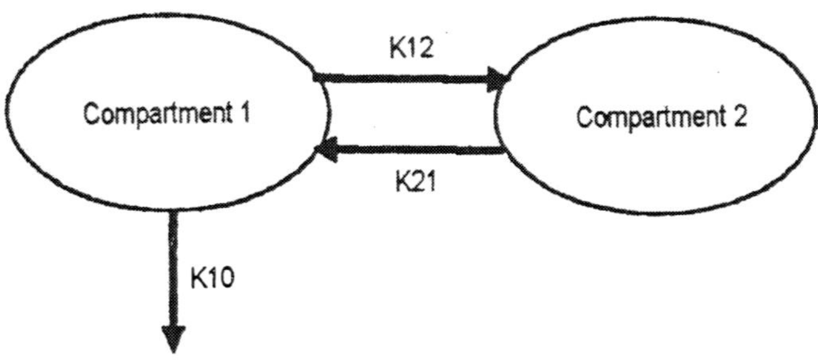

Fig. 16.1. A diagrammatic example of a two-compartment pharmacokinetic model.

Pharmacokinetics

Pharmacokinetics (PK) is the estimation and development of mathematical models that describe the time course of drug and metabolite levels in various regions of a subject's body as a function of some drug input function, most often route and dose. PK models can be characterized as compartmental, noncompartmental, linear, and nonlinear. PK models are often described with figures illustrating the location of each compartment, as a geometric shape, and drug movement between compartments represented by arrows. Most models are parametrized in terms of clearances, apparent volumes, and rate constants; other models may not be founded on compartments; and still others may be physiologically based. Once data are assembled, the PK modeler determines which model best describes the data, which may involve the determination of the number of compartments that should be applied to the model or whether the model follows dose-dependent PK. These models can then be used to estimate the expected drug levels that would be the result of competing dosing strategies. PK models have their greatest utility when they are employed in conjunction with pharmacodynamic models.

Pharmacodynamics

Pharmacodynamic (PD) models are mathematical representations of the relationship between either the drug input function (dose and route) or the measured drug concentration and time, and some response variable (biomarker or surrogate) such as granulocyte count or tumor load. When selecting a PD model one must address:

1. What shape is the drug level–response relationship?
2. What are the response kinetics?
   (a) How long does the response take to develop (i.e., reach steady state for a given drug input/concentration); Is the PD effect immediate, delayed, or cumulative?
   (b) How long does the response last after the drug is discontinued?
3. Should the response be related to drug dose or concentration?
4. Which mathematical description best describes the relationship between the input function and the response variable?
5. Should the PD model be derived from known underlying mechanisms of action or estimated by empirical functions?
6. Are there time-varying (circadian) or state-varying (tolerance, induction) factors that affect the response?
7. Does the baseline effect need to be included in the model?

Commonly employed time-invariant PD models include the linear model (Eq. 1), the simple E_{max} model (Eq. 2), and the sigmoid E_{max} model (Hill equation, Eq. 3). More recently, indirect pharmacologic response models have been popular for modeling state- or time-varying pharmacologic responses. For the E_{max} and Hill equation, E_{max} represents the maximum possible effect. That is, as the drug level approaches infinity, the effect asymptotically approaches E_{max}. EC_{50} is the drug level at which 50% of E_{max} is observed and is a measure of the sensitivity to the drug. The lower the EC_{50} the more sensitive the system.

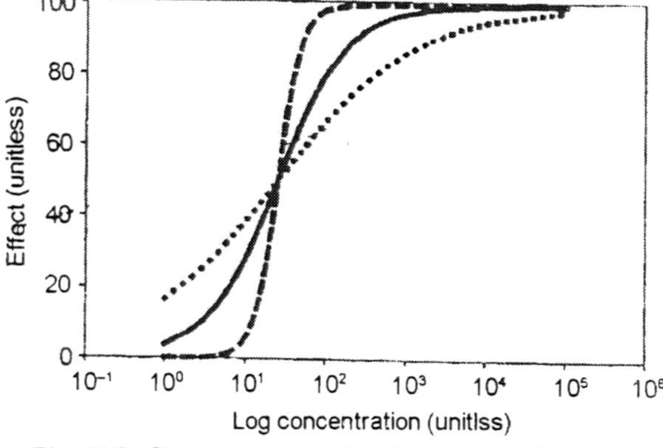

Fig. 16.2. Concentration vs effect for a simple E_{max} model.

$$\text{Effect} = \text{Constant} \times \text{conc.} \quad \ldots(1)$$

$$\text{Effect} = \frac{E_{max} \times \text{conc.}}{EC_{50} + \text{conc.}} \quad \ldots(2)$$

A modification of the simple E_{max} model is the sigmoid E_{max} model, which is sometimes referred to as the Hill equation. This model adds an exponential exponential component to the drug level and the EC_{50} (Eq. 3). Figure 16.3 shows the shape of a model where the EC_{50} is 25, E_{max} is 100, and gamma (the exponential) is 3.5.

The sigmoid E_{max}. (Hill equation) model is

$$\text{Effect} = \frac{E_{max} \times \text{conc.}^{\gamma}}{EC_{50}^{\gamma} + \text{conc.}^{\gamma}} \quad \ldots(3)$$

Careful consideration must be given when selecting a PD model. Although the above approaches to modeling PD responses are appealing, real-life pharmacology is more complex than described by formulas. Additional factors that must be considered in the model are tolerance effects, placebo effects, circadian rhythms, and drug interactions.

In time-invariant or stationary PD systems, a one-to-one correspondence exists between drug level at the effect site (C_e) and the effect (E). Often drug effects can be adequately described by time-invariant PK/PD, however, there are many drug effects that cannot. Frequently, drugs used in the treatment of cancers fall into this category of state- or time-varying PD. State-varying PD refers to PD parameters that change as an explicit function of the state of another aspect of the system/cascade (e.g., amount of enzyme, receptor, precursor, cofactor, or transporter such as multidrug resistance [MDR, P-glycoprotein]), which means that the observed effect is not simply the result of drug concentration, but rather some combination of the drug concentration and one or more of these states). Typical examples of state- varying PK/PD include drug tolerance, drug resistance, and enzyme induction or inhibition. Time-varying PK/PD, chrono-PK/PD, simply refers to PK/PD parameters that change as an explicit function of time (e.g., baseline effect or drug metabolism changes as a function of circadian rhythms or cell cycle). Because circadian rhythms and cell-cycle changes are presumably related to underlying changes in a state or states of the system, they could be referred to as state-varying as well. State-varying changes are directly linked to drug action, whereas the states of time-varying systems are primarily driven by genetic or internal biological clocking mechanisms. Although some drugs can alter a system's internal biological clock.

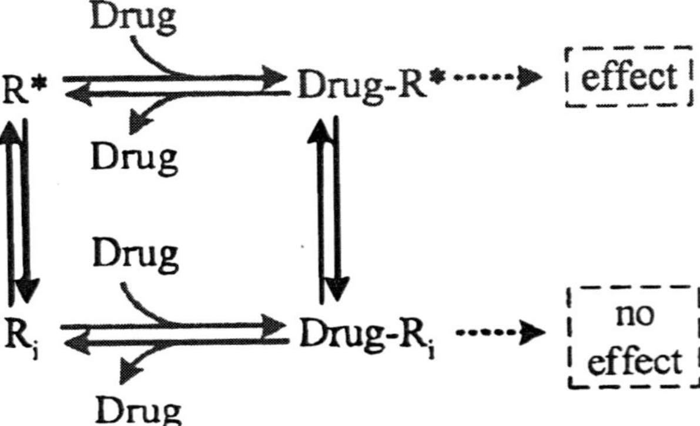

Fig. 16.3. The four-state receptor desensitization model. R and R_i are the receptors in the active and inactive states.*

Although extensive literature exists describing the occurrence of drug tolerance, the literature contains significantly fewer references describing its quantitative time course (development and recovery kinetics). Drug tolerance is a reversible decrease in drug effect in the presence of constant drug level. The timely reversible aspect of drug tolerance distinguishes it from drug resistance. Reversible decreased effect means that within the normal time frame of therapy the effect returns toward the drug-naïve state on cessation of drug input, whereas drug resistance, for example multidrug resistance (MDR), is usually the result of genetically driven alterations to the cells that are more permanent relative to the duration of therapy. Although systems experiencing drug resistance may ultimately return to the naïve state, the length of time to do so generally makes dosing regimens based on these kinetics impractical and clinically irrelevant.

Drug Tolerance Models

The mathematical distinctions between various models provide insight into differentiating between underlying mechanisms of tolerance. For example, some models of tolerance are restricted to identical onset and recovery rates, while others allow asymmetrical onset and recovery rates. The first model is known as receptor desensitization. This model, which has great modeling diversity, was first developed 1957 by Katz and Thessleff. Figure 16.3 shows the four different states of the drug receptor: (1) active with no drug bound, (2) active with drug bound, (3) desensitized with no drug bound, and (4) desensitized with drug bound. Although this model is capable of describing the kinetics of various tolerance mechanisms, pragmatically, its modeling robustness is tempered by its mathematical complexity.

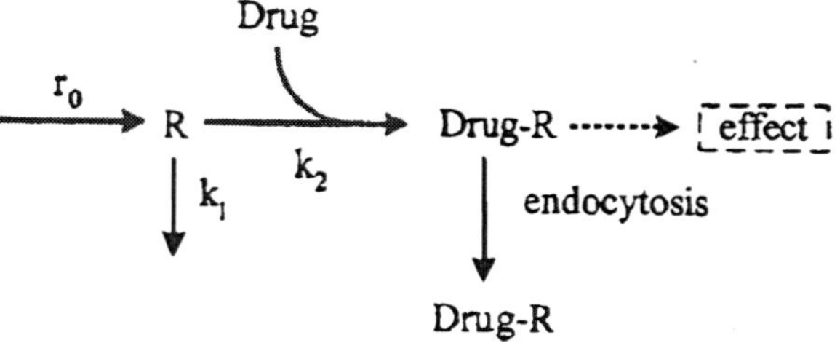

Fig. 16.4. The receptor down-regulation model.

The second model is the receptor down-regulation model. In this model, drug action is often initiated by the binding of drug to a cell surface receptor. On binding with cell surface receptors, the drug–receptor complexes are endocytosed into the cell, leaving fewer total receptors on the cell surface, thus leading to decreased sensitivity to the drug. Mathematically, this model can be expressed as

$$\frac{d[\mathrm{R}]}{dt} = r_0 - (k_1 + k_2[\mathrm{drug}])[\mathrm{R}] \qquad \ldots(4)$$

where R is the receptor, r_0 is the zero-order rate constant describing production, k_1 is a first-order rate constant describing constitutive receptor removal, and k_2 is the second-order rate constant describing receptor loss due to endocytosis-mediated down-regulation. In this model, the receptor concentration moves between two different steady-states $[\mathrm{R}]_{ss(1)} = r_0/k_1$ and $[\mathrm{R}]_{ss(2)} = r_0/(k_1 + k_2\,[\mathrm{drug}])$, corresponding to the naïve state and tolerant state, respectively. Because $[\mathrm{drug}] \geq 0$, two constraints of this model are apparent: (1) the rate of tolerance development ($k_1 + k_2$ [drug]) will always be greater than the rate of recovery k_1; and (2) this model is asymmetrical with respect to tolerance development and recovery.

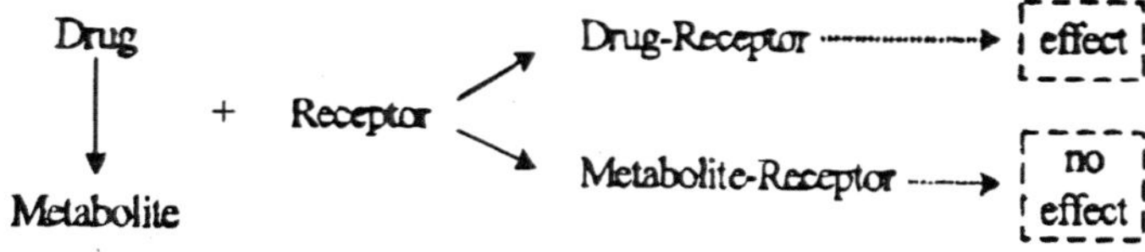

Fig. 16.5. Antagonistic activity model. In this model, the drug is converted to a metabolite that can also bind to the receptor.

The third model, which is mathematically a subset of the receptor desensitization model, is tolerance due to antagonistic activity. The antagonistic activity can be caused by one or more of the following: (1) one or more metabolites of the parent drug; (2) one or more metabolites of another drug, or even another drug, being used concomitantly; and (3) the production of some factor that leads to a decrease in the receptor binding affinity or the total amount of receptor protein. The antagonism can be competitive and/or non-competitive. This model requires symmetry between the onset and offset of tolerance, which is its most prominent constraint. The following two equations show competitive and noncompetitive antagonistic inhibition tolerance:

$$\text{Effect} = \frac{E_{\max} C_e}{C_{50}\left(\dfrac{T_{50} + T}{T_{50}}\right) + C_e} \qquad \ldots(5)$$

$$\text{Effect} = \frac{E_{\max}\left(\dfrac{T_{50}}{T_{50} + T}\right) C_e}{C_{50} + C_e} \qquad \ldots(6)$$

where E_{max} is the asymptotic maximal effect, C_e is the drug concentration at the effect site, C_{50} is the drug concentration leading to 50% of E_{max} in the absence of tolerance, T is the amount of tolerance, and T_{50} quantifies the relationship between C_e at steady-state and T.

A fourth model of tolerance is embodied in the indirect PD response models proposed by Jusko, specifically models I and IV, according to their nomenclature. Their four models are based upon the premise that "a measured response (R) to a drug may be produced by indirect mechanisms". The following two modified equations show the four possible models:

I. INHIBITION - k_{in}

k_{in} → Response (R) → k_{out}

IC_{50}

$$\frac{dR}{dt} = k_{in}\left(1 - \frac{Cp}{IC_{50} + Cp}\right) - k_{out} \cdot R$$

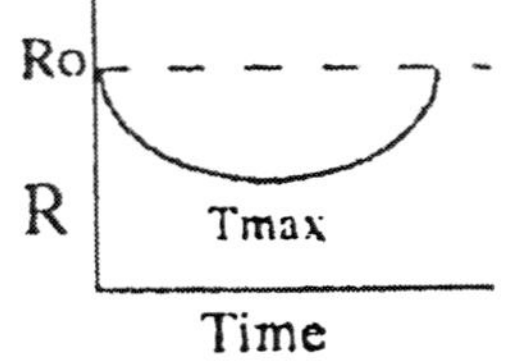

II. INHIBITION - k_{out}

k_{in} → Response (R) → k_{out}

IC_{50}

$$\frac{dR}{dt} = k_{in} - k_{out}\left(1 - \frac{Cp}{IC_{50} + Cp}\right) \cdot R$$

R
Tmax
Ro
Time

III. STIMULATION - k_{in}

k_{in} → Response (R) → k_{out}

EC_{50}

$$\frac{dR}{dt} = k_{in}\left(1 + \frac{Emax \cdot Cp}{EC_{50} + Cp}\right) - k_{out} \cdot R$$

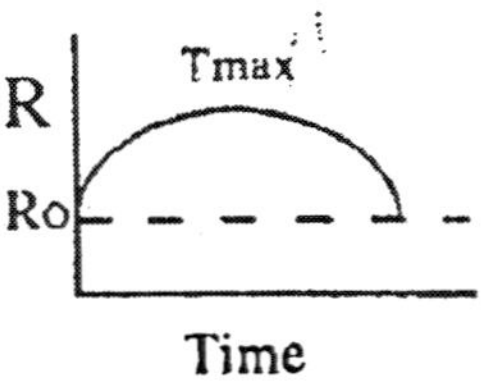

IV. STIMULATION - k_{out}

k_{in} → Response (R) → k_{out}

EC_{50}

$$\frac{dR}{dt} = k_{in} - k_{out}\left(1 + \frac{Emax \cdot Cp}{EC_{50} + Cp}\right) \cdot R$$

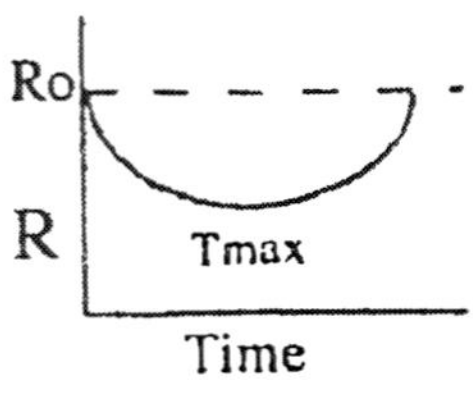

Fig. 16.6. The four fundamental types of pharmacodynamic indirect response models.

$$\frac{dR}{dt} = k_m V(S_{1...n}, t) - k_{out} R \qquad ...(7)$$

$$\frac{dR}{dt} = k_m - k_{out} W(S_{1...n}, t) R \qquad ...(8)$$

The functions $V(S_{1...n}\,t)$ and $W(S_{1...n}\,t)$ can be stimulatory or inhibitory, depending on the specific drug response. Only two of these four models describes drug tolerance: when V is inhibitory (model I) and/or W is stimulatory (model IV). Model 1 corresponds to a drug-related loss of a precursor necessary for the measured effect, while model IV corresponds to a system where the drug causes an increased removal rate of receptor, similar to the down-regulation model. This model has been used to model leukopenia secondary to cancer chemotherapy.

The fifth model of tolerance involves variations of an adaptive systems approach, which is familiar to the engineering discipline. Despite some major differences between competing systems approach models, the primary assumption made in all models is that the body seeks to maintain homeostasis and drugs disturb that homeostasis or trigger counter-regulatory mechanisms. Mandema and Wada proposed an elegant tolerance model based on physiological changes, both molecular and cellular. Although their model is quite sophisticated, it appears to be the only model that can account for within-systems and between-systems adaptation and should have applicability for MDR models in the future.

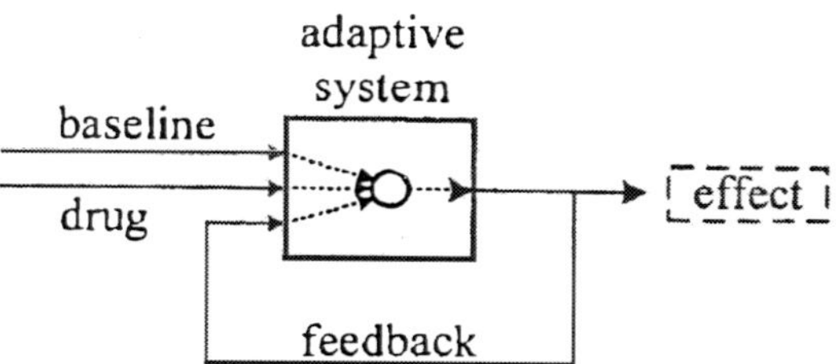

Fig. 16.7. Adaptive systems tolerance model. In this model, the baseline, disturbance (drug) and the output (effect feedback combine together to produce an overall effect.

When modeling drug tolerance, one of the above five general models should be sufficient to describe the kinetic onset and offset of tolerance. When choosing a tolerance model, one should ask several questions: (1) Is the pharmacological mechanism known for the drug being studied? (2) Is the rate of tolerance development and recovery symmetrical or asymmetrical with respect to time? (3) Does the drug of interest really undergo pharmacological tolerance or are the data simply the result of a tissue distribution artifact or PK sampling artifact? (4) Will an empirical model, not based on a specific mechanism, be sufficient for the intended purpose(s)? The answers to these questions will guide the choice of an appropriate drug-tolerance model.

Finally, two PK phenomena that can confound the interpretation of drug-tolerance data are (1) when the body establishes a steady state relationship between C_p and C_e more quickly than the establishment of a steady state between the site of drug administration and drug sampling site; and (2) when the drug causes an increase in its own clearance by inducing the enzyme responsible for the drug's metabolism, known as enzyme autoinduction.

Outcomes Models

An outcomes model relates some input function, biomarker, or surrogate endpoint (dose, drug serum concentration, tumor load, or lymphocyte count, MDR) to a terminal subject effect such as cure or no cure, improved vs worsened, survival, or disease progression. Outcomes models can be time to event models such as Kaplan–Meier curves for which hazard functions can be estimated. There are several hazard functions such as Weibull functions and Gompertz models that are differential equations that when integrated link the PD biomarker to the outcome in a time-dependent manner. Discrete outcomes can also be modeled as logistic regression or discriminant function models where the biomarker at some exact moment in time is related to an outcome. The disease progression model has recently been shown to be useful in relating drug administration to outcomes. Other models that should be considered are disease tolerance models that can be applied to such outcomes as tumor or viral load. MDR has a profound impact on outcomes because it is a major variable related to the failure of cancer chemotherapy. Recently, the presence of MDR-associated protein (MRP) was identified in resistant small-cell lung cancer cell lines. Several proteins have been associated with drug resistance including P-glycoprotein (Pgp) overexpression, p110 major vault protein, enzymes in the glutathione metabolic pathways, and DNA topoisomerases. The most common mechanism of MDR is the overexpression of Pgp and this is present in cancers with intrinsic resistance such as colon, renal, and pancreatic cancers. Pgp causes MDR by increasing the removal of chemotherapeutic agents from cancer cells. Drugs are being developed to inhibit the activity of Pgp. In the future it will be necessary to develop outcomes models that take into account the mechanism of MDR and the effect of those agents that counter the mechanisms of MDR and thus sensitize the cancer to drug.

Although outcomes models are important, they are less often available for use or application than are PK or PD models and therefore their development is one of the greatest areas of need in PM.

Population Models

Population modeling is the study of sources and correlates of variability of dependent variables (drug concentration or biomarkers) among individuals who are the target patient population receiving clinically relevant doses of a drug of interest. Therefore, covariates such as demographic variables (size or gender) are related to either PK or PD parameters such as clearance or E_{max}. As with other models, typical values for subjects are estimated, but most significantly with population models the between- and within-subject random effects are also estimated. Three approaches to estimating population models have been described. In recent years population models have become popular because of their broad applicability to drug development and a guidance on population pharmacokinetics has been issued by the Food and Drug Administration.

In the standard two-stage approach, one first estimates the individual model parameters for each subject. To implement this approach several observations per subject (usually eight or more) must be obtained and the individual parameters of the model estimated in the first of the two stages. In the second stage, the population parameters are estimated as the mean of all the individual parameters; the dependencies of the parameters on covariates can also be estimated by standard statistical approaches such as regression and in the final step the between-subject variability is estimated. When this approach is taken, the typical population parameter estimates are usually without bias; however, the variance and covariance parameters are inflated. The global two-stage approach has been proposed to improve the two-stage approach through bias correction for the random effects (covariance) and differential weighting of individual data according to the data's quality and quantity. The naive pooled data (NPD) approach is simple and is executed by pooling all the data across individuals to estimate the population parameters. This approach does not yield a characterization of the between-individual variability and therefore its ability to project the range of expected outcomes is limited. Although the NPD has worked well for population PK model estimation, it has not been valid for the E_{max} PD model because it does not account for the fact that different patients have different EC_{50s} and for the sigmoid E_{max} PD model, the estimate of γ is low.

The nonlinear mixed effects modeling approach has great utility for population model estimation. The nonlinear mixed-effects approach to population modeling can be used to obtain typical parameter estimates, between-subject variability, and unexplained residual variability, and relate PM parameters to covariates. It has great value when only sparse data have been or can be obtained, as for many pediatric studies, and the standard two- stage approach cannot be used because individual parameter estimates cannot be estimated directly. However, maximum *a posteriori* Bayesian (MAP Bayesian) estimates of individual subjects parameters can be generated from this approach. The nonlinear mixed effects approach was developed from the recognition that if PM models were to be developed in populations of investigated patients, practical considerations dictate that data should be collected under conditions that are not as restrictive as traditional study designs. This approach considers the study group as the unit of analysis rather than the individual and it functions even when data are sparse, fragmentary, and unbalanced. This approach has been used successfully to estimate PK, PD, and outcomes models of many different types.

Valid PM models developed from the nonlinear mixed-effects approach are especially useful for extrapolation to help understand the results of various competing study strategies. With these types of models the expected range of results of competing dosing strategies, differing patient populations, duration of study, and so forth can be investigated by Monte Carlo simulations.

Role of Real-time Modeling

For drug development there is always pressure to complete the process as expeditiously as possible. Real-time data collection and modeling can aid in lessening the time for drug development so that downstream segments can be impacted by the knowledge discovered from the PM models. Real-time data analysis and model development results in expeditious knowledge discovery, and can help identify potential problems in the analysis at an early stage of data collection.

Necessity of Planning

The complexities of drug development and the pivotal role of PM models point to the importance of planning. Both a macro-plan for the entire drug development process and a micro-plan for individual projects or studies must be in place. The macro-plan identifies (1) important questions that need to be answered, (2) the application and intended use of the PM model, (3) which covariates need to be studied, and (4) and possible drug–drug interaction.

Micro-planning at the level of the individual project or study must also take place. Plans must be in place for data management, data collection, quality assurance of the data, and staff training for data collection. A plan for data analysis and model validation must also be in place.

Use of Simulation

Monte Carlo simulation is a technique that is useful for the construction of clinical trials in the drug development process. Recent advances in computational performance, the appearance of new simulation software targeting clinical trials, and improved methods for estimating PM models have streamlined the execution of Monte Carlo simulations. Monte Carlo simulation provides an excellent avenue for application of the developed PM models. Simulation of clinical trials provides a means of evaluation of the impact of various dosing strategies, various compliance patterns, patient selection strategies, competing trial structures, competing outcomes measures, and competing statistical methods with all stochastic elements in the trial execution model on power, informativeness, efficiency, and robustness of a clinical trial. One large pharmaceutical company has reported that the early integration of PM

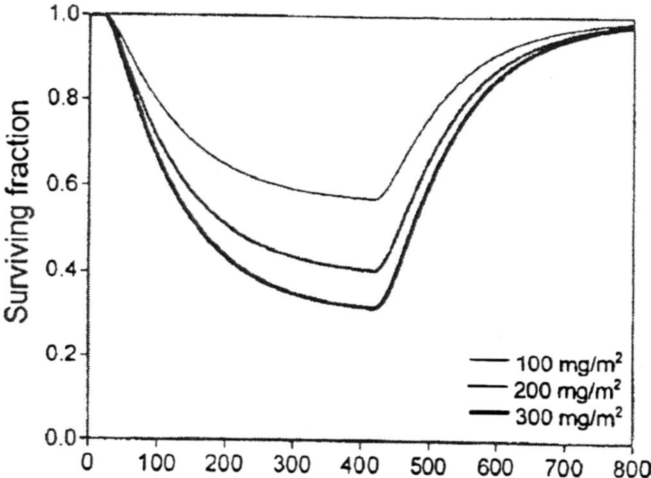

Fig. 16.8. Model projected time course of leukocyte survival after different doses of paclitaxel.

models via simulation resulted in development time-savings, regulatory concurrence, and a perceived value that outweighed costs.

For a simulation, three types of models are defined: the covariate model, the input–output model, and the execution model. The covariate model creates simulated individuals after defining the distribution of variables such as age, gender, weight, renal function, and so forth. The input–output models are the main place where the PM models enter into the simulation process. Here the trial structure, PK, PD, and outcomes models are defined in terms of both their typical parameter values and the variability of the parameters and also the residual random variability of the model. The execution model for a simulation deals with patient and practitioner behaviors during the execution of the trial, describing dropouts, compliance, and missing samples. Simulation provides a powerful tool for evaluating a broad range of assumptions and clinical trial structures on the eventual power, efficiency, informativeness, and robustness or any proposed study.

Dose Ranging Trials

For most therapeutic categories, dose-ranging studies have as their objective identifying a dose that is effective while avoiding toxicity or adverse effects. In contrast, for cancer chemotherapeutic agents dosing is limited by the maximum tolerated dose (MTD), because, for these agents, toxic and therapeutic effects cannot be separated by a dosing strategy. Targeting the MTD as the optimal dose in humans has implications for the dose ranging study. For efficiency it would be best if the initial dose in humans could begin at the highest yet safe dose with escalation occurring as rapidly as safety concerns will allow.

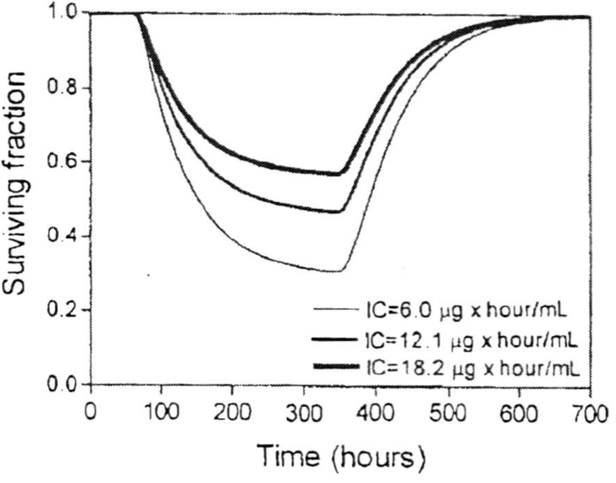

Fig. 16.9. Model based predictions of time course of leukocyte survival at different assumptions of IC.

First time in man (FTIM) studies and early clinical studies are targeted at identifying the MTD, single- and multiple-dose pharmacokinetics, and gender plus food effects on drug disposition. As such, these studies are initial attempts at dose ranging. Initially these FTIM studies require allometric scaling from animals to humans. Historically, this scaling has been on a mg/m^2 basis, but this can be improved on because of substantial interspecies differences in drug disposition and metabolism; and a stronger relationship between concentration and drug effect has been demonstrated when compared to dose alone. For example, it has been demonstrated that the MTD/LD_{10} ratio ranged from 0.1 to 6, whereas the AUCMTD/$LAUC_{10}$ ranged from 0.1 to 3.3, where LD_{10} is the lethal dose at which 10% of the animals died, AUCMTD is the area under the concentration–time curve at the maximum tolerated dose for humans, and $LAUC_{10}$ is the AUC at which 10% of the animals died. When the highest and lowest extremes were eliminated from the data, it was demonstrated that the MTD/LD_{10} ratio ranged from 0.4 to 5, whereas the AUCMTD/ $LAUC_{10}$ ranged from 0.6 to 1.3. Therefore, an exposure expressed as a function of concentration and time (e.g., the area under the concentration–time plot [AUC]) greatly improves on dose.

Early human trials for cancer chemotherapeutic agents have often been lengthy. The time taken to complete these trials is the number of dose escalations times the duration of each cycle. The typical drug here requires 12 cycles and 2 mo at each cycle; thus, 2 yr can be spent in this early clinical development stage. Collins et al. have stated, "The primary disadvantages of these lengthy trials are readily appreciated. Not only are the trials very resource intensive, but most of the patients receive doses with no potential for biological activity. Consequently, these studies are discouraging to both the investigator and the patient."

Collins et al. have proposed that murine and human biological effects occur at similar concentrations. Their proposed approach is based on exposure as a function of AUC rather than straight dose and is as follows:

1. Assume the murine $LAUC_{10}$ = human AUCMTD.
2. Determine the murine LD_{10} (current routinely done in toxicology protocols).
3. Determine the murine AUC at LD_{10}; this is the murine $LAUC_{10}$.
4. Begin human testing at a safe starting dose (1/10th the LD_{10}). This must be done because at the beginning of the FTIM study the pharmacokinetics in man are not yet known.
5. Estimate the AUC and pharmacokinetics at the starting dose in humans; this is routinely done for FTIM studies.
6. Set out an escalation strategy based on the initial AUC in humans and the target AUC, which in this case is the murine $LAUC_{10}$.

The above approach was applied to eight drugs. For four of the eight drugs, 2–12 cycles (average = 8 cycles) were eliminated, resulting in 4–24 mo time savings (average = 16 mo) in development while in no case was the time devoted to development increased. These studies not only result in time savings, but also fewer subjects are enrolled to complete early development. Thus there is a positive direct and indirect impact on expenditures.

Finally, delivery schedules must be considered when approaching early clinical development. There are some toxicities that are dependent on the maximum concentration (C_{max}) achieved during a dosing cycle. If a toxicity is C_{max} dependent, then a strategy must be laid out that takes this into account. It may be that a prolonged or continuous infusion could result in the desired AUC exposure and therefore efficacy while not exceeding the threshold C_{max} that would result in toxicity.

Applying PM Models

As PM knowledge is generated the intended use of the model must be kept in mind because the intended use of a model will influence the attitude and modeling approaches used by the pharmacometrician at the various stages of the modeling process. The intended use will determine what covariates are considered important and which parameters are of primary concern.

Models can be applied in several ways. Typical or average parameter estimates from models can be used to estimate typical values for dependent variables such as serum drug concentrations, typical exposures; typical biomarker effects such as tumor load or granulocyte count; or PK parameters such as area under the concentration–time curve. Issues that could be addressed with this type of model would be:

1. What would be the typical concentration–time profile for several different dosing approaches or for different types of patients?
2. What would be the typical biomarker as a function of patient type or differing dosing strategies?
3. What would be the expected concentration–time area under the curve for a capsule to be swallowed vs a buccal preparation design to avoid first-pass metabolism?

To estimate these types of variables from the model one simply applies the typical model parameters (clearance, apparent volume, etc.) and then inserts the missing elements such as dose and/or time to estimate the typical dependent variable. Models characterized by only typical values and applications estimating only average outcomes lack broad applicability and result in suboptimal understanding of the variable being studied (e.g., dose). Models containing random effects in addition to typical values have broader applications when compared to the models without random effects. These are the population models mentioned previously that contain typical values, between-subject random effects, and residual random effects. With these models not only can the typical result be projected but also the range of expected outcomes. These projections require not only models but also the implementation of Monte Carlo simulations. Simulations can be implemented in any of a number of software programs such as the Pharsight Trial Simulator or the NONMEM program with the simulation subroutine. These are implemented by supplying the software with the typical PM model values along with the random effects. In the end, a vector of concentrations or biomarkers' outcomes is generated and at each time point these could be ranked as the 10th, median, and 90th percentile concentrations observed. Therefore rather than estimate the typical concentration as a function of dose, one could go further and suggest a dosing strategy, then estimate the typical concentration, the 90th percentile concentration, and the 10th percentile concentration and even plot these as a function of time after dose.

A powerful use of PM models is their application for evaluation of the structure and strategy of confirming clinical drug trials. The PK, PD, and outcomes links models can be applied to understand the implications of various dosing strategies, patient compliance, patient population selection, dropout rates, duration of the study, and so forth on the power, robustness, efficiency, and informativeness of the trial. One may be interested in a strategy with four dosing levels for a pivotal confirming study. We would now wish to address the effect on power that would occur by adopting such a strategy. Adopting four levels of dosing has the advantage of adding a learning element to the confirming study. This may be valuable as one would not like the dose to be lowered after the drug has already entered the marketplace, and studying several levels of dosing ought to result in choosing an optimal dose. If the lower dose is equally effective as the higher dose, then it would be chosen as the standard of care. If the lower dose is less effective than the high dose, the administration of the low dose would be unethical, as the documentation of the inappropriateness of the lower dose has occurred. In the simulation one would specify in the software program the typical and random effects for the PK, PD, and linking parameters; an execution model would be employed by specifying the number of subject, patient compliance, dropout rates, duration of the study, and so forth; and finally a covariate model (distribution of gender, weights, etc.) would be specified. Power would then be calculated by determining how often the treatment was superior to the placebo after running 200 simulations. That is, if for these simulations the drug effect was greater than the placebo effect in 192 of the 200 simulations, then the power was estimated to be 0.96.

The cost of drug development has continued to escalate and is currently very high with no prospect of decreasing. PM offers an opportunity for knowledge-based drug development by developing models and applying them to clinical trial construction via Monte Carlo simulation. Application of knowledge-based PM models will result in powerful, efficient, informative, and robust clinical trials.

An Example of PM Model Application

Bruno et al. have provided an example of population pharmacokinetic (PPK) model application to clinical oncology drug development. The study was done in patients with non-small-cell cancer. In this example PPK was prospectively integrated into the clinical development of docetaxel. The integration was done so that exposure to the drug could be estimated and related to clinical outcome and adverse events. A PPK model was estimated from data obtained in 24 Phase II studies and MAP-Bayesian estimates of drug clearance and exposure were obtained for each subject.

Once the clearance and exposure was estimated for each subject, several PK parameters were estimated for each subject. A high AUC was noted to be a significant predictor of clinical response (time to progression [TTP]), where patients with the higher exposures had a prolonged TTP even after adjustment for other covariates. AUC was also noted to be a predictor of febrile and grade 4 neutropenia. However, the most significant predictor of febrile neutropenia was clearance, so that a 50% decrease in the clearance (CL) increased the odds by threefold.

It was noted further that patients with liver disease had a 27% lower CL than subjects without liver disease. This fact, combined with the association of low CL with febrile neutropenia, motivated a further analysis. Of the 1366 patients in the entire clinical database, 54 were noted to have elevated liver function tests. These 54 patients were further documented to have a threefold increase in the incidence of febrile neutropenia when compared with patients who had normal liver function tests.

The results of the PM analysis influenced the European Summary of Product Characteristics. On the basis of the PM analysis, a 25% decrease in dosing was recommended. Interestingly, in the US package insert there is no downward adjustment in this patient subgroup, but rather a complete avoidance is recommended in patients with liver function tests > 1.5 times the upper limit of normal. In contrast, the European guideline recommends that "Dosage should be reduced in hepatic impairment and hepatic function should be monitored." The docetaxel PM model development and application showed how the identification of subgroup differences led to a further analysis that when interpreted in light of the PPK model resulted in dosage modification in a subgroup. These findings were carried forward and recommended to the regulatory authorities. Thus, the analysis and application of these results impacted the safety, efficacy, and drug labeling.

Drug development has become unacceptably costly both in terms of money and in time expended. Most of the expenditures (both time and money) are applied to clinical development. It has been reported that increasing the approval rate from 21% to 25% and the efficiency of drug development by 19% would decrease the cost from $802 million to $560 million for each drug entering the marketplace. One important tool that will aid in decreasing the cost of development is changing from empirical boiler plate development to knowledge-based development. Without thoroughly applying PM, knowledge-driven drug development is not possible. The essential elements of PM have been presented so that they can be applied to knowledge-driven drug development in the oncology drug therapeutic arena or any therapeutic class in general.

17

Regional Therapy of Cancer

Many individuals afflicted with solid organ malignancies suffer from recurrence of disease limited to a particular region or organ of the body that is not amenable to surgical resection. For these individuals systemic combination chemotherapy may offer palliative benefits and, except for ovarian carcinoma, is rarely curable. Moreover, the maximum doses of systemically administered chemotherapeutic agents are almost invariably limited by the occurrence of severe systemic toxicity. Regional cancer treatments are those that are directly delivered to a cancer-bearing organ or region of the body. The rationale for such therapies is to intensify treatment to the site of a progressively growing cancer while minimizing or potentially eliminating unnecessary systemic toxicity. For many patients with peritoneal carcinomatosis secondary to gastrointestinal or ovarian carcinoma or mesothelioma, tumor progression in the peritoneum is the sole or life-limiting component of disease, and clinical evaluation of various forms of regional treatments for individuals afflicted with this condition have been long reported. One such therapy is continuous hyperthermic peritoneal perfusion (CHPP), which is administered during a laparotomy at the time of maximum tumor debulking and is administered with a recirculating hyperthermic circuit throughout the peritoneal cavity using a perfusate containing one or more types of chemotherapy.

A second form of regional therapy that has been in clinical use for almost 50 yr is vascular isolation and perfusion of either the limb (ILP) or the liver (*isolated hepatic perfusion* or IHP). For individuals with in transit melanoma or high-grade unresectable sarcoma of the extremity, ILP with *tumor necrosis factor* (TNF) and melphalan has been in use as either a primary curative modality or as a limb salvage procedure. For individuals with unresectable malignancies confined to the liver, IHP has been used and shown to be associated with response rates of up to 75%. Vascular isolation and perfusion therapy is administered with an extracorporeal bypass circuit consisting of a heat exchanger, oxygenator, roller pump, and reservoir in which a saline-based perfu sate containing packed red blood cells (PRBCs) and one or more therapeutic agents are administered directly through the vascular bed of the cancer-bearing region or organ of the body.

Continuous Hyperthermic Peritoneal Perfusion

CHPP has been administered to patients with peritoneal carcinomatosis secondary to a variety of malignancies including gastrointestinal cancers, mesothelioma, and ovarian cancer. The treatment parameters, chemotherapeutics, degree of hyperthermia, and duration of treatment vary from one institution to another to some degree, but several overarching considerations of CHPP treatment apply.

Patients with small-volume or completely resected peritoneal carcinomatosis appear to be the best candidates for CHPP. Peritoneal tumor implants must be exposed to sufficient doses of chemotherapeutic agents and hyperthermia at the center of the tumor to result in cell death. Because delivery of agents to tumor via CHPP is primarily by diffusion, tumor implants with a diameter > 6 mm are not likely to receive a tumoricidal dose. This was demonstrated by Dikhoff et al., who showed that cisplatin (CDDP) given intraperitoneally resulted in a fairly constant and high level of drug at a 3 mm depth into tumor, but CDDP concentrations decreased to 20% of tumor surface concentrations at a depth of 5 mm. Therefore, small implants such as those < 6 mm in diameter have the best theoretical likelihood of responding to intraperitoneal therapy.

A second potential limitation of intraperitoneal therapy is incomplete distribution of the therapeutic solution to all the serosal surfaces. This has largely been overcome by using technical maneuvers during CHPP that physically promote distribution of the perfusate such as gentle agitation or manipulation of the abdominal contents during treatment.

At laparotomy the peritoneal cavity is explored thoroughly and the nature and extent of the operative procedure are tailored based on the number, size, and location of peritoneal implants. In some circumstances when peritoneal disease is confined to a particular region of the abdomen, selective peritonectomy can be performed. Because tumors distributed in the peritoneal cavity are frequently limited to the serosa and not deeply infiltrative in nature, peritonectomy can be performed on the visceral and parietal peritoneum. Implants located on the serosa of the viscera can be excised or ablated with electrocautery. Some advocate a formal abdominal peritonectomy be performed to reduce the tumor burden as much as possible. However, the extent of peritonectomy that is necessary to optimize the therapeutic effects of the subsequent CHPP and patient outcome has not been definitively established. When larger tumor masses are encountered segmental resection of stomach, small bowel, large bowel, or omentectomy with or without splenectomy may be indicated. Once adequate tumor debulking has been accomplished, inflow and outflow catheters are positioned at either end of the peritoneal cavity. Typically the inflow catheters are placed at the upper portion of the abdominal cavity over the dome of the liver and left upper quadrant and the outflow catheters are placed in the pelvis. Several intraperitoneal temperature probes are positioned to document uniform and sufficient heating of the peritoneal surfaces during treatment. The abdominal fascia is then temporarily closed and catheters are connected to a perfusion circuit consisting of a reservoir, roller pump, and heat exchanger. Some have advocated using an open "*coliseum*" technique in which the fascia of the abdominal cavity is suspended from a self-retaining retractor and a plastic seat is securely attached to the fascia. A small slit is then made in the plastic cover to allow the surgeon's double-gloved hand access to the abdominal cavity for gentle manipulation of the perfu sate. Because all the surfaces of the peritoneal cavity must be exposed to perfu sate, great care is taken to lyse all intraperitoneal adhesions and ensure that the peritoneal surfaces are adequately exposed. For the closed CHPP technique, which is employed at the National Cancer Institute (NCI) and other institutions, the perfusion is initiated with saline that is heated until satisfactory perfusion parameters have been established and the peritoneal cavity has been adequately warmed. The therapeutic agent is then administered into the reservoir bag and CHPP is continued for an additional 90 min.

Because the peritoneal cavity acts as a heat sink, flow rates of the perfusate should be high enough to achieve uniform and adequate intraperitoneal hyperthermia. In our experience, this requires 1- to 1.5-L per minute flow rates through the peritoneal cavity. The patient should have a cooling blanket placed prior to the procedure and arms should be abducted on arm boards to allow both the cooling blanket and ice bags to be applied as necessary to maintain a core (esophageal) temperature of < 40°C. The therapeutic agent used at the NCI is CDDP at a dose of 250 mg/m^2, the maximum safe tolerated dose established in an initial Phase I study . To minimize the likelihood of renal toxicity from systemically absorbed CDDP, sodium thiosulfate is administered systemically as described by Howell et al. and urine output is increased using intravenous hydration and diuretics as necessary. Because CDDP is a large hydrophilic compound, it is less permeable across an intact peritoneal membrane than small lipophilic compounds. The estimated clearance across the peritoneal cavity during CHPP has been calculated to be approx 18 mm/min, which compares favorably to the absorbed plasma clearance of CDDP of 329 mm/min.

Pharmacokinetics

The two most common agents used in CHPP are CDDP and mitomycin C. Both of these agents offer a pharmacological advantage when given via a perfusion in the peritoneal cavity. The pharmacokinetic advantage of cisplatin given to 27 patients via CHPP. The concentration of CDDP in the perfusate over time, represented by the area under the curve of the concentration over time graph (AUC), was 3518 ± 1402 mg·min/mL compared with 287 ± 212 mg·min/mL in the plasma. The ratio of perfusate to plasma CDDP concentrations at each time point ranged from 4.6 to 119, with a median of 14. The 14-fold greater perfusate concentration compared to systemic concentration illustrates the favorable regional pharmacokinetics achieved via CHPP. These data were supported further by Cho and co-workers, who analyzed pharmacokinetics of CDDP at doses between 100 and 450 mg/m² administered via CHPP in 56 patients. They found that the percentage of total CDDP present in perfu sate at the end of CHPP was about 28% of the total dose.

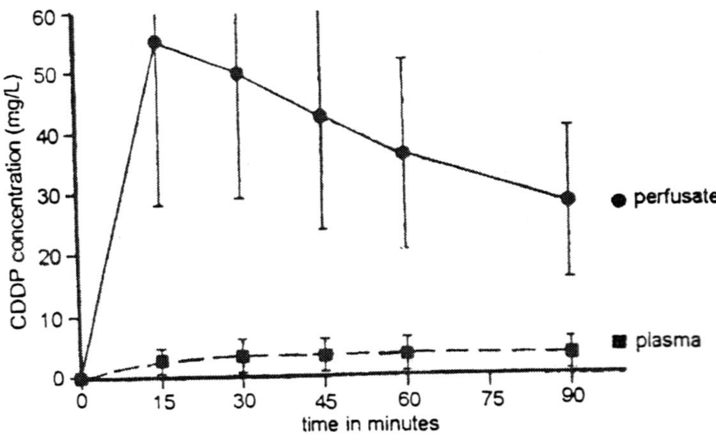

Fig. 17.1. Cisplatin concentration is perfusate and plasma over time in 27 patients undergoing CHPP at a dose of 250 mg/m².

TNF is an endogenously produced protein that has remarkable antitumor activity in murine models. Its use as a systemic anticancer agent resulted in remarkable disappointment, as humans are exceedingly sensitive to the toxic side effects of the protein. In multiple Phase I and Phase II trials of intravenously administered TNF, significant toxicity, most commonly hypotension, was encountered at doses that were insufficient to produce any significant antitumor activity. However, regional administration of TNF has been surprisingly well tolerated, particularly when systemic levels of the protein can be largely reduced or eliminated. Several Phase I trials of recombinant TNF administered intraperitoneally as a dwell show that the protein was well tolerated at doses up to 350 μg/m². Of note, concentrations of TNF in ascitic fluid were detectable up to 24 h after infusion and the estimated intraperitoneal half-life of the protein was between 8 and 12 h. No consistent serum levels of the protein could be detected in these trials. The reason for this is not entirely understood but may be related to the fact that the protein forms naturally occurring homotrimers that may limit systemic absorption from the peritoneal cavity. Resolution of malignant ascites was observed in a significant number of individuals, indicating that the protein may have exerted meaningful antitumor activity following this form of intracavitary administration.

Based on these data a Phase I trial of escalating dose TNF administrated with CDDP via CHPP was conducted at the NCI. In that trial 250 mg/m² of CDDP was administered with TNF at 0.1–0.3 mg/L of perfusate. At the first dose escalation of TNF (0.3 mg/L) severe dose-limiting nephrotoxicity was encountered and the maximum safe tolerated doses of CDDP and TNF given in combination were

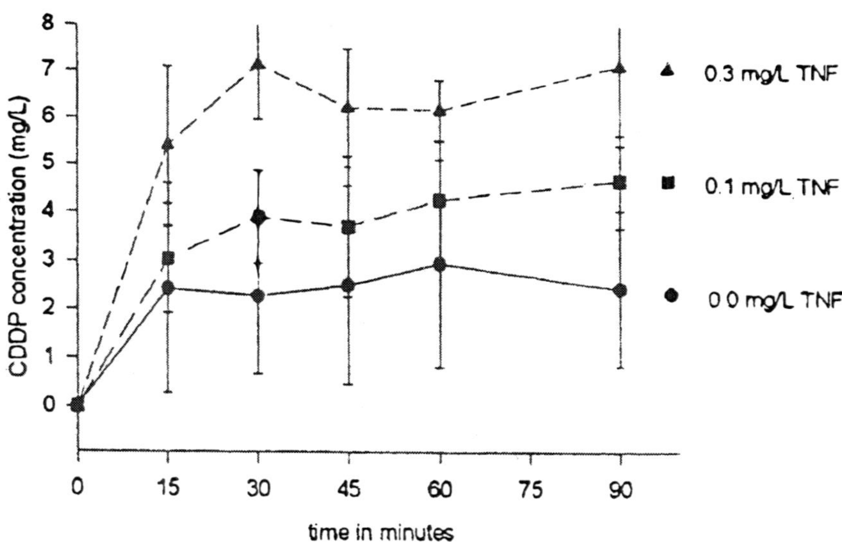

Fig. 17.2. Cisplatin perfusate concentrations over time in patients undergoing CHPP with increasing doses of TNF.

determined to be 250 mg/m^2 and 0.1 mg/L, respectively. The perfusate AUC for TNF was > 4000-fold higher than plasma AUC. Interestingly, there was a 1.6-fold higher plasma CDDP AUC in two patients treated at 0.3 mg/L of TNF compared to seven patients receiving 0.1 mg/L TNF and a 2.5-fold higher plasma CDDP AUC compared to the four patients who received no TNF at an equivalent dose of CDDP. Taken together, these data indicate that the dose-limiting renal toxicity observed with the combination therapy may have been related to some inflammatory changes secondary to TNF within the peritoneal cavity that promoted absorption of CDDP and resulted in higher systemic concentrations.

Mitomycin C showed an advantage similar to CDDP when administered via CHPP. Serial perfusate and plasma AUCs were determined for five patients with pancreatic or gastric cancer treated by laproscopic CHPP with both cisplatin and mitomycin C. The AUC of MMC in perfusate was 389 ± 181 mg·min/mL compared to 18 ± 2 mg·min/mL in the plasma and represents a 22-fold higher dose in perfusate compared to serum. As would be expected, systemic toxicity is minimal, with no grade 3 or 4 toxicities.

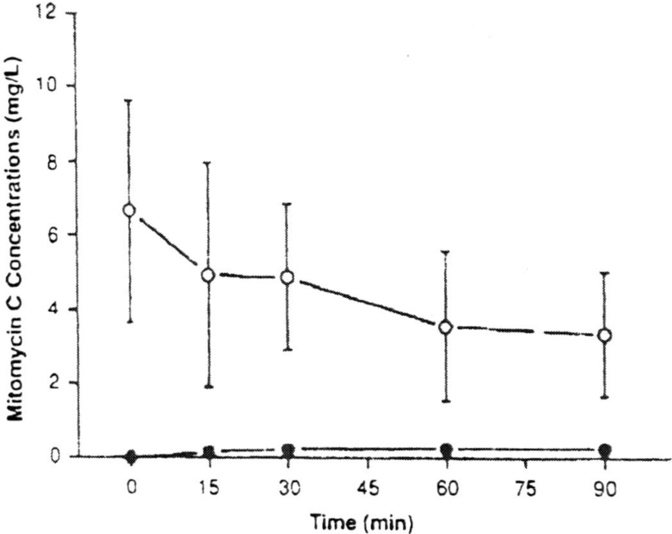

Fig. 17.3. Mitomycin C concentrations in perfusate (open circles) and plasma (filled circles) over time in patients undergoing CHPP at a dose of 10 mg/L.

Clinical Results with CHPP

The first reported CHPP, or the use of a recirculating infusion system to deliver hyperthermia and chemotherapy to the abdominal compartment, was performed in 1980 by Spratt et al. in a 35-yr-old male with pseudomyxoma peritoneii. However, most of the early studies of this technique come from the Japanese experience using CHPP for prophylactic or therapeutic treatment after resection for gastric cancer. Koga et al. reported the first multiarm clinical trial of CHPP as prophylaxis against abdominal carcinomatosis in 60 patients with gastric cancer. All patients underwent gastric resection with curative intent and were then randomized to receive no further treatment or CHPP with mitomycin C at 8–10 mg/L. Results from the subset analysis of 47 patients with serosal invasion by pathology showed a trend toward better survival at 3 yr in the CHPP treated group (83%) vs the standard therapy group (67%). In a similar trial, Fujimoto et al. selected 59 patients with gastric cancer to receive CHPP with perfusate containing mitomycin C at 10 mg/L vs no further treatment after resection. At 1-yr follow-up, overall survival was significantly different at 80% for the CHPP-treated patients compared to 34% for the nonperfused controls. Moreover, in patients with peritoneal carcinomatosis, median posttreatment survival was 1 yr whereas the median survival for those who received CHPP had not been reached at the 3-yr follow-up. Hamazoe et al. treated 82 gastric cancer patients with gross serosal invasion but no peritoneal implants with either CHPP using mitomycin C or no further treatment after curative surgery. The CHPP-treatment group had a trend toward lower incidence of peritoneal recurrence compared to the nonperfused control group ($p = 0.08$), but no statistically significant difference in survival at 5 yr (64% vs 53%). Fujimura et al. treated 31 patients with peritoneal carcinomatosis from gastric cancer using CHPP with 200 mg/m^2 of CDDP and 20 mg/m^2 of mitomycin C; subsequently, 12 patients underwent second-look laparotomy which showed four complete responses (CR) and one partial response (PR) with an overall response rate of 41%. In patients with a CR or PR, overall survival at 2 yr was 50% compared with 0% of the nonresponders. Fujimura et al. followed this study with a three-arm randomized trial initially reported in 1994 comparing CHPP with CDDP/mitomycin C, continuous normothermia peritoneal perfusion (CNPP) with CDDP/mitomycin C vs surgery alone in 139 patients receiving curative surgery for T2–T4 gastric cancer. The perfusate in CHPP-treatment group was heated to 42–43°C whereas that of the CNPP-treatment group remained at 37°C. Overall survival at 5 yr was 61% for CHPP, 43% for CNPP, and 42% for surgery alone.

More recent result of Phase II and I clinical trials of CHPP for a variety of tissue histologies other than gastric cancer have been reported. After treating 84 patients with peritoneal carcinomatosis from a variety of primary sites including colon ($n = 38$), appendix ($n = 22$), or stomach ($n = 19$) with CHPP using mitomycin C, Loggie et al. reported a median survival of 14.6, 31.1, and 10.1 mo, respectively. The NCI reported the results of CHPP with CDDP on 18 patients with primary peritoneal mesothelioma. This cohort experienced a 26-mo progression-free survival and overall 2-yr survival of 80%, with nine out of ten patients having resolution of their ascites. In a Phase I trial of CHPP using carboplatin on six patients with residual epithelial ovarian cancer after standard debulking, Steller et al. reported five of six patients had no evidence of disease at a median follow-up of 15 mo. In summary, CHPP shows promise as a treatment option for peritoneal carcinomatosis for a wide variety of histologies. The administration of hyperthermia and chemotherapy to the peritoneal cavity, the minimal systemic absorption of these agents, and the resulting decrease in systemic toxicity make this an attractive treatment that certainly warrants further investigation.

Vascular Isolation and Perfusion

Vascular isolation and perfusion is a specialized operative procedure used to physically isolate blood flow to and from an organ or extremity to deliver chemotherapy, biological agents, and hyperthermia to a region of the body at doses higher than would otherwise be tolerated systemically. In general, the main artery and vein supplying blood to the region are prepared by dissecting and ligating all collateral vessels, cannulated, and connected to an extracorporeal bypass machine to circulate agents under hyperthermic conditions. In the liver, isolated hepatic perfusion (IHP) is performed for isolated unresectable hepatic metastases or primary hepatocellular carcinoma. In the extremity, isolated limb perfusion (ILP) has been utilized for metastatic extremity melanoma or unresectable high-grade sarcoma

Isolated Hepatic Perfusion

There are both advantages and disadvantages to IHP when compared with other types of systemic and regional cancer therapies for unresectable cancers of the liver. IHP allows for the delivery of higher doses of agents directly to the liver than systemically tolerated, but, as a regional treatment, does not treat occult disease outside of the liver. Unlike surgical resection or regional ablative techniques such as radiofrequency ablation, cryotherapy, or ethanol injection, IHP can be used to treat large (>5 cm) deposits, bilobar disease, and potentially micrometastases. Although chemoembolization or infusion of chemotherapy into the hepatic artery through implantable pumps or percutaneous catheters can minimize systemic toxicity and treat the entire organ, these techniques still rely on the first-pass effect to remove the agent from the circulation. However, IHP allows for complete isolation of the vascular supply from the systemic circulation; therefore, the dose of therapeutic agent is limited only by the tissue tolerance of normal hepatic parenchyma. Also, at the end of the perfusion the circuit is flushed with normal saline to remove residual therapeutic agents from the hepatic vasculature and further decrease systemic exposure. IHP also effectively delivers potentially tumoricidal levels of hyperthermia uniformly to the liver. However, IHP is a technically challenging procedure to perform and provides one relatively short exposure to the hyperthermia and chemotherapy, necessitating the use of a highly efficacious agent.

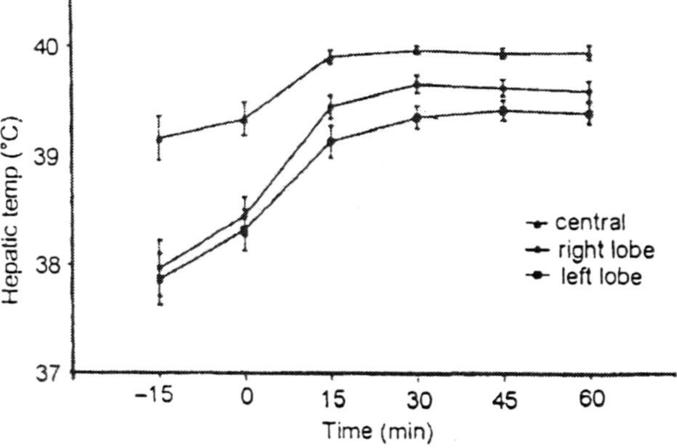

Fig. 17.4. Intrahepatic temperature levels during IHP showing prompt and uniform distribution of hyperthermia throughout the hepatic parenchyma during treatment.

Initially, a right subcostal incision is made and the abdomen is explored to exclude extrahepatic metastases. Except for limited periportal lymphadenopathy which can be completely dissected, if no other extrahepatic disease is found then the incision is extended and the liver is mobilized. Complete dissection and identification of the arterial and venous structures are performed to ensure that all collateral flow from the hepatic to systemic system is controlled. This involves mobilizing the retrohepatic inferior vena cava (IVC) and ligating the right adrenal vein, phrenic veins, and IVC tributaries to the retroperitoneum. The gallbladder is removed to prevent chemotherapy-induced postoperative cholecystitis. The porta hepatis is throughly dissected and all palpable lymphadenopathy is removed. The common hepatic artery, proper hepatic artery, and the gastroduodenal artery (GDA) are isolated. The GDA is cannulated for hepatic inflow. A catheter is advanced through a saphenous vein cut down into the IVC just below the renal veins and another in the portal vein. These two catheters are attached via veno-veno bypass pump to a catheter in the axillary vein shunting IVC and portal venous blood to the axillary vein. The infrahepatic IVC is isolated and a catheter place in the retrohepatic IVC to collect the venous outflow from the perfusion. Probes are placed in the right and left lobes of the liver to monitor temperature. The perfusion is performed with outflow from the retrohepatic IVC and inflow into the hepatic artery via the GDA. The perfusion circuit consists of a roller pump membrane oxygenator, and heat exchanger. The temperature and pH of the perfusate are monitored. After completion of a 1-h perfusion, the liver is flushed via the GDA and the portal vein. The catheters are removed, the vasculature repaired, and the incision closed.

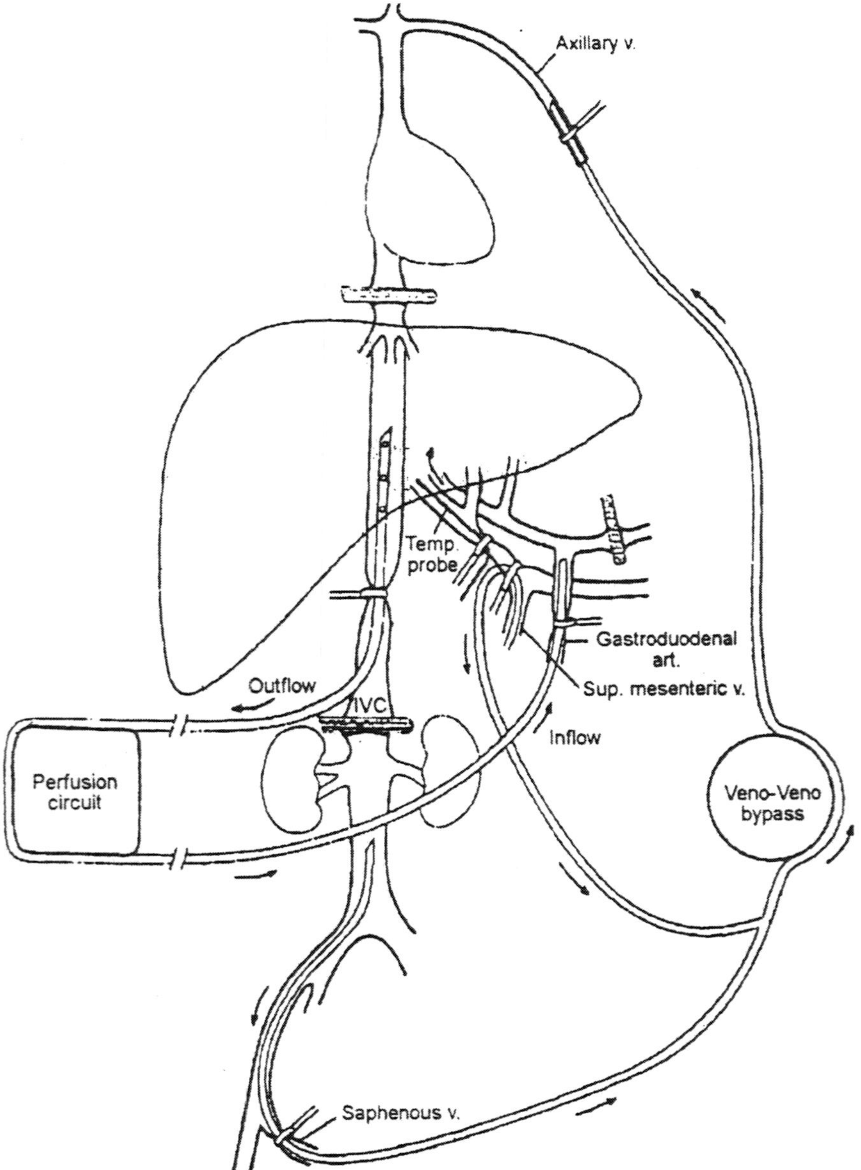

Fig. 17.5. Schema showing setup of the IHP circuit.

Pharmacokinetics

Despite the technical challenges of this procedure, the application of IHP for the delivery of therapy for liver metastases is particularly attractive because complete vascular isolation allows dose escalation and removes the need for drug elimination via the first pass effect. The most common agents used in IHP currently are TNF and melphalan and some centers have previously used 5-fluorouracil (5-FU), mitomycin C, or CDDP. In a Phase I trial of IHP at the NCI using TNF and melphalan with an alternating dose escalation design, hepatic venoocclusive disease occurred at a melphalan dose of 2 mg/kg body weight and dose-limiting coagulopathy was seen at 1.5 mg of TNF. The maximum safe tolerated doses are therefore 1.5 mg/kg of melphalan and 1 mg of TNF.

In the past, leakage of perfusate into the systemic circulation was monitored by using a radioactive tracer technique. However, the liver is an ideal organ for isolated perfusion, and in 50 patients undergoing IHP we detected a small leak in only two, both of which were easily corrected by adjusting vascular clamps. Enzyme-linked immunosorbent assay (ELISA) was used to measure TNF levels in the cohort of 50 patients from samples of serum and perfusate taken every 15 min during perfusion. TNF levels in the perfusate rise within the first 15 min and stay consistently elevated throughout the length of the perfusion. However, serum TNF levels are undetectable at all time points, indicating no systemic leak. The decrease in melphalan concentration over time is presumably due to hydrolysis of drug under hyperthermic conditions, which has been demonstrated in mock perfusion and no consistently measurable systemic levels could be identified.

Clinical results of IHP

The first reported IHP on human subjects was performed by Ausman in 1961 at Roswell Park Cancer Institute in Buffalo, NY. Five patients received normothermic IHP with nitrogen mustard and although no response data were recorded, two of the five patients were long-term survivors, indicating some treatment response. No further studies were reported using this technique until 20 yr later. In 1984, Aigner et al. used a 1-h hyperthermic IHP with 700–1100 mg of 5-FU to treat 32 patients. Although they did not report response data, median survival with IHP alone was only 8 mo and with IHP plus intraarterial chemotherapy it was only 12 mo. Treating six patients with a 4-h IHP with hyperthermia of 42.5°C alone, Skibba and Quebbeman demonstrated radiographic evidence of central tumor necrosis in five of six evaluable patients. Schwemmle et al. treated 50 patients with 1-h IHP using moderate hyperthermia to 39.5°C and two chemotherapeutic regimens, 5-FU alone or 5-FU, mitomycin C, and CDDP. They reported an overall response rate of 68% and complete response (CR) of 18% but used criteria such as decreased carcinoembryonic antigen (CEA) levels and nonstandard radiographic criteria to determine response

There was a significant treatment and operative mortality of 10–25% in these early studies. Most of these reports represented results of a single initial institutional experience with this technique in patients who frequently had very advanced conditions. Because the treatment risks are relatively high and the early results were equivocal, IHP has not been used except in a limited number of centers worldwide.

Within the last 10 yr, several European and United States clinical centers have reported their experiences with IHP. After treating 29 patients with melphalan and CDDP with a 1-h IHP at 40°C, Hafstrom reported a partial response (PR) rate of 20% and had five patients who survived 3 yr. Van de Velde and co-workers reported the results of 1-h normothermic IHP using either mitomycin C or melphalan, with overall response rates of 28% and 41%, respectively. De Vries from the Netherlands treated eight patients with TNF and melphalan with a 1-h hyperthermic IHP and five of six patients experienced a PR (80%) but treatment had a 33% treatment-related mortality. Using melphalan and escalating doses of TNF in a 1-h hyperthermic IHP, Hafström et al. treated 11 patients, resulting in a 27% PR rate (3/11) but a high treatment mortality of 18%. Oldhafer and co-workers from Germany reported a 50% RR and no mortality from six patients treated with TNF and melphalan in a 1-h hyperthermic IHP. The largest series comes from the NCI where Alexander and colleagues treated 50 patients with 1-h hyperthermic IHP with melphalan and TNF with an overall response rate of 75% and mortality of 4%. Median duration of response was 9 mo, but some responses continued beyond 3 yr. In summary, IHP provides regional delivery of chemotherapeutic agents to the liver, but is technically challenging and has significant associated morbidity and mortality. Response rates are somewhat variable; current Phase III trials comparing hepatic arterial infusion (HAI) + IHP vs HAI alone in patients with colorectal cancer liver metastases may help to answer these continuing questions.

Isolated Limb Perfusion

ILP of the lower extremity is most commonly performed via the external iliac vessels and of the arm via the axillary vessels. However, the femoral, popliteal, or brachial vessels are also used in certain circumstances. With respect to lower extremity ILPs, the level of perfusion should be based on the distribution of the disease and technical considerations such as patient body habitus or a history of prior surgery in the iliac or femoral region. The rate of inguinal nodal recurrence in melanoma patients who received femoral or iliac perfusion was comparable (25 vs 32%, respectively) indicating that perfusion through the more proximal iliac vessels does not eradicate inguinal lymph node micrometastases.

Using a lower abdominal "*transplant*" incision, a retroperitoneal approach to the iliac vessels is made. The external iliac artery and vein are dissected distally and all venous tributaries and arterial branches arising proximal to, or under, the inguinal ligament are ligated and divided. Proximally the hypogastric vein is ligated *in situ* as it may contribute to increased systemic leak rates. The external iliac vessels are cannulated and a Steinmann pin is anchored into the anterior superior iliac spine and an Esmarch tourniquet is snugly wrapped at the root of the extremity. The heat exchanger and external warming blankets are used to maintain tissue temperatures in the range of 38.5–40.0°C.

The extracorporeal perfusion circuit is comprised of a roller pump, heat exchanger, and oxygenator. The circuit is typically primed with 700 mL of balanced salt solution, 1 U of packed red blood cells, and 1500 U of heparin. The resultant hematocrit of approx 25% provides adequate tissue oxygen tension, and perfusing at a higher hematocrit confers no additional benefit in preventing regional toxicity. Flow rates in the range of 50 mL/L of limb volume/min are desirable and adjusted depending on line pressure, reservoir volume, or the presence of systemic leak based on intraoperative monitoring.

Continuous intraoperative monitoring to assess perfusate leak into the systemic circulation is being used more routinely and is an important component of isolated perfusion therapy when one considers that perfusate doses of melphalan and tumor necrosis factor are at least 10-fold greater than maximally tolerated systemic doses. Careful monitoring of leak may reduce the severity of systemic complications and improve response rates in the limb. Standard protocols using ^{131}I-radiolabeled albumin or ^{99m}Tc labeled red blood cells have been described for continuous intraoperative monitoring of leak during isolated limb perfusion. A gamma detection camera is positioned over the precordium so the heart serves as a stable reservoir of blood to measure radioactivity leak. The detection system provides continuous assessment of leak rates and can discriminate a leak of $< 1\%$. Leak rates using this system have been shown to correlate with measured leak of TNF or melphalan from the perfusate and the development of systemic toxicity.

Pharmacokinetics

The dose of melphalan that is typically administered in ILP is based on limb volume and 10–13 mg/L are associated with acceptable transient side effects but significant antitumor efficacy. The disposition of melphalan in the perfusion circuit is influenced by several factors. First, there can be systemic leakage of the drug during limb perfusion and several investigators have shown that leak rates of $> 5\%$ occur in approx 10% of patients. If there is systemic leakage, then several maneuvers can be performed to reverse or slow the efflux of melphalan into the systemic circulation such as altering the flow rate of the perfusion circuit. Typically, isolated limb perfusion is performed for 30 min under hyperthermic conditions alone and then after tissue temperatures are approx 38.5°C melphalan is added slowly into the arterial line of the perfusion circuit over 5 min. The perfusion continues for an additional 60 min and then the perfusate is flushed from the extremity to remove residual melphalan prior to reestablishing the native blood flow to the extremity. We have analyzed melphalan concentrations in the perfusion circuit in 18 individuals undergoing lower extremity ILP with melphalan with or without 3–4 mg of TNF at the NCI. The data show that peak melphalan concentrations are observed immediately after the drug is administered and decrease progressively over the course of the perfusion. It is also known that melphalan undergoes spontaneous hydrolysis under hyperthermic condition, which may account for the decrease in concentrations in the perfusate observed over time.

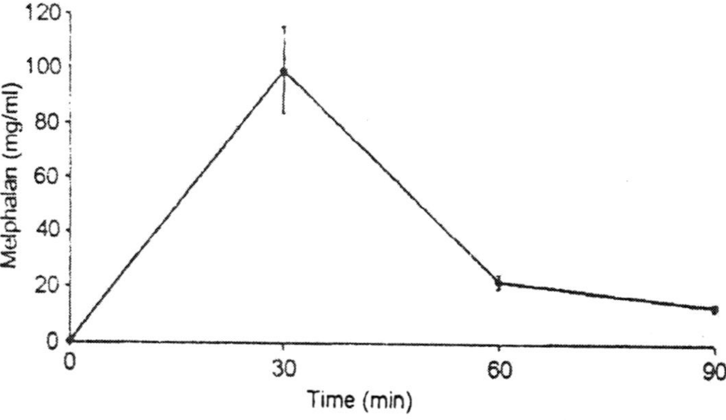

Fig. 17.6. Melphalan concentrations over time in patients undergoing a hyperthermic lower extremity ILP with 10 mg/L of limb volume of melphalan with (n=9) or without (n=9) TNF.

Klasse and co-workers reported melphalan tissue concentrations for patients undergoing ILP for melanoma arising in the lower extremity. They found a direct correlation between increasing tumor concentrations of melphalan and the AUC of the drug in the perfusion circuit. On the other hand, muscle concentrations were directly correlated with peak melphalan concentrations, suggesting that a lower peak level but a sustained higher AUC will be associated with better efficacy in minimal regional toxicity. As a consequence, several investigators administered the total dose of melphalan in the perfusion circuit as divided doses at time 0 and then at 30 min into the perfusion treatment. Concentrations of melphalan within tumor are likely due to the fact that melphalan is a phenylalanine derivative and is actively taken out by cells of melanocyte origin. The concentration of TNF in the perfusion circuit, in contrast to melphalan concentrations, remain largely stable and indicate that there is very little degradation or absorption of the cytokine into tissues over the course of the treatment. It is known that patients who have leak of perfusate > 1% peak systemic concentrations of TNF occur within 4 h of treatment. The systemic exposure to low doses of TNF is associated with a variety of cardiovascular and metabolic alterations that have been well characterized but are easily managed with fluid hydration and close monitoring during the first 24 h after treatment.

Current results with ILP for extremity melanoma or sarcoma

In the initial report from Liènard and Lejuenne, results from 29 patients treated with ILP using a combination of TNF, melphalan, and hyperthermia for in-transit melanoma or high- grade sarcoma of the extremity were presented. The overall response rate in that initial trial was 100%, with 89% of patients having a complete response to treatment. In subsequent reports from various institutions, including a follow-up report from Lienard and Lejuenne of a larger series of patients, the complete response rates were lower and ranged between 70% and 79%. A prospective random assignment trial was initiated at the NCI and subsequently expanded to a multiinstitutional study but was closed prematurely in 1997 owing to a lack of available clinical grade TNF in the United States. The results of that trial showed no difference in overall or complete response rates between the groups. It is also noteworthy that in several trials of ILP using melphalan alone, complete response rates between 56% and 82% have been reported. A prospective random assignment trial comparing melphalan and TNF with melphalan alone administered via ILP for in-transit melanoma of the extremity was closed in Europe because of low accrual, suggesting a bias that for most patients with this histology, TNF does not substantially contribute to efficacy compared with melphalan alone.

ILP has been used for patients with unresectable high-grade extremity sarcoma for palliation, for potential cure in cases of multifocal disease, and as a neoadjuvant therapy to convert an unresectable lesion to a resectable one. Most data reported on ILP using chemotherapeutics alone indicate limited antitumor activity against this histology. After the initial reports by Liènard and Lejuenne using the combination of TNF, melphalan, and hyperthermia as a neoadjuvant treatment for high-grade unresectable sarcoma, a multi-institutional trial using this regimen for patients with condition was conducted in Europe and the results reported in two papers by Eggermont and co-workers. In more than 219 patients, the overall clinical and pathologic response rate was > 80% and the limb salvage rate was 84%. Based on these results TNF is now licensed for administration via ILP for high- grade sarcoma in Europe, but no trials are currently being conducted in the United States.

Regional delivery of hyperthermia and chemotherapy for patients with disease confined to the treatment field has shown promise as well as a decreasing treatment-related mortality. CHPP is being used to treat abdominal carcinomatosis for a wide variety of sources, with long-term results still pending. Vascular isolation techniques have become safer, and may present an option for the treatment of isolated liver, limb, lung, or renal disease. The pharmacokinetic advantage of these regional treatments has been well established and continuing clinical evaluation will further define the best clinical applications of these therapies.

INDEX